# BRAD W. NEVILLE, DDS

Professor and Director

Division of Oral & Maxillofacial Pathology

Department of Stomatology

College of Dental Medicine

Medical University of South Carolina

Charleston, South Carolina

# DOUGLAS D. DAMM, DDS

Professor of Oral & Maxillofacial Pathology

University of Kentucky College of Dentistry

Lexington, Kentucky

# DEAN K. WHITE, DDS, MSD

Professor and Head of Oral & Maxillofacial Pathology

University of Kentucky College of Dentistry

Lexington, Kentucky

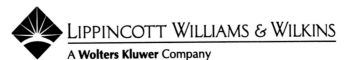

LIPPINCOTT WILLIAMS & WILKINS
A **Wolters Kluwer** Company
Philadelphia • Baltimore • New York • London
Buenos Aires • Hong Kong • Sydney • Tokyo

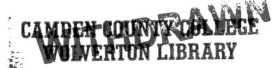

*Editor:* Tim Hiscock
*Managing Editor:* Tanya Lazar
*Project Editor:* Robert D. Magee

351 West Camden Street
Baltimore, Maryland 21201-2436 USA

Rose Tree Corporate Center
1400 North Providence Road
Building II, Suite 5025
Media, Pennsylvania 19063-2043 USA

The publisher is not responsible (as a matter of product liability, negligence or otherwise) for any injury resulting from any material contained herein. This publication contains information relating to general principles of medical care which should not be construed as specific instructions for individual patients. Manufacturers' product information and package inserts should be reviewed for current information, including contraindications, dosages and precautions.

*Printed in the United States of America*

First Edition, 1991

**Library of Congress Cataloging-in-Publication Data**
Neville, Brad W.
    Color atlas of clinical oral pathology / Brad W. Neville, Douglas D. Damm,
Dean K. White.—2nd ed.
       p.    cm.
    Rev. ed. of: Color atlas of clinical oral pathology / Brad W. Neville . . . [et al.]. 1991.
    Includes bibliographical references and index.
    ISBN 0–683–30208–6
    1. Mouth—Diseases—Atlases.  2. Radiography—Atlases.   I. Damm, Douglas D.
II. White, Dean K.    III. Title.
   [DNLM:  1. Mouth Diseases atlases.    WU  17  N523c 1998]
RK287.C65    1998
617.5′2207—dc21
DNLM/DLC
for Library of Congress                           98–3616
                                            CIP

*The publishers have made every effort to trace the copyright holders for borrowed material. If they have inadvertently over-looked any, they will be pleased to make the necessary arrangements at the first opportunity.*

To purchase additional copies of this book, call our customer service department at **(800) 638-0672** or fax orders to **(800) 447-8438.** For other book services, including chapter reprints and large quantity sales, ask for the Special Sales department.

Canadian customers should call **(800) 665-1148,** or fax **(800) 665-0103.** For all other calls originating outside of the United States, please call **(410) 528-4223** or fax us at **(410) 528-8550.**

**Visit Williams & Wilkins on the Internet:** **http://www.wwilkins.com** or contact our customer service department at **custserv@wwilkins.com.** Williams & Wilkins customer service representatives are available from 8:30 am to 6:00 pm, EST, Monday through Friday, for telephone access.

                                                       00
3 4 5 6 7 8 9 10

To our colleagues, many of whom have shared these cases with us.

# PREFACE

Over the past decade, the area of diagnostic pathology has undergone dramatic changes. Newer techniques such as immunochemistry, in situ hybridization, polymerase chain reaction, and flow cytometry have revolutionized the way in which diseases are diagnosed. However, despite these advances in laboratory technology, the diagnosis of disease still remains primarily in the realm of the clinician. Many diagnoses are made solely on a clinical basis; for lesions that require biopsy, a clinical differential diagnosis is an important step leading to the decision to obtain a tissue sample. Even after a laboratory diagnosis is made, the clinician must correlate these results with the clinical findings to best determine patient treatment.

With these thoughts in mind, our goal in this second edition of **Color Atlas of Clinical Oral Pathology** is the same: to provide the reader with a large body of high-quality color photographs and radiographs to assist in the diagnosis of oral diseases. The book has been designed mainly with the dental profession in mind, including the general dentist, the specialist, and the dental hygienist. In addition, this atlas should prove useful to other members of the health care community, especially those in areas such as otolaryngology and dermatology who also treat oral diseases.

The age-old adage that a picture is worth a thousand words is particularly true for this type of book; therefore, we have opted to include more pictures rather than more words. The reader is referred to standard texts of oral and maxillofacial pathology for more detailed discussions and references. We have attempted to be comprehensive, including as many diseases as possible without becoming overly esoteric. Added emphasis has been given to more commonly occurring disorders, since these are the diseases most likely to be encountered by the clinician. No photomicrographs have been included in this book. Although, as oral and maxillofacial pathologists, we recognize the importance of histopathology in the overall understanding of disease processes, we think the purpose of this atlas and its usefulness to the clinician are better served by limiting it to clinical photographs and radiographs.

In this second edition, we have attempted to thoroughly update both the text and references. In addition, a total of 181 new illustrations have been included, and 22 new entities have been added. The section on acquired immunodeficiency syndrome has been expanded, and a separate chapter on allergies and immunologic diseases has been added.

The task of writing this second edition was made sadder by the death of one of our original authors, Dr. Charles A. Waldron. Our thoughts were always with Chuck as we worked on this second edition; many of the written words on the following pages still reflect his thoughts and ideas, either directly or indirectly through his teachings to us.

*Charleston, SC*                                                                    Brad W. Neville
*Lexington, KY*                                                                  Douglas D. Damm
*Lexington, KY*                                                                    Dean K. White

# ACKNOWLEDGMENTS

Obviously, any undertaking of this nature reflects more than just the work of its authors. We are deeply indebted to our many friends and colleagues who have shared cases with us for use in this book. We have attempted to be as thorough as possible in listing credit for those shared cases. However, if anyone's name has been inadvertently omitted, please accept our sincerest apologies.

We wish to thank Sharon Zinner, Tanya Lazar, Bob Magee and Tim Hiscock at Williams & Wilkins for all of their considerable help and patience in the production of this book. Special praise goes to Mr. Thomson Rast at the Medical University of South Carolina for his help in preparing many of the radiographic prints. Finally, our families deserve a more personal thanks for their love, understanding, and support during the preparation of this atlas.

# CONTENTS

# chapter 1
# DEVELOPMENTAL DISTURBANCES OF THE
# ORAL AND MAXILLOFACIAL REGION

## DOUBLE LIP

**Fig. 1.1**

Double lip refers to a linear fold of excess hyperplastic tissue along the mucosal surface of the lip. Typically, the process involves the upper lip bilaterally, but it may be unilateral or affect the lower lip. When bilateral, the enlargements often have a "cupid's bow" appearance. Most examples are congenital but do not become evident clinically until after teeth eruption. A minority of the cases are acquired and associated with Ascher syndrome, an oral habit or trauma. The cause of Ascher syndrome has not been determined definitively, but affected patients classically present with double lip, blepharochalasis, and nontoxic thyroid enlargement. The blepharochalasis usually occurs in the upper lids and presents as a sagging fold of tissue located between the eyebrow and the edge of the lid. The thyroid enlargement normally is present by the second decade of life but, in some patients, may be found only on thyroid scan. In cases of double lip that are problematic, either functionally or aesthetically, excision is indicated. Recurrence has been documented only in the acquired forms.

## COMMISSURAL LIP PITS

**Fig. 1.2**

Commissural lip pits are congenital invaginations of the surface mucosa of the vermilion of the lip at the commissure. The process may be unilateral or bilateral and seems to be inherited as an autosomal-dominant disorder. These pits are not rare and, in a male prevalence study, were detected in approximately 20% of blacks and 12% of whites. Usually, the invagination is 1 to 2 mm in diameter, may be as deep as 4 mm, and is lined by stratified squamous epithelium. Occasionally, minor salivary gland ducts empty into the pits, and mucus can be expressed from these invaginations. Commissural lip pits create no adverse symptoms, are not objectionable cosmetically, and require no therapy.

## PARAMEDIAN LIP PITS

**Fig. 1.3**

Paramedian lip pits are congenital invaginations of the vermilion of the lip that typically are found on the lower lip on either side of the midline. The pits vary in size and may be as large as 3 mm in diameter and 2.5 cm in depth. Communication with the underlying minor salivary glands is seen, and mucin may be present in the pits. Paramedian lip pits are rare and thought to be autosomal dominant with variable expressivity. Although these pits may be seen as an isolated finding, they are present in combination with cleft lip or palate in 70 to 80% of patients (van der Woude syndrome). Patients with isolated paramedian lip pits should be counseled concerning the 15 to 29% risk of having a child with a cleft lip or palate. These pits are a characteristic feature of the popliteal pterygium syndrome and may occur as a finding in the orofaciodigital syndrome, type I. Other alterations reported to occasionally occur in association with paramedian lip pits include hypodontia, ankyloglossia, syndactyly, equinovarus foot deformity, and congenital heart disease. Aesthetically objectionable examples are treated by surgical excision with inclusion of the surrounding minor salivary glands.

### ► Figure 1.1
**DOUBLE LIP**
Linear fold of hyperplastic tissue of the upper lip in a patient with Ascher syndrome. (Courtesy of Dr. R. C. Zeigler.)

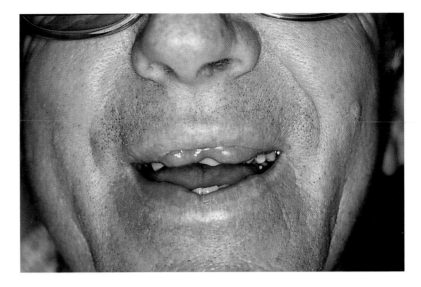

### ► Figure 1.2
**COMMISSURAL LIP PITS**
Surface mucosal invagination of the right corner of the mouth.

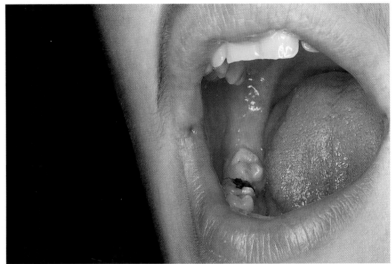

### ► Figure 1.3
**PARAMEDIAN LIP PITS**
Bilateral invaginations of the vermilion highlighted with gutta percha points.

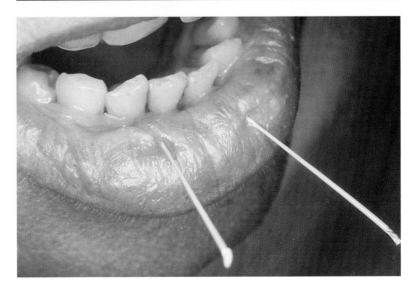

## CLEFT LIP

**Fig. 1.4**

Cleft lip is a relatively common defect of the lateral upper lip characterized by failure of the tissue processes to fuse during embryonic life. It may occur as an isolated defect or as a component of a variety of hereditary syndromes. Midline clefts of the upper or lower lip also rarely occur. The cleft may extend through the soft tissue and involve the maxillary alveolar ridge as deep as the incisive canal. The cleft may involve only the free portion of the upper lip (incomplete cleft) or extend to involve the nostril on that side (complete cleft). Unilateral or bilateral involvement can be seen. Cleft lip occurs in combination with cleft palate approximately twice as often as it is seen as an isolated defect and is more frequent among males. Whites are affected more often than blacks, and the reported prevalence in the general population ranges from 1.00 to 1.82 per 1000 live births. Cleft lips are usually repaired surgically before the affected infant is 6 weeks of age to avoid difficulties in nursing.

## CLEFT PALATE

**Fig. 1.5**

Cleft palate is a defect in which the lateral halves of the palate fail to fuse during embryonic development. It may be localized to the uvula, or it may involve the soft palate alone or both the hard and soft palate. The frequency of combined cleft palate and cleft lip is double that of isolated cleft palate. From a hereditary basis, isolated cleft palate is a separate entity from isolated cleft lip or combined cleft lip and cleft palate. As a group, these disorders exhibit a multifactorial inheritance pattern in which both hereditary and environmental factors seem to be involved. Combined cleft lip and cleft palate is more common in boys, whereas isolated cleft palate occurs more frequently in girls. Corrective surgery is usually successful and is scheduled after 18 months of age.

## BIFID UVULA

**Fig. 1.6**

Bifid uvula (cleft uvula) is division of the uvula into two lobes; it represents the mildest form of cleft palate. The size of the division may vary from minimal to complete separation of the uvula into two halves. The prevalence is greater in males than in females, and the disturbance exhibits a familial pattern similar to that of isolated cleft palate. Association with submucous clefts, eustachian tube hypoplasia, and aplasia of the salpingopharyngeal folds has been documented. Because of the association with submucous clefts, affected patients should be evaluated for hypernasality; removal of the adenoids should be avoided due to the risk of inducing hypernasality. Evaluation of otologic status also is recommended secondary to an increased prevalence of middle ear disease in patients with cleft palate. Bifid uvula also has been reported to occur in patients with craniofacial dysostosis and frontometaphyseal dysplasia. No treatment is necessary.

▶ **Figure 1.4**
**CLEFT LIP**
Bilateral complete cleft of the upper lip.
(Courtesy of Dr. Joel Cooper.)

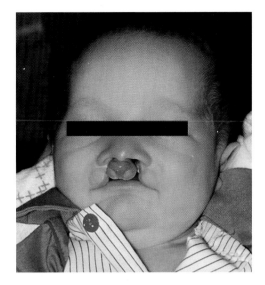

▶ **Figure 1.5**
**CLEFT PALATE**
Isolated cleft palate.

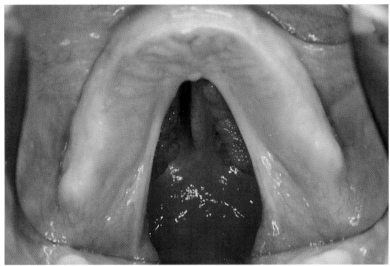

▶ **Figure 1.6**
**BIFID UVULA**
Incomplete division of the uvula into two
lobes.

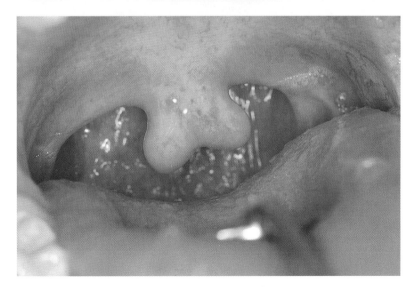

## LATERAL PALATAL FISTULA

### Fig. 1.7

Lateral palatal fistulas are epithelial-lined channels through the soft palate that interconnect the oral cavity and oropharynx or nasopharynx. Typically, these tracts are congenital, but they also may be acquired secondary to rupture of a peritonsillar abscess or surgical complications. Most congenital examples are bilateral and symmetrical, with familial cases having been documented. Congenital lateral palatal fistulas have been seen in association with absence or hypoplasia of the palatine tonsils, preauricular fistulas, hearing loss, and strabismus. The defect is thought to be secondary to a developmental abnormality of the second branchial pouch. No treatment is required.

## FORDYCE GRANULES

### Figs. 1.8 and 1.9

Fordyce granules are sebaceous glands located on the oral mucosa and the vermilion of the lips. These glands have been noted in the buccal mucosa and vestibules in approximately 80% of the adult population and should be considered normal structures. Although these glands begin to appear in many patients during the first decade of life, a significantly lower prevalence has been documented in the pediatric population. The granules also may occur on the anterior tonsillar pillar, the alveolar ridge, the gingiva, the palate, and the tongue but are uncommon in these locations and should be considered ectopic when discovered in these sites. Fordyce granules appear as multiple yellow maculopapular lesions typically smaller than 2 mm. The extent of involvement increases with age and is more pronounced in males than in females. Hyperplasia and neoplasia of the glands have been documented rarely, and biopsy is recommended for patients with abnormally large Fordyce granules or granules exhibiting continued growth. Otherwise, these sebaceous glands create no problems and require no therapy.

### Figure 1.7
**LATERAL PALATAL FISTULA**

Epithelial-lined tract of the right side of the soft palate joining the oral cavity and the nasopharynx. This adult patient had a tonsillectomy as a teen.

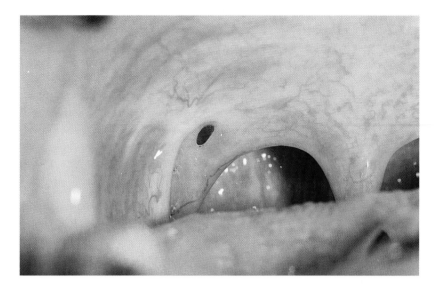

### Figure 1.8
**FORDYCE GRANULES**

Multiple yellow papules of the right buccal mucosa.

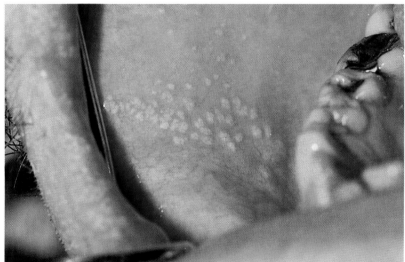

### Figure 1.9
**FORDYCE GRANULES**

Multiple closely spaced papules of the vermilion border of the upper lip.

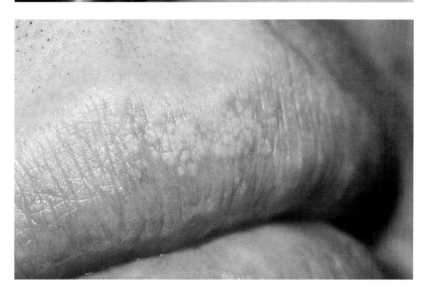

## Figs. 1.10 and 1.11

Leukoedema is a variation of oral mucosa in which the involved tissue appears white or gray with a filmy, opalescent hue. The tissue may be thickened sufficiently to form prominent wrinkles. Usually, it is seen on the buccal mucosa bilaterally, but adjacent mucosa also may be involved. Although the alteration seems to be more prevalent among adults, leukoedema is not rare in newborns. The process is much more common in blacks, with one study of newborns documenting a fivefold increased prevalence. Numerous publications have suggested that many instances of leukoedema represent an acquired alteration related to local low-grade irritants such as poor oral hygiene, spicy foods, and tobacco. There is conflicting evidence concerning the acquired form, and this may represent a clinically similar but somewhat different process.

When the involved area is stretched, the white appearance usually disappears or becomes hardly noticeable. When the stretched mucosa is relaxed, the typical features reappear. No treatment is necessary, but leukoedema must be distinguished from other mucosal alterations that may appear white.

## LINGUAL THYROID

## Fig. 1.12

Lingual thyroid is a developmental abnormality in which thyroid tissue is present in the base of the tongue between the circumvallate papillae and the epiglottis. Postmortem studies have demonstrated this ectopic tissue in 10% of individuals, but the prevalence of grossly visible lesions is only 1:10,000. Symptoms related to the abnormality rarely arise at any age, but hyperplasia may occur in response to an increased metabolic demand brought on by stress such as puberty, pregnancy, menopause, trauma, or infection. A female predominance of 7:1 is seen, with the most common symptoms being hemorrhage, dysphagia, dysphonia, and dyspnea. Approximately 70% of affected patients exhibit some hypothyroidism. Carcinoma may arise within lingual thyroid, but the rate of malignant transformation is no greater than that seen in normally placed glands.

Computed tomography, magnetic resonance imaging, and radionuclide scans with technetium 99m and radioactive iodine aid in arriving at a definitive diagnosis and in investigating the presence of cervical thyroid. The initial therapeutic approach in symptomatic patients is administration of suppressive exogenous thyroid hormone. Surgical removal is performed in patients who worsen during medical treatment. During surgical removal, accidental loss of the parathyroid glands does not occur because they follow a different path of descent and still will be located in their normal cervical position. If surgically removed, autotransplantation to another body site has been performed in an attempt to maintain functional thyroid tissue. Due to unpredictable results, ablation with radioactive iodine is reserved for poor surgical candidates or those who refuse surgery.

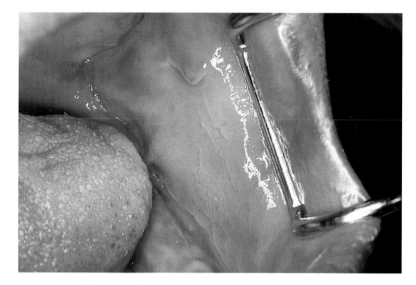

**Figure 1.10**
**LEUKOEDEMA**
White opalescent appearance of buccal mucosa with thin folds.

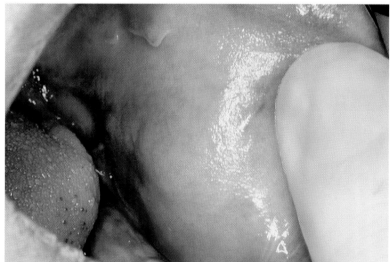

**Figure 1.11**
**LEUKOEDEMA**
Same patient as in Figure 1.10 with clearing of white appearance when buccal mucosa is stretched.

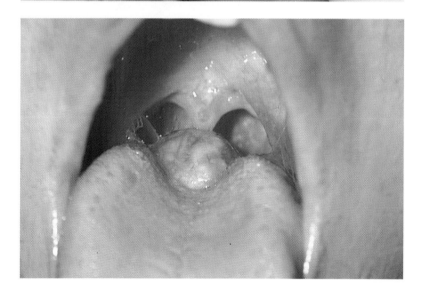

**Figure 1.12**
**LINGUAL THYROID**
Exophytic mass of the posterior tongue. (Courtesy of Dr. Jerry Bouquot.)

## ANKYLOGLOSSIA

**Fig. 1.13**

Ankyloglossia is limited tongue movement secondary to improper attachment to the floor of the mouth, with the majority of patients demonstrating a familial pattern. The restriction of movement may be due to a shortened lingual frenum or a more anterior attachment between the free end of the tongue and the floor of the mouth. Ankyloglossia may be partial or total, with the latter exhibiting complete fusion between the tongue and the floor of the mouth. Recent investigations in infants have demonstrated a correlation between ankyloglossia and an upper-forward displacement of the epiglottis and larynx, with resultant varying degrees of dyspnea and difficulties in nursing. An association with sudden infant death syndrome has been proposed. In addition, the abnormal tongue position is thought to affect the growth and development of the skull, with a resultant increased prevalence of high-arched palate and Angle class III malocclusion. In older patients, the most common presenting symptoms include sucking or swallowing problems, speech difficulties, and mechanical problems such as the inability to lick the lips or play a wind instrument.

Secondary to past overtreatment, a significant reduction in the number of patients receiving treatment has been seen, with many practitioners refusing to consider surgical intervention. Frenotomy is deemed appropriate for infants who reveal related dyspnea or significant associated nursing difficulties and for older patients with ankyloglossia-related symptoms. Surgically cutting the anterior connective tissues (the lingual frenum if present) and the front bundles of the genioglossal muscles corrects the anterior deviation of the tongue, epiglottis, and larynx.

## HAIRY TONGUE

**Fig. 1.14**

Hairy tongue is an unusual condition characterized by elongation and hyperkeratosis of the filiform papillae, resulting in a hairlike appearance. The elongated papillae usually exhibit brown, yellow, or black pigmentation, but occasionally they are white. The process often is misdiagnosed as candidiasis but typically does not respond to treatment with antifungal medications. These changes must be separated from those of pseudohairy tongue, in which there is discoloration of the dorsal surface of the tongue but no elongation of the filiform papillae. The most commonly affected region is the midline just anterior to the circumvallate papillae, but sometimes most of the dorsal surface is involved. Most patients are asymptomatic, but occasionally patients complain of irritation, gagging, malodor, or an altered taste.

Although the cause is uncertain, most affected patients are heavy smokers. Hairy tongue also has been associated with use of oxidizing agents, poor oral hygiene, vitamin deficiency, gastrointestinal disturbances, general debilitation, and radiation therapy and less certainly with the overgrowth of microorganisms or antibiotic therapy. A variety of therapeutic measures ranging from topical corticosteroids to salicylic acid have been used, but the most common approach is frequent use of a mechanical tongue scraper to promote desquamation of the papillae. Recently, isolated case reports have documented successful use of tretinoin, which is thought to decrease cohesiveness of the superficial epithelium, resulting in increased desquamation.

## FISSURED TONGUE (SCROTAL OR PLICATED TONGUE)

**Fig. 1.15**

Fissured tongue (scrotal or plicated tongue) is a textural variation of the surface of the tongue that exhibits a prevalence of approximately 2 to 5%. Classically, a central groove is present along the midline of the dorsal surface, with an arborization of smaller grooves from this main fissure. Heredity seems to affect the development of the grooves, but local environmental factors also may contribute to the process. It is not uncommon for patients with fissured tongue also to demonstrate geographic tongue (erythema migrans). In addition, patients who have orofacial granulomatosis may demonstrate fissured tongue in addition to facial edema, facial paralysis, and cheilitis granulomatosa; this has been termed Melkersson-Rosenthal syndrome (see Figs. 6.10 to 6.12). Typically, fissured tongue is asymptomatic, except when debris becomes lodged within deep grooves. Mechanical removal of the debris resolves the symptoms.

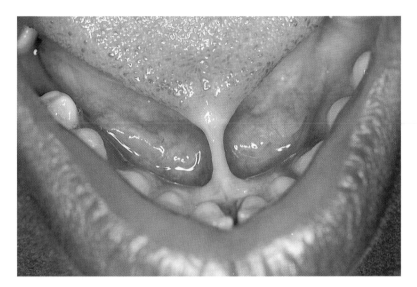

### Figure 1.13
**ANKYLOGLOSSIA**
Short lingual frenum attaching the tip of the tongue to the floor of the mouth.

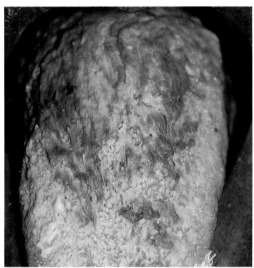

### Figure 1.14
**HAIRY TONGUE**
Dorsal surface of the tongue exhibiting brown and elongated filiform papillae. (Courtesy of Dr. Robert Strohaver.)

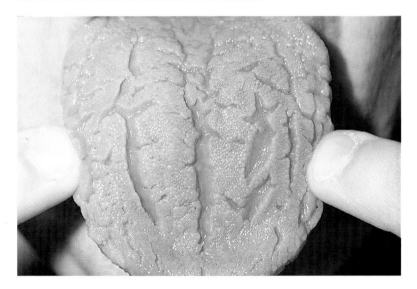

### Figure 1.15
**FISSURED TONGUE**
Dorsal surface of the tongue with numerous invaginations of the surface epithelium.

## HYPERPLASTIC LYMPHOID AGGREGATES

**Figs. 1.16 and 1.17**

Hyperplastic lymphoid aggregates are submucosal accumulations of benign reactive lymphoid tissue that occur in locations other than the tonsillar fauces and the areas of the foliate papillae. Some authors refer to these nodules as ectopic tonsils, but not all of these aggregates occur in patients with Waldeyer's ring. Although hyperplastic lymphoid tissue is most frequent on the soft palate or oropharynx, it is not uncommon in the floor of the mouth. Cases in the buccal mucosa, gingiva, and tongue have been reported also.

The typical lymphoid aggregate presents as a nodular elevation of the surface mucosa; the elevation is usually approximately 3 mm in diameter. The color varies from pink to amber to pale yellow. Multiple lesions are not rare. Occasionally, lymphoid aggregates develop central areas of bright yellow coloration that, on biopsy examination, often prove to be lymphoepithelial cysts or epithelial-lined crypts filled with desquamated keratin. Occasionally, isolated hyperplastic lymphoid aggregates present as firm submucosal nodules and vary sufficiently from the typical presentation to mimic neoplasia. Many of these aggregates appear in the buccal mucosa. Excisional biopsy is the treatment of choice for these deeper lesions if they fail to resolve on their own.

## MINERALIZATION OF THE STYLOHYOID LIGAMENT

**Fig. 1.18**

Commonly, the stylohyoid ligament undergoes partial mineralization. The alteration typically begins in the upper part of the ligament, but the changes may occur in isolated segments or extend to involve the entire ligament. When significant mineralization is present, a radiopaque extension of the stylohyoid process is seen posterior to the ramus of the mandible on a panoramic radiograph. Prevalence studies present conflicting information, but the detection of the process seems to increase with age, and there is a slight predominance among females. Secondary to an increasingly high prevalence reported in a few studies of older patients, some investigators believe the mineralization represents a variation of normal anatomy.

Rarely, complete mineralization of the stylohyoid ligament has been associated with difficulties in intubation and, in other patients, significant clinical symptoms. In symptomatic patients, the classic pattern of presentation has been termed Eagle syndrome, and it exhibits a sharp pain felt in the tonsillar region, the base of the tongue, posterior to the angle of the mandible or the temporomandibular joint. Typically, it occurs on mandibular movement or from turning the head or neck. Many cases follow tonsillectomy, which often produces scar tissue over the area of the mineralized ligament. Some patients exhibit syncope when they quickly turn their heads and the ligament places pressure on the external carotid (carotid artery syndrome). In these patients, surgical resection resolves the symptoms, but only after a thorough medical evaluation to rule out other possible causes.

▶ **Figure 1.16**
**HYPERPLASTIC LYMPHOID AGGREGATES**
Multiple small pink lymphoid aggregates of the soft palate.

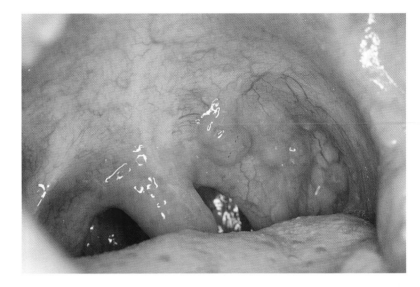

▶ **Figure 1.17**
**HYPERPLASTIC LYMPHOID AGGREGATES**
Two dark pink nodules in the floor of the mouth on either side of the lingual frenum.

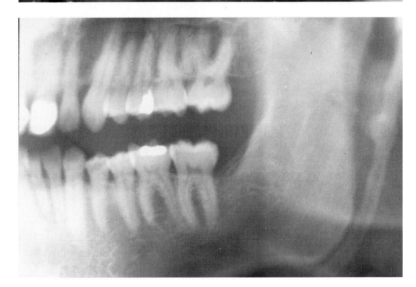

▶ **Figure 1.18**
**MINERALIZATION OF THE STYLOHYOID LIGAMENT**
Radiopaque stylohyoid ligament seen immediately posterior to the mandibular ramus.

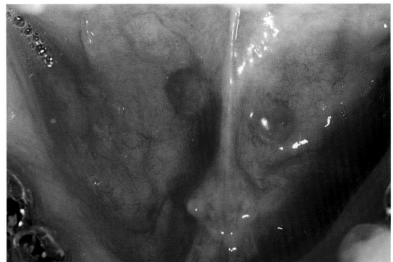

## BUCCAL EXOSTOSES

### Fig. 1.19

Exostoses are localized outgrowths of the cortical surface of a bone. The enlargements may consist of dense lamellar bone or demonstrate a normal-thickness cortex with underlying bone marrow and medullary bone. These nonneoplastic proliferations frequently affect the jaws, and the most common patterns are torus palatinus and torus mandibularis (see Figs. 1.20 to 1.23).

Although frequent, buccal exostoses are noted less often than are tori. Typically, these outgrowths present as a bilateral row of exophytic bone along the facial surface of the alveolar ridges, usually at the midroot level. The enlargements may involve only the posterior dentition or may extend to the contralateral quadrant, with involvement of the anterior regions of the jaw. Either one or both arches may be affected, and concurrence with tori is not rare. Unilateral involvement of an isolated portion of the alveolar ridge occurs less commonly and may be related to localized irritation or inflammation. Such solitary exostoses have arisen underlying skin and mucosal grafts. Surgical removal is reserved for exostoses affecting aesthetics, periodontal therapy, or dental prostheses.

## TORUS PALATINUS

### Figs. 1.20 and 1.21

Torus palatinus is one of the more common forms of exostosis that affects the jaws. These tori arise in the midline of the palate and present in a variety of shapes, varying from sessile enlargements to discrete nodules to larger nodules that often are subdivided into several lobes. The protuberance usually is localized and found in the mid-third of the palate but may enlarge and fill the entire vault, with extension above the level of the alveolar ridges. The elevation either consists entirely of dense cortical bone or presents as an outer layer of lamellar bone with underlying cancellous bone and abundant fatty marrow. The overlying mucosa is normal or pale in color. Secondary ulceration from trauma is not rare.

Palatal tori exhibit a predominance among females and seem to be affected by both genetic and environmental influences. The enlargement is not a static or progressively enlarging lesion but a dynamic process that constantly is responding to environmental and functional factors, especially those of masticatory stress. The prevalence is higher among middle-aged patients, with smaller numbers noted in both younger and older groups. Most palatal tori do not create significant radiographic alterations, with the diagnosis made from the clinical presentation. Most palatal tori require no treatment, but the enlargements occasionally are removed when they interfere with the construction of dental appliances, affect speech, become constantly traumatized, or bother the patient. Recurrence is not expected but theoretically is possible due to the dynamic nature of the process.

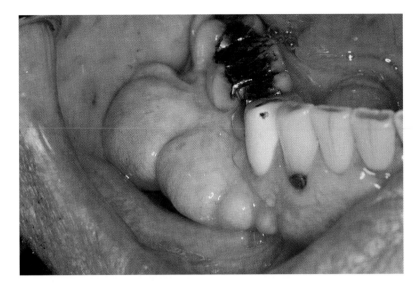

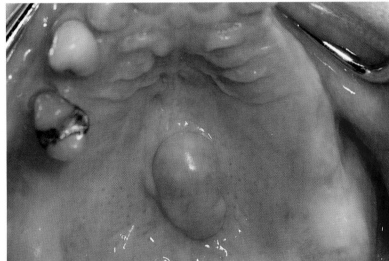

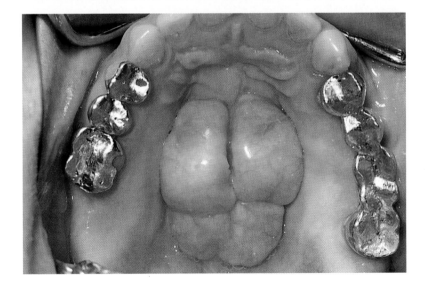

### Figs. 1.22 and 1.23

Torus mandibularis is another common pattern of exostosis that affects the jaws and presents as an enlargement of the lingual surface of the mandible, usually located above the mylohyoid line adjacent to the mandibular bicuspids. The mass may consist entirely of dense lamellar bone or may demonstrate a cap of cortical bone overlying cancellous bone and fatty marrow. These tori typically are bilateral, but occasionally they are unilateral. They vary widely in size and shape, with individual tori presenting as single sessile masses, lobulated growths, or multiple separate enlargements. The overlying mucosa may be normal, atrophic, or secondarily ulcerated from trauma. With large tori, periapical radiographs of the anterior dentition typically reveal the overlying cortical enlargements. Radiographs of the body of the mandible vary according to the degree of compact bone present within the torus. Little evidence will be noted in those with a significant amount of cancellous bone and marrow. In contrast, those consisting primarily of compact bone demonstrate areas of increased density typically overlying the bicuspids. The radiopacities may be confused with other signs of disease, but when they are combined with the clinical presentation, the diagnosis is obvious.

Like its palatal counterpart, torus mandibularis is a dynamic process that exhibits a hereditary predisposition but is influenced by environmental and functional factors, especially masticatory stress. Its presence has been correlated positively to the number of functioning teeth. The prevalence peaks during early adulthood and declines during senescence, suggesting that resorption remodeling occurs secondary to decreased masticatory stress. Unlike torus palatinus, mandibular tori demonstrate an increased prevalence in males. The presence of either a palatal or a mandibular torus is associated with an increased prevalence of a torus of the opposing arch. Treatment is required only when the enlargements constantly are traumatized or when they interfere with speech or with construction of a dental prosthesis. Although theoretically possible, recurrence is not expected.

### Fig. 1.24

Subpontine exostosis (subpontic hyperostosis) represents a unique nonneoplastic proliferation of cortical bone that so far occurs exclusively in the premolar-molar area of the mandible underlying pontics of fixed partial dentures. The crestal cortical expansion may arise within a few months or many years after placement of the prosthesis. Typically, the process stabilizes after a period of slow enlargement; but, rarely, the growth continues until displacement of the prosthesis occurs. Clinically, expansion of the alveolar ridge between the abutments is noted and often fills the space beneath the pontic, creating difficulties in oral hygiene. These exostoses radiographically present as opaque enlargements that are continuous with the adjacent cortical bone and often form a dome-shaped extension toward the overlying pontic. On occasion, the crestal portion forms a saucer-shaped indentation that conforms to the inferior portion of the pontic. Histopathologic examination of removed samples reveals dense, vital lamellar bone.

Concurrence with mandibular tori is high (more than 40%), suggesting that similar factors may be involved in the initiation of the process. Like other forms of exostoses, the exact cause is unknown. Most likely it arises from a combination of heredity and localized environmental factors, such as inflammation or altered masticatory stresses created by the prosthesis. Surgical excision is recommended when the enlargement displaces the prosthesis or creates difficulties in oral hygiene. Recurrences have been reported. In one patient with recurrence, spontaneous resolution occurred after removal of the prosthesis, which ultimately was replaced with a single tooth implant and crown.

▶ **Figure 1.22**
**TORUS MANDIBULARIS**
Bilateral enlargements of the lingual surface of the mandible.

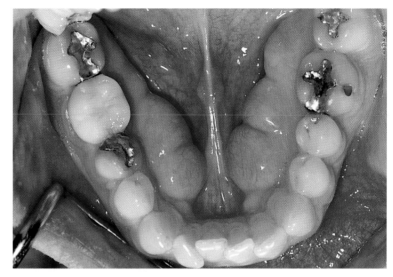

▶ **Figure 1.23**
**TORUS MANDIBULARIS**
Bilateral radiodensities overlying the apices of the mandibular teeth. (Courtesy of Dr. L. R. Bean.)

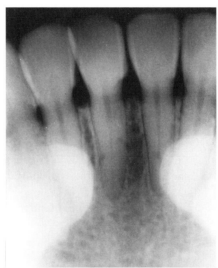

▶ **Figure 1.24**
**SUBPONTINE EXOSTOSIS**
Radiopaque expansion of crestal bone immediately beneath pontic of a fixed partial denture.

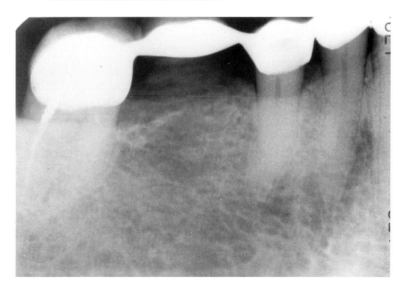

## LINGUAL VARICOSITIES

**Fig. 1.25**

Lingual varicosities are dilated tortuous veins that occur on the ventral surface of the tongue. The affected veins typically are noted as numerous dark blue to purple nodules located between the central sublingual veins and the lateral border of the tongue. Due to an increased prevalence in older adults, varicosities seem to be secondary to the aging process, with the alteration being noted in the majority of patients older than 60 years. The occurrence of lingual varicosities in individuals younger than 60 years has been associated with a significantly higher prevalence of cardiopulmonary disease. The presence of lingual varicosities has been found to directly correlate with the presence of varicosities in the legs.

## SOLITARY AND THROMBOSED VARICOSITIES

**Figs. 1.26 and 1.27**

Intraoral varicosities commonly occur in sites other than the ventral tongue, with the upper and lower lip, buccal mucosa, and mucobuccal folds affected most frequently. On occasion, these superficial dilated veins may develop a thrombus; often, at that time, the varix is more obvious clinically and is easily discovered. These thrombosed varicosities present as dark blue or purple, firm, nontender, and freely movable submucosal masses. Typically, a solitary varix requires no therapy unless the clinical diagnosis is in doubt. Thrombi within oral varicosities may dissolve, undergo rechannelization, or exhibit dystrophic calcification (phlebolith). Due to their small size, they are of little clinical significance but occasionally are excised to confirm the diagnosis or to alleviate related symptoms such as mild tenderness or swelling.

**▶ Figure 1.25**
**LINGUAL VARICOSITIES**
Multiple dark blue nodules of the ventral surface of the tongue.

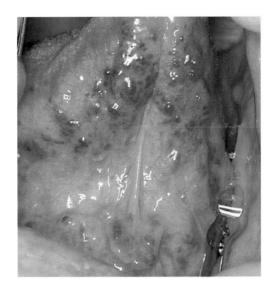

**▶ Figure 1.26**
**MUCOSAL VARIX**
Soft, dark blue nodule of the left buccal mucosa. Note blue vein leading to the area of dilation.

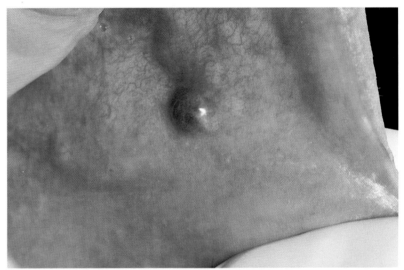

**▶ Figure 1.27**
**THROMBOSED VARIX**
Firm dark blue nodule of the lower lip on the right side.

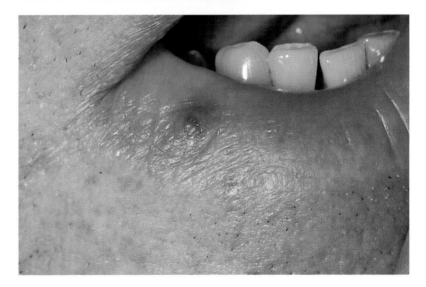

**Figs. 1.28 and 1.29**

The nasopalatine duct cyst (median anterior maxillary cyst incisive canal cyst) is a developmental cyst that arises from remnants of the nasopalatine duct, which is enclosed within the incisive canal and normally disappears before birth. At birth, only vestigial epithelial strands are found within the incisive canal, and these strands represent the source of epithelium for this cyst. The nasopalatine duct cyst is the most common nonodontogenic cyst in the jaws, and it exhibits a slight predominance among males. Although the majority of nasopalatine duct cysts are discovered secondary to related symptoms, many are found during routine radiographic examination. The classic presentation is a symmetrical ovoid or heart-shaped radiolucency above or between the roots of the maxillary central incisors. At times, enlarged lucencies in the area have been stated to represent an enlarged incisive foramen, but the average diameter of this structure is approximately 3 mm.

A majority of patients are symptomatic and usually present with swelling, pain, drainage, or tooth movement. On occasion, these cysts may be present completely within the soft tissue of the incisive papilla (cyst of the incisive papilla), and secondary inflammation, pain, and swelling are not uncommon. Occasionally, intraosseous examples may present clinically as anterior midline palatal swellings that can perforate the cortical bone and drain thin fluid or pus. Larger cysts rarely may enlarge to such an extent as to produce both palatal and facial swelling with possible drainage on either side of the alveolus. Histopathologically, the cysts demonstrate a lining of stratified squamous epithelium, cuboidal epithelium, columnar epithelium, pseudostratified ciliated columnar epithelium, or a combination of any of these.

Although nasopalatine duct cysts seem to demonstrate limited growth potential, all symptomatic lesions and those larger than 6 mm in diameter should be removed and submitted for histopathologic examination. Many other cystic and solid tumors, especially odontogenic keratocysts, can mimic nasopalatine duct cysts, and definitive diagnosis cannot be made from the clinical and radiographic features alone. With thorough curettage, recurrences are uncommon. Rare carcinomatous transformation has been reported.

## MEDIAN PALATAL CYST

**Fig. 1.30**

The median palatal cyst is a fissural cyst that develops from entrapped epithelium along the fusion line of the palatal processes of the maxilla. This cyst is so uncommon that many pathologists deny its existence, and it has been removed from the most recent World Health Organization listing of nonodontogenic cysts of the jaws. Despite this, extremely rare examples may occur. Many cases diagnosed in the past actually represent superiorly positioned nasopalatine duct cysts. The diagnosis of median palatal cyst must be made from a correlation of the clinical, radiographic, and histopathologic features. Because median palatal cysts arise at the level of the palatal vault, all patients demonstrate a clinically evident swelling in the midline of the hard palate.

Radiographically, the cyst typically presents as a midline unilocular radiolucency in the palate posterior to the apices of the maxillary central incisors, a pattern also produced by superiorly located nasopalatine duct cysts. In its path from the incisive papilla to the nasal cavity, the nasopalatine duct courses superiorly and slightly posteriorly. Superiorly positioned nasopalatine duct cysts typically mimic the radiographic pattern of median palatal cysts; however, due to its superior location, no clinically evident swelling of the palate is noted until the cyst reaches significant size. Histopathologically, median palatal cysts typically are lined by stratified squamous epithelium; however, cuboidal, columnar, and ciliated pseudostratified columnar epithelium may be seen. The diagnosis of median palatal cyst should be made with caution and requires compatible histopathologic features, clinically evident midline swelling of the palate, and no anatomic possibility of communication with remnants of the nasopalatine duct. This rare cyst should be removed surgically.

▶ **Figure 1.28**
**NASOPALATINE DUCT CYST**
Small radiolucency between the roots of
vital maxillary central incisors.

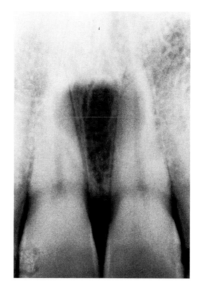

▶ **Figure 1.29**
**NASOPALATINE DUCT CYST**
Large radiolucency in the midline of the
anterior maxilla. (Courtesy of Dr. Richard
Marks.)

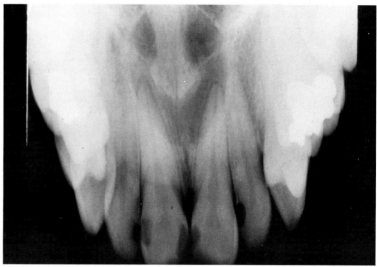

▶ **Figure 1.30**
**MEDIAN PALATAL CYST**
Midline radiolucency of the palate.

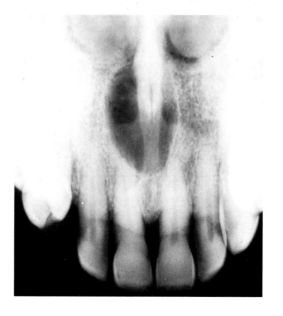

## NASOPALATINE DUCT CYST MIMICKING A MEDIAN PALATAL CYST

**Figs. 1.31 and 1.32**

As mentioned previously, reports of patients with persisting nasopalatine ducts have demonstrated that the ducts typically course superiorly and slightly posteriorly from the incisive canal on their path toward the nasal cavity. Nasopalatine duct cysts that arise from a portion of the duct located close to the nasal cavity may present radiographically as a median palatal cyst. Examples of nasopalatine duct cysts have been seen that present radiographically as median palatal cysts but on surgery communicate with the incisive canal. Many lesions called median palatal cysts may represent posteriorly located nasopalatine duct cysts.

## PERIAPICAL CYST PRESENTING AS SO-CALLED "GLOBULOMAXILLARY CYST"

**Fig. 1.33**

The globulomaxillary cyst classically was described as a fissural cyst that developed along the fusion line of the globular and maxillary processes. The cyst typically presented as a unilocular radiolucency located between the roots of the maxillary cuspid and the lateral incisor, with divergence of the roots of these adjacent teeth. Several reports have appeared during the past two decades that cast serious doubt on this entity, with reviews of the embryologic evidence failing to show epithelial entrapment within the mesenchyme of the area. Evaluations of radiographically diagnosed globulomaxillary cysts fail to reveal any fissural cysts, with most examples representing periapical inflammatory lesions, odontogenic keratocysts, or other odontogenic tumors. After a thorough review of the available facts, the World Health Organization chose to delete globulomaxillary cyst from the list of jaw cysts in its 1992 classification.

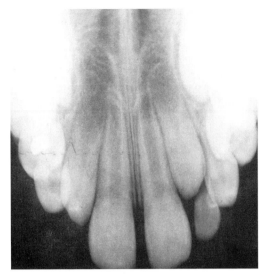

► **Figure 1.31**
**NASOPALATINE DUCT CYST MIMICKING A MEDIAN PALATAL CYST**
Midline radiolucency of the posterior palate. On surgery, the cyst communicated with the incisive canal.

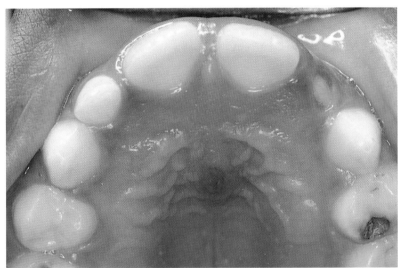

► **Figure 1.32**
**NASOPALATINE DUCT CYST MIMICKING A MEDIAN PALATAL CYST**
Erythematous enlargement in the midline of the anterior palate. This is the clinical presentation of the previous radiograph (Fig. 1.31).

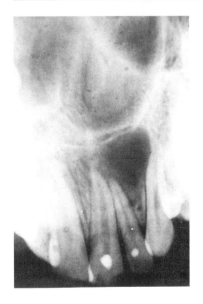

► **Figure 1.33**
**PERIAPICAL CYST PRESENTING AS SO-CALLED "GLOBULOMAXILLARY CYST"**
Radiolucency between the apices of the maxillary lateral and cuspid. The surgical specimen revealed an apical periodontal cyst and the lateral incisor was shown to be nonvital.

# NASOLABIAL CYST (NASOALVEOLAR CYST, KLESTADT CYST)

## Figs. 1.34 and 1.35

The nasolabial cyst (nasoalveolar cyst, Klestadt cyst) presents as a soft-tissue swelling of the maxillary anterior mucolabial fold that is off the midline and causes elevation of the ala of the nose on that side. This cyst is external to the bone but may produce cupping of the underlying cortical plate. Although computed tomography, magnetic resonance imaging, and ultrasonography may be used to confirm the cystic nature and define its relationship to surrounding structures, some investigators consider these procedures an unnecessary waste of time and money. An approximate 3:1 female predominance is noted, and slightly more than 10% of the cases are bilateral. The cyst occasionally is lined by stratified squamous epithelium, but it usually demonstrates pseudostratified columnar epithelium that can be ciliated, often with goblet cells.

Classically, the cyst was said to have arisen from entrapped epithelium along the fusion line of the globular, lateral nasal, and maxillary processes; however, subsequent investigations of the embryologic findings have failed to demonstrate ectoderm entrapment in this area. This cyst is in the area of the naso-optic fissure, and proliferation of the nasolacrimal duct has been seen at this site. The high percentage of linings that demonstrate pseudostratified columnar epithelium, often with cilia or goblet cells, is compatible with origin from primitive ductal or glandular structures. The most likely origin is from the nasolacrimal duct or minor salivary gland ducts. Treatment is surgical removal.

# SURGICAL CILIATED CYST (POSTOPERATIVE MAXILLARY CYST)

## Fig. 1.36

The surgical ciliated cyst (postoperative maxillary cyst) presents as a unilocular radiolucency that occurs in the maxilla adjacent to the sinus or nasal cavity but separated from it. The cyst is lined by ciliated pseudostratified columnar epithelium that may exhibit inflammation and squamous metaplasia. Classically, the cyst arises following a Caldwell-Luc operation and is thought to develop from a fragment of sinus lining that becomes entrapped within the adjacent bone of the maxilla and subsequently develops into a cyst. Epithelial entrapment with subsequent cyst formation also has been reported following tooth extraction, facial bone trauma, and orthognathic surgery. Pain, tenderness, and enlargement of the area may be seen. Treatment is surgical enucleation; recurrences are unusual.

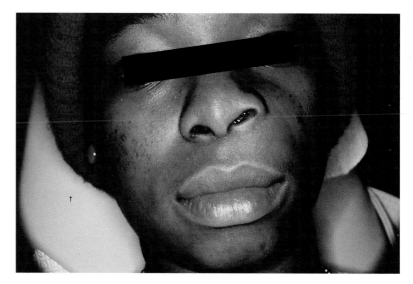

▶ **Figure 1.34**
**NASOLABIAL CYST**
Enlargement of the left side of the upper lip, which has superiorly displaced the adjacent ala of the nose. (Courtesy of Dr. J. C. Weir.)

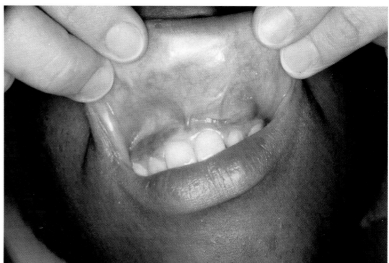

▶ **Figure 1.35**
**NASOLABIAL CYST**
Enlargement of the upper lip on the left side, which has filled the mucolabial fold. (Courtesy of Dr. J. C. Weir.)

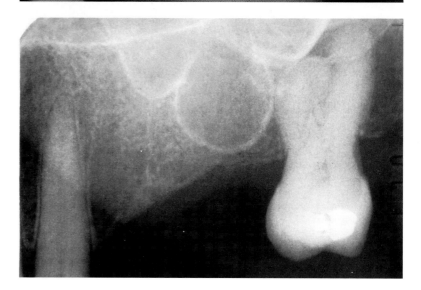

▶ **Figure 1.36**
**SURGICAL CILIATED CYST**
Well-defined radiolucency mesial to the maxillary second molar.

## POSTERIOR LINGUAL MANDIBULAR CORTICAL DEPRESSION (STAFNE DEFECT, SUBMANDIBULAR GLAND DEPRESSION, LATENT BONE CYST, STATIC BONE CYST)

**Fig. 1.37**

The posterior lingual mandibular cortical depression (Stafne defect, submandibular gland depression, latent bone cyst, static bone cyst) presents as a radiolucency of the posterior mandible below the level of the inferior alveolar canal. Most cases typically are well circumscribed and unilocular. Occasionally, examples are bilocular, multilocular, irregular, or associated with buccal expansion. Although most cases are unilateral, bilateral involvement is also seen. The change rarely is documented in children and, on detection in adulthood, may slowly enlarge for several years. The prevalence discovered in radiographic surveys usually is less than 0.05%, with a predominance among males.

The definitive cause has not been determined, but the lesion seems to arise from pressure of adjacent soft tissue on the lingual surface of the mandible with the resultant development of a lingual cortical depression of variable depth. Although the concavity may contain only fat or connective tissue, the submandibular gland typically fills the space. The diagnosis may be confirmed by computed tomographic scan or by demonstrating the presence of intralesional ductal elements on sialogram. In one patient exhibiting spontaneous pain, removal of the involved submandibular gland resulted in resolution of the symptoms and disappearance of the radiographic abnormality. In asymptomatic patients, no treatment is required.

## ANTERIOR LINGUAL MANDIBULAR CORTICAL DEPRESSION

**Fig. 1.38**

Although rare compared with posterior concavities, anterior lingual cortical depressions containing salivary gland tissue also have been documented. Typically, these defects are filled with lobules of sublingual gland and present more difficult diagnostic dilemmas because they do not create a distinctive radiographic pattern. Anterior mandibular concavities present as circumscribed or ill-defined radiolucencies that typically are superimposed over the teeth or in a periapical location. Although usually unilateral, bilateral cases have been documented. In contrast to those reported in the posterior mandible, anterior concavities do not cluster in one anatomic location and can be scattered from the area of the central incisor to the second bicuspid. Cortical expansion and associated symptoms typically are not seen.

Standard radiographic results provide few clues to the definitive diagnosis; in a review of 25 patients, only one investigator considered a salivary gland depression during initial radiographic review. An anterior lingual mandibular cortical depression should be considered in the differential diagnosis of any interradicular or periapical radiolucency associated with vital teeth within the anterior mandible. Although expensive, computed tomographic and magnetic resonance imaging scans are able to confirm the diagnosis without surgical intervention. Once appropriately diagnosed, no therapy is required.

## EPSTEIN'S PEARLS

**Fig. 1.39**

Epstein's pearls are common congenital, keratin-filled cysts that occur in the palatal raphe area. In one review of 420 neonates, these cysts were present in 56%. They are thought to arise from epithelial remnants present along the line of fusion of the palatal halves. Epstein's pearls should not be confused with the dental lamina cysts of the newborn that occur on the alveolar ridge from rests of dental lamina or with Bohn's nodules that occur between the midline and the maxillary alveolar ridge from rests of salivary gland epithelium. No treatment is required, and the cysts rupture and disappear spontaneously during the first few months of life.

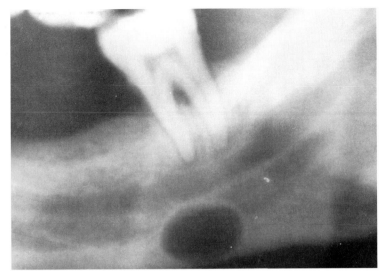

**Figure 1.37**
**POSTERIOR LINGUAL MANDIBULAR CORTICAL DEPRESSION**
Radiolucency of the posterior mandible below the level of the inferior alveolar canal. (Courtesy of Dr. H. E. Ownby.)

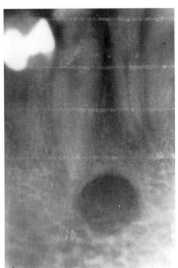

**Figure 1.38**
**ANTERIOR LINGUAL MANDIBULAR CORTICAL DEPRESSION**
Radiolucency apical to the right mandibular cuspid and lateral incisor. (Courtesy of Dr. L. R. Bean.)

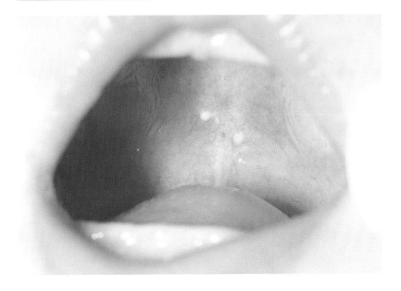

**Figure 1.39**
**EPSTEIN'S PEARLS**
Multiple white papules adjacent to the median palatal raphe in a newborn.

## Figs. 1.40, 1.41, and 1.42

Epidermoid cysts are slow-growing, benign cystic lesions lined by stratified squamous epithelium that exhibits a well-defined granular cell layer and the formation of orthokeratin. Skin appendageal structures and intramural teratomatous elements are not present. These cysts occur most commonly on the skin of the face, scalp, neck, and trunk and present as normal-colored nodules that usually are bound to the overlying skin. Occasionally, they may be found on the oral mucosa with a widespread distribution of locations. Intraoral epidermoid cysts present as yellow or normal-colored submucosal nodules. Most of the cysts occur spontaneously, but some may occur after trauma (epithelial inclusion cysts).

Not infrequently, the cyst may rupture and spill its keratinous contents into the surrounding connective tissue. The released keratin elicits a foreign body reaction with numerous multinucleated giant cells; this reaction may become sufficiently intense to produce total destruction of the cyst lining. Inflammation of these cysts can produce pseudocarcinomatous hyperplasia.

In rare cases, persistent enlargement of epidermoid cysts arising in the floor of the mouth has resulted in significant breathing difficulties. In addition, needle aspiration or incisional biopsy may result in secondary infection and rapid enlargement, with similar breathing difficulties. In deeply seated lesions, magnetic resonance imaging has proved beneficial in localizing the anatomic location and narrowing the clinical differential diagnosis. Surgical excision is the therapy of choice. Rare reports of carcinoma developing within these cysts exist, but some of these may represent pseudocarcinomatous hyperplasia. Numerous epidermoid cysts are known to occur in Gardner syndrome (see Figs. 11.11 and 11.12).

Enlargement with yellowish coloration of the skin on the posterior surface of the right ear. (Courtesy of Dr. Kevin Riker.)

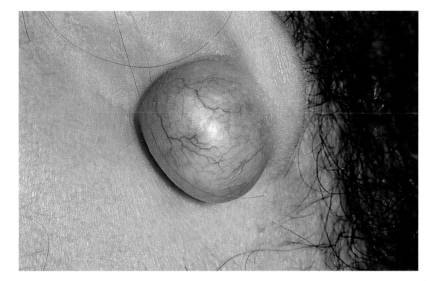

▶ **Figure 1.41**
**EPIDERMOID CYST**
Intraoperative photograph taken during removal of the cyst depicted in Figure 1.40. (Courtesy of Dr. Kevin Riker.)

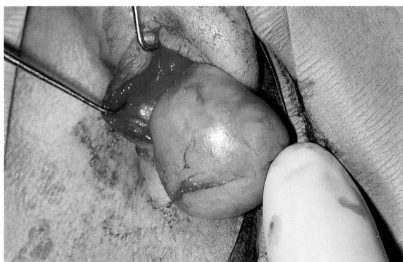

▶ **Figure 1.42**
**EPIDERMOID CYST**
Yellow nodule of the mucosa of the upper lip.

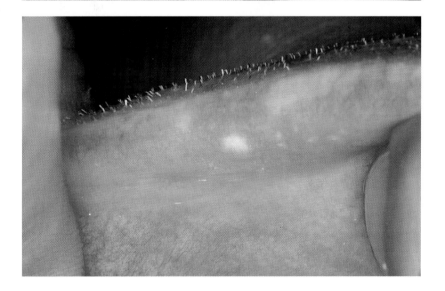

### Figs. 1.43 and 1.44

The dermoid cyst is a slowly growing benign cystic lesion lined by stratified squamous epithelium that exhibits a well-defined granular cell layer, the formation of orthokeratin, and associated skin appendageal structures (sebaceous glands, sweat glands, or hair follicles). If the lining or mural tissue contains mesodermal or endodermal elements (bone, respiratory epithelium, gastrointestinal lining, etc.), the cyst would be classified most appropriately as a teratoid cyst and not as a dermoid cyst.

In the head and neck area, the most common location for dermoid cysts is in the midline of the floor of the mouth or in the submental region. The cysts that arise between the genioglossal and geniohyoid muscles protrude into the floor of the mouth, and those that develop between the geniohyoid and mylohyoid muscles present as submental swellings. Lateral lesions also occur and typically are found in the space above the mylohyoid and lateral to the base of the tongue.

Magnetic resonance imaging is beneficial in localizing the anatomic position, arriving at an appropriate differential diagnosis, and planning the surgical approach. Significant enlargement is possible and has been associated with obstructive sleep apnea and other breathing difficulties. Treatment is surgical excision.

## THYROGLOSSAL TRACT CYST

### Fig. 1.45

The cervical thyroid develops from an epithelial proliferation that migrates from the site that ultimately becomes the foramen cecum of the tongue to its final position on either side of the anterior trachea. The thyroglossal tract cyst (thyroglossal duct cyst) arises from epithelial remnants anywhere along this developmental path. These cysts typically present as asymptomatic midline swellings that display vertical movement with tongue protrusion and swallowing. The majority of cases present below the hyoid bone as a midline neck swelling, with approximately 70% arising before the patient reaches age 20 years. Less frequently, the mass occurs in the neck above the hyoid or in the musculature of the tongue. On occasion, the cyst may be associated with a draining sinus, pain, airway obstruction, dysphonia, dysphagia, coughing, or choking.

The cyst is lined by stratified squamous epithelium or ciliated, pseudostratified columnar epithelium; the wall may contain inflammatory cells, mucous glands, or thyroid follicles. Although associated thyroid agenesis is rare, documentation of normal thyroid is recommended. The treatment of choice is the Sistrunk procedure, which results in a recurrence rate of less than 5% and involves surgical removal of the cyst, the tract connecting the cyst to the foramen cecum, and the central portion of the hyoid bone. Carcinoma arising within a thyroglossal tract cyst is extremely rare.

▶ **Figure 1.43**
**DERMOID CYST**
Midline submental mass. (Courtesy of
Dr. J. E. Haubenreich.)

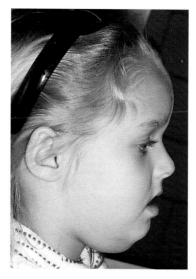

▶ **Figure 1.44**
**DERMOID CYST**
Large midline mass of the floor of the
mouth that results in posterior displacement
of the tongue. (Courtesy of Dr. E. R.
Costich.)

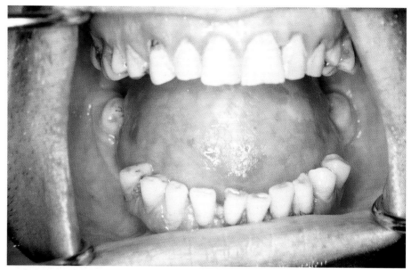

▶ **Figure 1.45**
**THYROGLOSSAL TRACT CYST**
Midline neck mass.

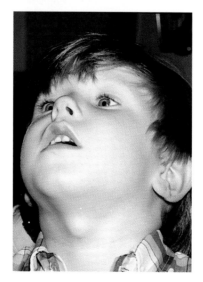

## Figs. 1.46 and 1.47

The lymphoepithelial cyst arises from epithelium entrapped within lymphoid tissue. This cyst presents as a superficial submucosal mass that is yellow or whitish in coloration. The floor of the mouth is the most frequent location, but these cysts are not uncommon in areas that contain a large amount of lymphoid tissue, such as the posterior lateral border of the tongue, the soft palate, the tonsillar pillars, the oropharynx, and the ventral tongue. The entrapped epithelium may originate from salivary gland ducts or from the lining epithelium of surface invaginations or crypts that are not uncommon in oral lymphoid aggregates. Some investigators believe that many lymphoepithelial cysts are not true cysts but represent crypts of the surface epithelium that have become plugged with desquamated keratin. Typically, the lesion consists of a cystic structure lined by stratified squamous epithelium that normally is parakeratotic. The wall of the cyst contains mature lymphoid tissue with germinal centers, and the lumen is filled with desquamated parakeratin. The lumen may become so engorged with keratin that the cyst may feel firm to palpation. Surgical excision can be performed if the clinical diagnosis is in doubt.

## BRANCHIAL CLEFT CYST (CERVICAL LYMPHOEPITHELIAL CYST)

## Fig. 1.48

The branchial cleft cyst presents as an enlargement in the lateral aspect of the upper neck, usually along the anterior edge of the sternocleidomastoid muscle. Histopathologically, this cyst bears great resemblance to its intraoral counterpart, the lymphoepithelial cyst, and many prefer the term "cervical lymphoepithelial cyst." The lesion is thought to arise from epithelial remnants entrapped within cervical lymph nodes; salivary gland ducts or remnants of the branchial arches are thought to be the source of the epithelium. The cyst is lined by stratified squamous or respiratory epithelium, and the wall contains lymphoid tissue. Treatment is surgical removal. Rarely, squamous cell carcinoma arises within cervical lymphoepithelial cysts; in these cases, it is important to rule out a cystic metastasis from an occult primary such as nasopharynx.

> **Figure 1.46**
> **LYMPHOEPITHELIAL CYST**
> Yellow mucosal nodule of the floor of the mouth.

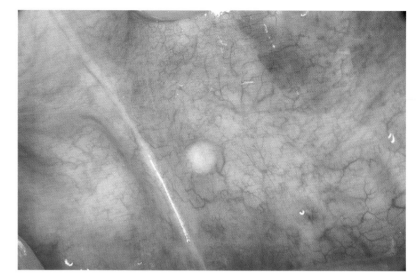

> **Figure 1.47**
> **LYMPHOEPITHELIAL CYST**
> Yellow mucosal nodule of the left tonsillar fauces. The medial normal-colored nodule represents a minor lymphoid aggregate.

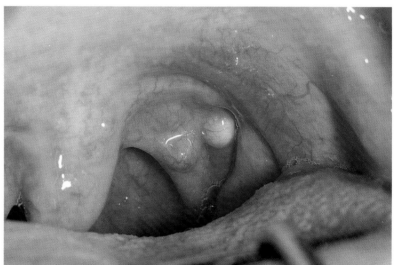

> **Figure 1.48**
> **BRANCHIAL CLEFT CYST**
> Left lateral neck mass just anterior to the sternocleidomastoid muscle.

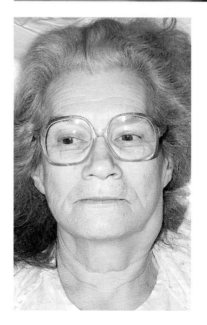

### Double Lip

Barnett ML, Bosshardt LL, Morgan AF. Double lip and double lip with blepharochalasis (Ascher's syndrome). Oral Surg Oral Med Oral Pathol 1972;34:727.

Benmeir P, Weinberg A, Neuman A, et al. Congenital double lip: report of five cases and a review of the literature. Ann Plast Surg 1992;28:180.

Kenny KF, Hreha JP, Dent CD. Bilateral redundant mucosal tissue of the upper lip. J Am Dent Assoc 1990;120:193.

Papanayotou PH, Hatziotis JC. Ascher's syndrome: report of a case. Oral Surg Oral Med Oral Pathol 1973;35:467.

### Commissural Lip Pits

Baker WR. Pits of the lip commissure in caucasoid males. Oral Surg Oral Med Oral Pathol 1966;21:56.

Chewning LC, Sullivan CJ, Bavitz JB. Congenital commissural and lower lip pits in the same patient: report of a case. J Oral Maxillofac Surg 1988;48:499.

Everett FG, Wescott WB. Commissural lip pits. Oral Surg Oral Med Oral Pathol 1961;14:202.

### Paramedian Lip Pits

Cervenka J, Gorlin RJ, Anderson VE. The syndrome of pits of the lower lip and/or cleft palate: genetic considerations. Am J Hum Genet 1967;19:416.

Cheney ML, Cheney WR, LeJeune FE. Familial incidence of labial pits. Am J Otolaryngol 1986;7:311.

Ord RA, Sowray JH. Congenital lip pits and facial clefts. Br J Oral Maxillofac Surg 1985;23:391.

Rintala AE, Ranta R. Lower lip sinuses, 1: epidemiology, microforms, and transverse sulci. Br J Plast Surg 1981;34:25.

Vélez A, Alamillos F-J, Deán A, et al. Congenital lower lip pits (Van der Woude syndrome). J Am Acad Dermatol 1995;32:520.

### Cleft Lip, Cleft Palate, and Bifid Uvula

Derijcke A, Eerens A, Carels C. The incidence of oral clefts: a review. Br J Oral Maxillofac Surg 1996;34:488.

Gorlin RJ. Facial clefting and its syndromes. Birth Defects 1971;7:3.

Meskin LH, Gorlin RJ, Isaacson RJ. Abnormal morphology of the soft palate, I: the prevalence of cleft uvula. Cleft Palate J 1964;1:342.

Shprintzen RJ, Schwartz RH, Daniller A, et al. Morphologic significance of bifid uvula. Pediatrics 1985;75:553.

Wharton P, Mowrer DE. Prevalence of cleft uvula among school children in kindergarten through grade five. Cleft Palate Craniofac J 1992;29:10.

### Lateral Palatal Fistula

Gorlin RJ, Cohen MM, Levin LS. Syndromes of the head and neck. New York: Oxford University Press, 1990;902–903.

Gorlin RJ, Goldman HM. Thoma's oral pathology. St. Louis: CV Mosby, 1970;46–47.

Miller AS, Brookreson KR, Brody BA. Lateral soft-palate fistula. Arch Otolaryngol 1970;91:200.

Neville BW, Damm DD, Allen CM, Bouquot JE. Oral & maxillofacial pathology. Philadelphia: WB Saunders, 1995;14–15.

### Fordyce Granules

Daley TD. Intraoral sebaceous hyperplasia: diagnostic criteria. Oral Surg Oral Med Oral Pathol 1992;74:343.

Fordyce JA. A peculiar affection of the mucous membranes of the lip and oral cavity. J Cutan Genito-Urin Dis 1896;14:413.

Halperin V, Kolas S, Jefferies KR, et al. The occurrence of Fordyce spots, benign migratory glossitis, median rhomboid glossitis and fissured tongue in 2,478 dental patients. Oral Surg Oral Med Oral Pathol 1953;6:1072.

Sedano H, Freyre IC, de la Garza ML, et al. Clinical orodental abnormalities in Mexican children. Oral Surg Oral Med Oral Pathol 1989;68:300.

Sewerin I. The sebaceous glands in the vermilion border of the lips and in the oral mucosa of man. Acta Odontol Scand 1975;33(Suppl 68):1-227.

## Leukoedema

Archard HO, Carlson KP, Stanley HR. Leukoedema of the human oral mucosa. Oral Surg Oral Med Oral Pathol 1968;25:717.

Axéll T, Henricsson V. Leukoedema: an epidemiologic study with special reference to the influence of to-bacco habits. Community Dent Oral Epidemiol 1981;9:142.

Friend GW, Harris EF, Mincer HH, et al. Oral anomalies in the neonate, by race and gender, in an urban setting. Pediatr Dent 1990;12:157.

Martin JL. Leukoedema: a review of the literature. J Natl Med Assoc 1992;84:938.

van Wyk CW, Ambrosio SC. Leukoedema: ultrastructural and histochemical observations. J Oral Pathol 1983;12:319.

## Lingual Thyroid

Batsakis JG, El-Naggar AK, Luna MA. Thyroid gland ectopias. Ann Otol Rhinol Laryngol 1996;105:996.

Baughman RA. Lingual thyroid and lingual thyroglossal tract remnants: a clinical and histopathologic study with review of the literature. Oral Surg Oral Med Oral Pathol 1972;34:781.

Declerck S, Casselman JW, Depondt M, et al. Lingual thyroid imaging. J Belge Radiol 1993;76:241.

Diaz-Arias A, Bickel JT, Loy TS, et al. Follicular carcinoma with clear cell change arising in lingual thyroid. Oral Surg Oral Med Oral Pathol 1992;74:206.

Reaume CE, Sofie VL. Lingual thyroid, review of the literature and report of a case. Oral Surg Oral Med Oral Pathol 1978;45:841.

Soni NK, Chatterji P. An unusual tumor mistaken as a lingual thyroid: a case report. J Laryngol Otol 1984;98:1055.

Williams JD, Sclafani AP, Slupchinsku O, et al. Evaluation and management of the lingual thyroid gland. Ann Otol Rhinol Laryngol 1996;105:312.

## Ankyloglossia

Masaitis NS, Kaempf JW. Developing a frenotomy policy at one medical center: a case study approach. J Hum Lact 1996;12:229.

Mathewson RJ, Siegel MJ, McCanna DL. Ankyloglossia: a review of the literature and a case report. J Dent Child 1966;33:238.

Mukai S, Mukai C, Asaoka K. Ankyloglossia with deviation of the epiglottis and larynx. Ann Otol Rhinol Laryngol 1991;100:3.

Mukai S, Mukai C, Asaoka K. Congenital ankyloglossia with deviation of the epiglottis and larynx: symptoms and respiratory function in adults. Ann Otol Rhinol Laryngol 1993;102:620.

Sato T, Iida M, Yamaguchi Y. A family with hereditary ankyloglossia complicated by heterochromia irides and a congenital clasped thumb. Int J Oral Surg 1983;12:359.

Wright JE. Tongue-tie. J Paediatr Child Health 1995;31:276.

## Hairy Tongue

Celis A, Little JW. Clinical study of hairy tongue in hospital patients. J Oral Med 1966;21:139.

Darwazeh AMG, Pillai K. Prevalence of tongue lesions in 1013 Jordanian dental outpatients. Community Dent Oral Epidemiol 1993;21:323.

Farman AG. Hairy tongue (lingua villosa). J Oral Med 1977;32:85.

Langtry JA, Carr MM, Steele MC, et al. Topical tretinoin: a new treatment for black hairy tongue (lingua villosa nigra). Clin Exp Dermatol 1992;17:163.

McGregor JM, Hay RJ. Oral retinoids to treat black hairy tongue (letter). Clin Exp Dermatol 1993;18:291.

Salonen L, Axéll T, Helldén L. Occurrence of oral mucosal lesions, the influence of tobacco habits and an estimate of treatment time in an adult Swedish population. J Oral Pathol Med 1990;19:170.

Sarti GM, Haddy RI, Schaffer D, et al. Black hairy tongue. Am Fam Physician 1990;41:1751.

## Fissured Tongue

Bànóczy J, Rigó O, Albrecht M. Prevalence study of tongue lesions in a Hungarian population sample. Community Dent Oral Epidemiol 1993;21:224.

Darwazeh AMG, Pillai K. Prevalence of tongue lesions in 1013 Jordanian dental outpatients. Community Dent Oral Epidemiol 1993;21:323.

Eidelman E, Chosack A, Cohen T. Scrotal tongue and geographic tongue: polygenic and associated traits. Oral Surg Oral Med Oral Pathol 1976;42:591.

Halperin V, Kolas S, Jefferis KR. The occurrence of Fordyce spots, benign migratory glossitis, median rhomboid glossitis, and fissured tongue in 2,478 dental patients. Oral Surg Oral Med Oral Pathol 1953;6:1072.

Kullaa-Mikkonen A, Sorvari T. Lingua fissurata: a clinical, steromicroscopic and histopathologic study. Int J Oral Maxillofac Surg 1986;15:525.

Sedano HO, Freyre IC, Garza de la Garza ML, et al. Clinical orodental abnormalities in Mexican children. Oral Surg Oral Med Oral Pathol 1989;68:300.

## Hyperplastic Lymphoid Aggregates

Adkins KF. Lymphoid hyperplasia in the oral mucosa. Aust Dent J 1973;18:38.

Doyle JL, Weisinger E, Manhold JH Jr. Benign lymphoid lesions of the oral mucosa. Oral Surg Oral Med Oral Pathol 1970;29:31.

Knapp MJ. Oral tonsils: location, distribution, and histology. Oral Surg Oral Med Oral Pathol 1970;29:155.

## Mineralization of the Stylohyoid Ligament

Aris AM, Elegbe EO, Krishna R. Difficult intubation stylohyoid calcification. Singapore Med J 1992;33:204.

Baddour HM, McAnear JT, Tilson HB. Eagle's syndrome. Oral Surg Oral Med Oral Pathol 1978;46:486.

Correll RW, Jensen JL, Taylor JB, et al. Mineralization of the stylohyoid-stylomandibular ligament complex: a radiographic incidence study. Oral Surg Oral Med Oral Pathol 1979;48:286.

Dwight T. Stylo-hyoid ossification. Ann Surg. 1907;46:721.

Eagle WW. Elongated styloid process: further observations and a new syndrome. Arch Otolaryngol 1948;47:630.

Ferrario VF, Sigurtá D, Daddona A, et al. Calcification of the stylohyoid ligament: incidence and morpho-quantitative evaluations. Oral Surg Oral Med Oral Pathol 1990;69:524.

Langlais RP, Miles DA, Van Dis ML. Elongated and mineralized complex: a proposed classification and report of a case of Eagle's syndrome. Oral Surg Oral Med Oral Pathol 1986;61:527.

O'Carroll MK. Calcification in the stylohyoid ligament. Oral Surg Oral Med Oral Pathol 1984;58:617.

## Exostoses, Torus Palatinus, and Torus Mandibularis

Eggen S, Natvig B. Relationship between torus mandibularis and number of present teeth. Scand J Dent Res 1986;94:233.

Eggen S, Natvig B, Gåsemyr J. Variation in torus palatinus prevalence in Norway. Scand J Dent Res 1994;102:54.

Gould AW. An investigation of the inheritance of torus palatinus and torus mandibularis. J Dent Res 1964;43:159.

Haugen LK. Palatine and mandibular tori: a morphologic study in the current Norwegian population. Acta Odontol Scand 1992;50:65.

Hegtvedt AK, Terry BC, Burkes EJ, et al. Skin graft vestibuloplasty exostosis. Oral Surg Oral Med Oral Pathol 1990;69:149–152.

King DR, King AC. Incidence of tori in three population groups. J Oral Med 1981;36:21.

Kolas S, Halperin V, Jefferis K, et al. The occurrence of torus palatinus and torus mandibularis in 2,478 dental patients. Oral Surg Oral Med Oral Pathol 1953;6:1134.

Pack ARC, Gaudie WM, Jennings AM. Bony exostosis as a sequela to free gingival grafting: two case reports. J Periodontol 1991;62:269.

Seah YH. Torus palatinus and torus mandibularis: a review of the literature. Aust Dent J 1995;40:318.

## Subpontine Exostosis

Appleby DC. Investigating incidental remission of subpontic hyperostosis. J Am Dent Assoc 1991;122:61.

Burkes EJ, Marbry DL, Brooks RE. Subpontic osseous proliferation. J Prosthet Dent 1985;53:780.

Cailleteau JG. Subpontic hyperostosis. J Endod 1996;22:147.

Mortin TH, Natkin E. Hyperostosis and fixed partial denture pontics: report of 16 patients and review of the literature. J Prosthet Dent 1990;64:539.

Ruffin SA, Waldrop TC, Aufdemorte TB. Diagnosis and treatment of subpontic osseous hyperplasia: report of a case. Oral Surg Oral Med Oral Pathol 1993;76:68.

Wasson DJ, Rapley JW, Cronin RJ. Subpontic osseous hyperplasia: a literature review. J Prosthet Dent 1991;66:638.

## Varicosities

Corbet EF, Holmgren CJ, Philipsen HP. Oral mucosal lesions in 65-74-year-old Hong Kong Chinese. Community Dent Oral Epidemiol 1994;22:392.

Ettinger RL, Manderson RD. A clinical study of sublingual varices. Oral Surg Oral Med Oral Pathol 1974;38:540.

Kaplan I, Moskona D. A clinical survey of oral soft tissue lesions in institutional geriatric patients in Israel. Gerodontology 1990;9:59.

Weathers DR, Fine RM. Thrombosed varix of oral cavity. Arch Dermatol 1971;104:427.

## Nasopalatine Duct Cyst

Abrams AM, Howell FV, Bullock WK. Nasopalatine duct cysts. Oral Surg Oral Med Oral Pathol 1963;16:306.

Allard RHB, de Vries K, van der Kwast WAM. Persisting bilateral nasopalatine ducts: a developmental anomaly. Oral Surg Oral Med Oral Pathol 1982;53:24.

Daley TD, Wysocki GP, Pringle GA. Relative incidence of odontogenic tumors and oral and jaw cysts in a Canadian population. Oral Surg Oral Med Oral Pathol 1994;77:276.

Neville BW, Damm DD, Brock T. Odontogenic keratocysts of the midline maxillary region. J Oral Maxillofac Surg 1997;55:340.

Swanson KS, Kaugers GE, Gunsolley JC. Nasopalatine duct cyst: an analysis of 334 cases. J Oral Maxillofac Surg 1991;49:268.

Takagi R, Ohashi Y, Suzuki M. Squamous cell carcinoma in the maxilla probably originating from a nasopalatine duct cyst: report of a case. J Oral Maxillofac Surg 1996;54:112.

## Median Palatal Cyst

Allard RHB, de Vries K, van der Kwast WAM. Persisting bilateral nasopalatine ducts: a developmental anomaly. Oral Surg Oral Med Oral Pathol 1983;53:24.

Courage GR, North AF, Hansen LS. Median palatine cysts. Oral Surg Oral Med Oral Pathol 1974;37:745.

Gardner DG. An evaluation of reported cases of median mandibular cysts. Oral Surg Oral Med Oral Pathol 1988;65:208.

Kramer IRH, Pindborg JJ, Shear M. International histological classification of tumours: histological typing of odontogenic tumours. 2nd ed. New York: Springer-Verlag, 1992:9.

Neville BW, Damm DD, Allen CM, Bouquot JE. Oral & maxillofacial pathology. Philadelphia: WB Saunders, 1995:27.

## The So-Called "Globulomaxillary Cyst"

Christ TF. The globulomaxillary cyst: an embryologic misconception. Oral Surg Oral Med Oral Pathol 1970;30:515.

D'Silva NJ, Anderson L. Globulomaxillary cyst revisited. Oral Surg Oral Med Oral Pathol 1993;76:182.

Kramer IRH, Pindborg JJ, Shear M. International histological classification of tumours: histological typing of odontogenic tumours. 2nd ed. New York: Springer-Verlag, 1992:9.

Wysocki GP. The differential diagnosis of globulomaxillary radiolucencies. Oral Surg Oral Med Oral Pathol 1981;51:281.

Wysocki GP, Goldblatt LI. The so-called "globulomaxillary cyst" is extinct. Oral Surg Oral Med Oral Pathol 1993;76:185.

## Nasolabial Cyst

Campbell RL, Burkes EJ Jr. Nasolabial cyst: report of a case. J Am Dent Assoc 1975;91:1210.

Chinellato LEM, Damante JH. Contribution of radiographs to the diagnosis of naso-alveolar cyst. Oral Surg Oral Med Oral Pathol 1984;58:729.

Curé JK, Osguthorpe JD, Tassel PV. MR of nasolabial cysts. Am J Neuroradiol 1996;17:585.

David VC, O'Connell JE. Nasolabial cyst. Clin Otolaryngol 1986;11:5.

Hynes B, Martin LC. Nasoalveolar cysts: a review of two cases. J Otolaryngol 1994;23:194.

Roed-Petersen B. Nasolabial cyst, a presentation of five patients with a review of the literature. Br J Oral Surg 1970;7:85.

Wesley RK, Scannell T, Nathan LE. Nasolabial cyst: presentation of a case with a review of the literature. J Oral Maxillofac Surg 1984;42:188.

## Surgical Ciliated Cyst

Gregory GT, Shafer WG. Surgical ciliated cysts of the maxilla: report of cases. J Oral Surg 1958;16:251.

Hayhurst DL, Moenning JE, Summerlin D-J, et al. Surgical ciliated cyst: a delayed complication in a case of maxillary orthognathic surgery. J Oral Maxillofac Surg 1993;51:705.

Yamamoto H, Takagi M. Clinicopathologic study of the postoperative maxillary cyst. Oral Surg Oral Med Oral Pathol 1986;62:544.

## Posterior Lingual Mandibular Cortical Depression

Ariji E, Fujiwara N, Tabata O, et al. Stafne's bone cavity: classification based on outline and content determined by computed tomography. Oral Surg Oral Med Oral Pathol 1993;76:375.

Correll RW, Jensen JL, Rhyne RR. Lingual cortical mandibular defects: a radiographic incidence study. Oral Surg Oral Med Oral Pathol 1980;50:287.

Hansson L. Development of a lingual mandibular bone cavity in an 11-year-old boy. Oral Surg Oral Med Oral Pathol 1980;49:376.

Shibata H, Yoshizawa N, Shibata T. Developmental lingual bone defect of the mandible: report of a case. Int J Oral Maxillofac Surg 1991;20:328.

Tsui SHC, Chan FFY. Lingual mandibular bone defect: case report and review of the literature. Aust Dent J 1994;39:368.

## Anterior Lingual Mandibular Cortical Depression

Barak S, Katz J, Mintz S. Anterior lingual mandibular salivary gland defect: a dilemma in diagnosis. Br J Oral Maxillofac Surg 1993;31:318.

Miller AS, Winnick M. Salivary gland inclusion in the anterior mandible: report of a case with a review of the literature on aberrant salivary gland tissue and neoplasms. Oral Surg Oral Med Oral Pathol 1971;31:790.

Salman L, Chaudhry AP. Malposed sublingual gland in the anterior mandible: a variant of Stafne's idiopathic bone cavity. Compendium 1991;12:40.

Ström C. An unusual case of lingual mandibular depression. Oral Surg Oral Med Oral Pathol 1987;64:159.

Tominaga K, Kuga Y, Kubota K, et al. Stafne's bone cavity in the anterior mandible: report of a case. Dentomaxillofac Radiol 1990;19:28.

## Epstein's Pearls

Cataldo E, Berkman MD. Cysts of the oral mucosa in newborns. Am J Dis Child 1968;116:44.

Fromm A. Epstein's pearls, Bohn's nodules and inclusion cysts of the oral cavity. J Dent Child 1967;34:275.

Rivers JK, Frederiksen PC. A prevalence survey of dermatoses in the Australian neonate. J Am Acad Dermatol 1990;23:77.

## Epidermoid Cyst

Cortezzi W, de Albuquerque BE. Secondarily infected epidermoid cyst in the floor of the mouth causing a life-threatening situation: report of a case. J Oral Maxillofac Surg 1994;52:762.

Gardner EJ. Follow-up study of a family group exhibiting dominant inheritance for a syndrome including intestinal polyposis, osteomas, fibromas and epidermal cysts. Am J Hum Genet 1962;14:376.

Potts M, Macleod RI, McLean NR, et al. The value of magnetic resonance imaging in the assessment of a sublingual epidermoid cyst. Dentomaxillofac Radiol 1992;21:102.

Turetschek K, Hospodka H, Steiner E. Case report: epidermoid cyst of the floor of the mouth: diagnostic imaging by sonography, computed tomography and magnetic resonance imaging. Br J Radiol 1995;68:205.

Zachariades N, Skoura-Kafoussia C. A life-threatening epidermoid cyst of the floor of the mouth: report of a case. J Oral Maxillofac Surg 1990;48:400.

## Dermoid Cyst

Goldman JM, Barnes DJ, Pohl DV. Obstructive sleep apnea due to a dermoid cyst of the floor of the mouth. Thorax 1990;45:76.

Howell CJT. The sublingual dermoid. Oral Surg Oral Med Oral Pathol 1985;59:578.

King RC, Smith BR, Burk JL. Dermoid cyst in the floor of the mouth: review of the literature and case reports. Oral Surg Oral Med Oral Pathol 1994;78:567.

Meyer I. Dermoid cysts (dermoids) of the floor of the mouth. Oral Surg Oral Med Oral Pathol 1955;8:1149.

Nagar H, Baratz M. Congenital sublingual teratoid cyst: case report. Int J Oral Maxillofac Surg 1993;22:44.

Oygür T, Dursun A, Uluoglu Ö, et al. Oral congenital dermoid cyst in the floor of the mouth of a newborn: the significance of gastroinstestinal-type epithelium. Oral Surg Oral Med Oral Pathol 1992;74:627.

### Thyroglossal Tract Cyst

Brereton RJ, Symonds E. Thyroglossal cysts in children. Br J Surg 1978;65:507.

Brown EG, Albernaz MS, Emery MT. Thyroglossal duct cyst causing airway obstruction in an adult. Ear Nose Throat J 1996;75:530.

Girard M, Deluca SA. Thyroglossal duct cyst. Am Fam Physician 1990;42:665.

Sturgis EM, Miller RH. Thyroglossal duct cysts. J La State Med Soc 1993;145:459.

Wampler HW, Krolls SO, Johnson RP. Thyroglossal-tract cyst. Oral Surg Oral Med Oral Pathol 1978;45:32.

Wigley TL, Chonkich GD, Wat BY. Papillary carcinoma arising in a thyroglossal duct cyst. Otolaryngol Head Neck Surg 1997;116:386.

### Lymphoepithelial Cyst

Buchner A, Hansen LS. Lymphoepithelial cysts of the oral mucosa. Oral Surg Oral Med Oral Pathol 1980;50:441.

Chaudhry AP, Yamane GM, Scharlock SE, et al. A clinicopathologic study of intraoral lymphoepithelial cysts. J Oral Med 1984;39:79.

### Branchial Cleft Cyst

Bhaskar SN, Bernier JL. Histogenesis of branchial cysts: a report of 468 cases. Am J Pathol 1959;35:407.

Howie AJ, Proops DW. The definition of branchial cysts, sinuses and fistulae. Clin Otolaryngol 1982;7:51.

Kenealy JFX, Torsiglieri AJ, Tom LWC. Branchial cleft anomalies: a five-year retrospective review. Trans Pa Acad Ophthalmol Otolaryngol 1990;42:1022.

Shankar L, Josephson R, Hawke M. The branchial cleft cyst. J Otolarngol 1991;20:62.

# chapter 2
# PATHOLOGY OF THE TEETH

## DENTAL FLUOROSIS

**Fig. 2.1**

When fluoride in the drinking water exceeds 1 ppm, changes can be seen in the structure of developing teeth secondary to defective or deficient enamel formation. In addition, clinically evident dental fluorosis has been detected in children living in areas using water with less than 1 ppm of fluoride. It has become evident that total fluoride intake comes from a combination of fluoride supplements, food sources, naturally released components, and man-made commercial emissions into the environment. In many instances, the actual fluoride intake greatly exceeds the recommended level and results in detectable dental changes. Significant ingestion of toothpaste by children younger than age 4 years has been correlated directly with fluorosis, even in nonfluoridated communities.

The dental changes vary significantly even at similar fluoride levels because of individual variations in fluoride intake. Changes from white opaque teeth, with or without brown-stained areas, to teeth that are extremely pitted and corroded in appearance are seen. The changes are usually generalized to all of the teeth; in mild cases, however, not all of the tooth surface may be involved. Although the teeth may be severely pitted, they are still resistant to caries. Cosmetic therapies include vital bleaching, veneers, or crowns.

## LOCALIZED ENVIRONMENTAL ENAMEL HYPOPLASIA (TURNER'S TOOTH)

**Figs. 2.2 and 2.3**

Localized infection or trauma to a deciduous tooth can affect the enamel formation of the underlying permanent tooth. It may involve either a disturbance in the matrix formation or calcification, depending on when the damage occurred. These teeth may exhibit only a slight area of discoloration, areas of pitting, or a totally irregular hypoplastic crown. The degree of malformation varies according to the severity of the injury and the stage of development of the permanent tooth. Coronal enamel maturation continues until eruption of the tooth; therefore, traumatic enamel alterations can arise long after cessation of ameloblastic activity. Coronal or radicular dilaceration also may occur.

The most commonly involved teeth are the maxillary central incisors secondary to physical trauma to the overlying deciduous teeth. Traumatic intrusion of the deciduous tooth is correlated with the highest prevalence of damage to the underlying permanent tooth and usually affects the facial surface of the permanent tooth due to the anatomic relationship between the deciduous apices and the adjacent crown. Similar coronal damage may occur in bicuspids secondary to periapical inflammatory disease of the overlying deciduous molars. These damaged permanent teeth are referred to as "Turner's teeth," and this type of environmental dental malformation is called "Turner's hypoplasia."

### Figure 2.1
**DENTAL FLUOROSIS**
Dentition exhibiting diffuse white and opaque enamel, with demonstrated areas of brown discoloration, in a patient with chronic ingestion of excess fluoride.

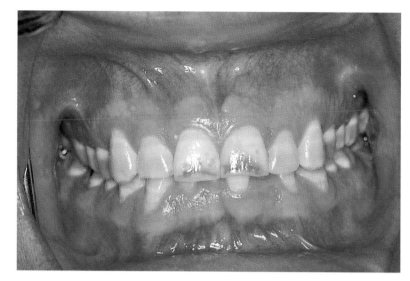

### Figure 2.2
**LOCALIZED ENVIRONMENTAL ENAMEL HYPOPLASIA**
Hypoplasia of the erupting permanent mandibular central incisors as a result of previous trauma to the deciduous incisors.

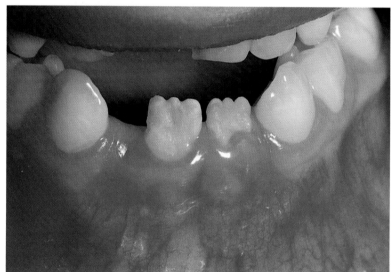

### Figure 2.3
**LOCALIZED ENVIRONMENTAL ENAMEL HYPOPLASIA**
Radiograph of incisors depicted in Figure 2.2. Note the developmental abnormality of the incisal enamel.

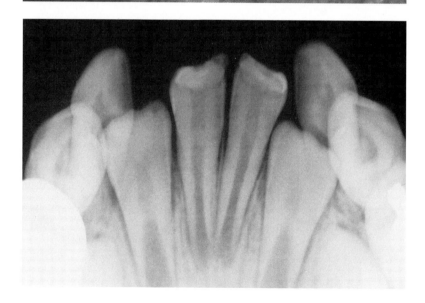

## Figs. 2.4, 2.5, and 2.6

Certain systemic problems can affect the sensitive ameloblasts and cause enamel hypoplasia more widespread than that seen in Turner's hypoplasia. Affected teeth may reveal pits or grooves as well as partial or total lack of enamel. In deciduous teeth, the most common pattern is a horizontal groove positioned at the level of the crown that was being developed at the time of injury. In the permanent dentition, one of the frequent patterns presents as areas of opacity, horizontal rows of pits, or linear defects present on the anterior teeth and the first molars. These teeth are formed during the first year of life; if the sensitive ameloblasts are damaged, hypoplasia or hypomaturation will be present in the enamel that was being formed at that time. The damage is bilaterally symmetrical and correlates well with the developmental pattern of the involved teeth. Less commonly, similar alterations of enamel may be present in the bicuspids and second molars if the inciting event occurs around the age of 3 years. A large number of factors are associated strongly with subsequent environmental enamel alterations. Before birth, a maternal history of smoking, higher prepregnancy weight, and lack of appropriate prenatal care are associated with an increased prevalence. Prematurity, low-birth weight, and prolonged intubation of the infant also are implicated. After birth, infections (especially the exanthematous diseases), malnutrition, congenital cardiac and renal disorders, hypocalcemia, hyperbilirubinemia, and significant exposure to tetracycline, antineoplastic therapy, or excessive fluoride can lead to enamel hypoplasia. Treatment of the altered teeth consists of repair with aesthetic resins, until the teeth fully erupt, and then evaluation to determine whether further restoration is required for cosmetic reasons and function.

**ENVIRONMENTAL ENAMEL HYPOPLASIA**
Horizontal rows of pits on the anterior
teeth. The maxillary central incisors have
been restored with acrylic resin. The
affected areas are symmetrical and
coincide with the portion of the teeth
formed at the time of ameloblastic
damage.

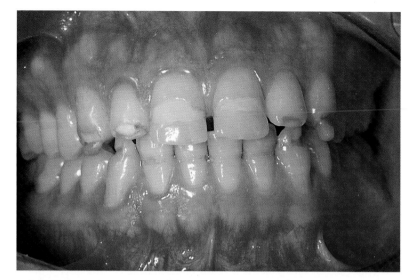

► **Figure 2.5**
**ENVIRONMENTAL ENAMEL HYPOPLASIA**
Posterior teeth of the patient depicted in
Figure 2.4. The bicuspids are free of
hypoplasia. Although not seen well in this
view, all of the first molars exhibited a
horizontal row of scattered pits in the
middle one-third of the crown.

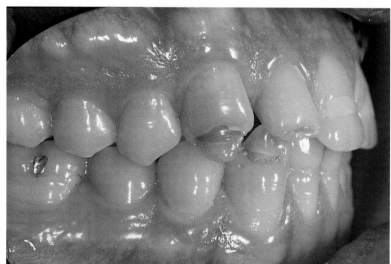

► **Figure 2.6**
**ENVIRONMENTAL ENAMEL HYPOPLASIA**
Horizontal enamel defects occurring in the
bicuspids and second molars in a patient
whose damage occurred at age 3 years.

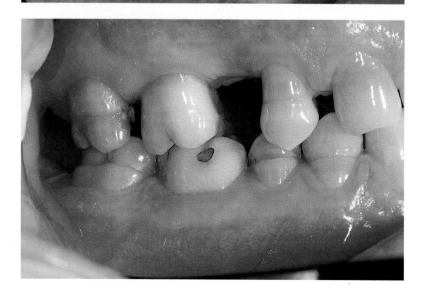

## RADIATION EFFECTS ON THE TEETH

### Fig. 2.7

Review of childhood cancer survivors has demonstrated that therapeutic radiation and, to a lesser extent, chemotherapy can induce developmental abnormalities of the dentition and craniofacial skeleton. The tooth germs are sensitive to such external stimuli and are easily damaged. The pattern and severity of the dental alterations are related to the child's age at the time of treatment, the form of therapy, and the dose and field of radiation. The most extensive findings are seen in patients receiving therapy between the ages of 3 and 5.5 years, the time of initial root formation for all permanent teeth except the second and third molars.

It is well documented that radiotherapy may produce both qualitative and quantitative dental abnormalities, whereas chemotherapy alone typically, but not always, creates only qualitative defects in enamel. The most frequently noted quantitative defects are white-to-cream–colored areas of enamel hypomaturation. The pattern of qualitative defects varies according to the timing of the injury. If crown calcification has not been completed, the tooth may be absent totally or be rudimentary. If the crown was formed but root development was not complete at the time of radiation, the tooth may exhibit short, pointed roots. Individual differences in the degree of developmental alterations between same-age patients receiving identical therapeutic regimens are evident.

## ABFRACTION OF TEETH

### Fig. 2.8

Abfraction (stress-induced cervical lesions) is the newest documented cause of noncarious cervical lesions in teeth and is added to the list that also includes abrasion, attrition, and erosion. As such, the diagnosis is being used in many situations, some of which may be inappropriate. Abfraction refers to the loss of cervical tooth structure secondary to repeated flexure of the tooth caused by occlusal stresses. It is thought that lateral occlusal forces bend the tooth with tensile stress concentrated in the cervical fulcrum area, leading to disruption of the enamel and dentin bonds. Once damaged, the area may be enlarged secondarily by abrasion, attrition, or erosion.

The typical lesion is a narrow and deep U- or wedge-shaped cervical concavity in enamel or dentin that exhibits sharp line angles and is located on the facial surface of the tooth at the fulcrum. There is a higher prevalence in mandibular teeth, most likely because of the lingual orientation of the arch. Definitive diagnosis requires not only compatible tooth defects but also demonstration of lateral occlusal forces during mastication or parafunctional movements.

Although restoration is not mandatory, most teeth benefit from appropriate interventions. Of primary importance is elimination of the abnormal occlusal forces; without such intervention, the restorative failure rate is high. Due to their ability to flex with teeth rather than debond, microfilled resins and composite glass ionomer restorative materials have been used in the restoration of these defects.

## ATTRITION OF TEETH

### Fig. 2.9

Attrition is the physiologic wearing away of tooth structure as a result of contact between adjacent teeth or with the teeth in the opposing arch. This wear can be found on the occlusal, incisal, or interproximal surfaces. With time, it may lead to a reduction in both the height of the teeth and the length of the arch. Both deciduous and permanent teeth may exhibit significant attrition. Severe degrees of attrition must be considered a pathologic process. At times, the distinction between attrition, abrasion, erosion, and abfraction is blurred.

Bruxism and other similar habits may accelerate the process. Increased tooth wear has been associated with increased bite force, decreased occlusal tactile sensitivity, and a decreased number of teeth. Males exhibit greater degrees of wear, and the process is more prevalent in late adulthood. Pathologic conditions such as dentinogenesis imperfecta and amelogenesis imperfecta also may result in increased attrition. Pulp exposures typically are not seen because the process proceeds slowly enough to allow for pulpal recession.

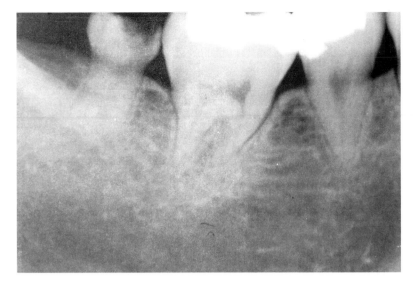

► **Figure 2.7**
**RADIATION EFFECTS ON THE TEETH**
Short, pointed hypoplastic root development in a patient who received therapeutic radiation to the area during the time of final root formation.

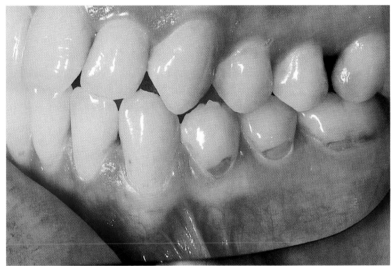

► **Figure 2.8**
**ABFRACTION OF TEETH**
Isolated and narrow U-shaped cervical concavities of the posterior mandibular dentition.

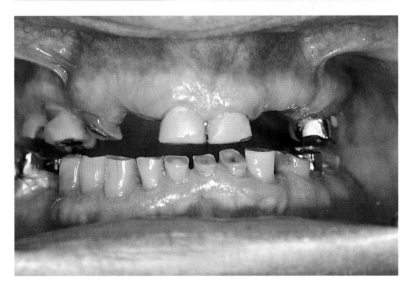

► **Figure 2.9**
**ATTRITION OF TEETH**
Dentition demonstrating diffuse and extensive loss in tooth height. Note the anterior mandibular incisors with exposed dentin and secondary dentin filling the coronal pulp chambers.

## Figs. 2.10, 2.11, and 2.12

Abrasion is the pathologic wearing away of tooth structure by some abnormal mechanical force. This most commonly occurs on exposed root surfaces and usually is related to a combination of age and an improper toothbrushing technique. Most of these patients practice very good oral hygiene but use a horizontal toothbrushing technique that has resulted in abnormal tooth wear. Abrasiveness of the dentifrice and bristle stiffness do not seem to be correlated strongly.

The exposed cementum and dentin of the facial root surfaces typically exhibit notching that is oriented horizontally and adjacent to the gingiva. In about 20% of the cases, it is most severe on the quadrants opposite the dominant hand because of a tendency to brush longer or to use greater force on that side. The pulp typically is not exposed because the process proceeds slowly enough to allow for pulpal recession. The tertiary dentin filling the old pulp canal often can be visualized. On rare occasions, the crown can be undermined so severely by the deep notching that all or part of the crown fractures off.

Abrasion also may occur on the incisal or proximal surfaces. These patterns of abrasion most often are related to habits or occupations that involve biting or habitual placement of foreign objects between the teeth. Nails, toothpicks, bobby pins, and tobacco pipes are common culprits. In some cases, abrasion may be diffuse and closely resemble attrition. These examples typically arise secondary to abrasives being present constantly in the mouth. Such lesions are associated with use of tobacco products (containing silica contaminants) and industrial exposure to sand, cement, or stone dust. In one ironic case, a dental technician developed severe anterior abrasion from chronic oral exposure to porcelain powder. In these cases, pulp exposure also is rare.

### Figure 2.10
**ABRASION OF TEETH**

Dentition demonstrating significant wear of the exposed facial root surfaces of the left side of both arches. The patient was right-handed and used a horizontal brushing technique.

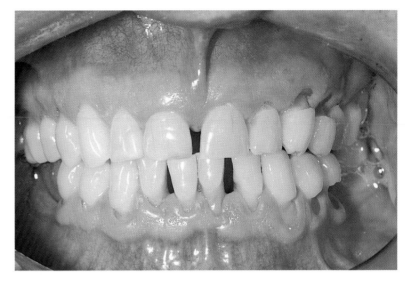

### Figure 2.11
**ABRASION OF TEETH**

Facial mirror view of the dentition on the left side of the patient described in Figure 2.10. Note the exposed dentin and pulp canals, which have filled with tertiary dentin.

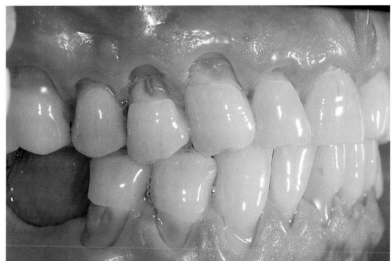

### Figure 2.12
**ABRASION OF TEETH**

Incisal wear present on the mandibular incisors from chronic placement of pipe stem while smoking.

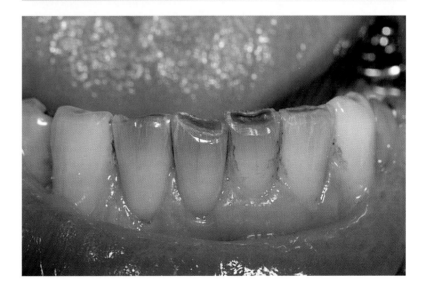

### Figs. 2.13, 2.14, and 2.15

Erosion is the pathologic loss of tooth structure resulting from chemical action that does not include a bacterial process. The causes of erosion can be subdivided into intrinsic, extrinsic, and idiopathic. Intrinsic factors are related to prolonged exposure of the oral cavity to gastric acid. Patients who regurgitate their stomach contents can exhibit significant dental erosion that often is prominent on the lingual surfaces of the teeth. This is not rare in bulimics, individuals with a hiatal hernia, and those receiving chemotherapy. One pattern of erosion that may occur in bulimics is known as "perimolysis." This pattern of erosion demonstrates loss of enamel on the occlusal surfaces with eventual relative elevation of any occlusal amalgam above the surface of the remaining tooth structure.

Extrinsic causes can be grouped into environmental, diet, medications, and lifestyle. Many cases related to extrinsic exposure can be explained easily by exposure to a highly acidic substance. Dental erosion is a well-recognized hazard associated with several occupations involving significant exposure to acidic chemicals. Swimmers have exhibited significant erosion secondary to low pH levels in their pools. Individuals who exhibit a large intake of highly acidic beverages or suck on citrus fruits frequently exhibit loss of tooth structure.

Many cases diagnosed as erosion are idiopathic. This category is becoming a "diagnostic dumping ground" for unexplained tooth loss that does not fit the criteria for the diagnosis of attrition or abrasion. A number of examples of cervical idiopathic erosion have been reassessed and appropriately diagnosed as abfraction. In some cases, definitive diagnosis is not possible; chemical action may be involved, but defensible proof is lacking.

Many patients with erosion exhibit a distinctive pattern of tooth loss in which the facial surfaces of the anterior teeth are affected predominantly. The area of loss is noted in the gingival one-third as a shallow, spoon-shaped depression of the enamel adjacent to the cementoenamel junction. Although the loss usually is located in these areas, posterior teeth and occlusal surfaces may be involved, with great variation in the size and shape of the damage. Often, because of dentin being destroyed more rapidly than enamel, the defects present as concave depressions of dentin surrounded by elevated rims of enamel. In some cases, this begins as a small pit at the cusp tip that may enlarge to destroy much of the coronal anatomy.

**Figure 2.13**
**EROSION OF TEETH**
Loss of facial enamel on the maxillary central incisors as a result of chronic lemon sucking.

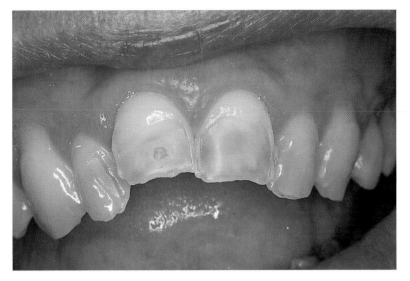

**Figure 2.14**
**EROSION OF TEETH**
Loss of occlusal enamel and dentin on the mandibular teeth of a bulimic patient. Note the amalgams slightly above the occlusal surface.

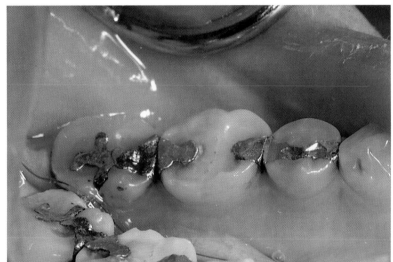

**Figure 2.15**
**EROSION OF TEETH**
Idiopathic loss of enamel and dentin on the occlusal and facial surfaces of the mandibular bicuspids. Widespread loss of tooth structure was noted on either or both the occlusal and facial surfaces of most of the teeth. There were no signs of abrasion or attrition.

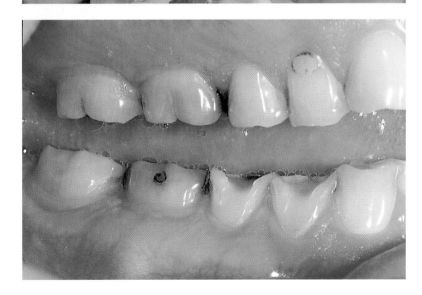

**Fig. 2.16**

If tetracycline is administered to pregnant women or to children younger than age 8 years, it may be incorporated into the dentin of developing teeth. Initially, this produces a yellow or gray-to-brown discoloration of the affected teeth. When exposed to ultraviolet light, the teeth will fluoresce a bright yellow. The color of the teeth is more brilliant immediately after eruption and becomes more brown with exposure to light. Long courses of the antibiotics normally are required to produce the staining. Occasionally, enamel hypoplasia also is seen; it is uncertain if these changes are caused by the drug or are secondary to the disorder that required use of the antibiotic. When the drug is required for a life-threatening problem, oxytetracycline or doxycycline should be used because they tend to produce less severe tooth staining.

Tooth discoloration is not restricted to the developing dentition of children. In patients using forms of tetracycline (especially minocycline) for long periods of time, significant discoloration of the teeth is possible in adults. This is thought to be due to incorporation into physiologic secondary dentin that continues to be deposited throughout life. In addition to tooth discoloration, minocycline use has also been shown to cause pigmentation of the bone, skin, nails, sclera, conjunctiva, and thyroid.

Mild cases of discoloration may be bleached externally. Although more severe cases may be bleached internally, most clinicians choose facial veneering with composite resins or porcelain. In teeth with significant enamel hypoplasia, complete crown coverage often is beneficial.

## EXTRINSIC STAINING OF TEETH

**Fig. 2.17**

Abnormal colorations of teeth may be due to intrinsic factors (tetracycline therapy, hyperbilirubinemia, etc.) or extrinsic influences. Frequently encountered extrinsic causes include bacterial stains, tobacco, foods/beverages, gingival hemorrhages, restorative materials, and medications. Common foods associated with significant staining of teeth include coffee, tea, and foods that contain abundant chlorophyll. Use of tobacco products often results in widespread discoloration of the pits and fissures, with more diffuse coverage occasionally noted. When the smooth surfaces are affected, the lingual portion of the mandibular incisors typically is involved initially and most extensively.

Recently, extrinsic staining has been associated with use of several popular oral antimicrobial mouthwashes. Chlorhexidine-containing and, to a lesser extent, essential oil/phenolic rinses have been associated with extrinsic staining. Accumulated evidence strongly suggests a dietary influence in the staining. Although many foods may be responsible, beverages such as tea, coffee, and red wine synergistically influence strongly the staining capability of these mouthwashes. Attempts to negate the staining characteristics of the antimicrobial rinses have been successful but have resulted in diminished antiplaque qualities.

## PINK TOOTH OF MUMMERY

**Fig. 2.18**

Pink tooth of Mummery refers to a rosy pink discoloration of the crown of a tooth, usually at the neck. Most frequently, this arises secondary to internal resorption in which the hyperplastic pulp tissue within the chamber enlarges at the expense of the coronal dentinal walls. On thinning of these walls, the pink, vascular pulp tissue may show through the thin enamel.

On occasion, a pink tooth may be seen secondary to undermining external resorption. One pattern of aggressive external resorption is termed "invasive or cervical resorption" and typically begins along the root surface in the cervical area below the epithelial attachment. Once initiated, the resorption can proceed in several directions and can extend coronally under the enamel, creating a pink discoloration of the crown.

▶ **Figure 2.16**
**TETRACYCLINE STAINING OF TEETH**
Dentition exhibiting diffuse grayish discoloration of the crowns. In addition, note the presence of environmental enamel hypoplasia on the cuspids and first bicuspids.

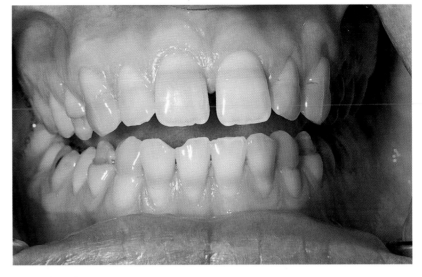

▶ **Figure 2.17**
**EXTRINSIC STAINING OF TEETH**
Dentition exhibiting diffuse brown surface staining secondary to long-term use of betel quid.

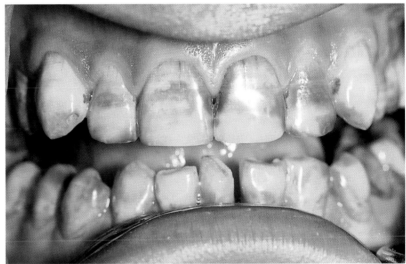

▶ **Figure 2.18**
**PINK TOOTH OF MUMMERY**
Diffuse red discoloration of the maxillary left central incisor. (Case courtesy of Dr. Sheila Porter.)

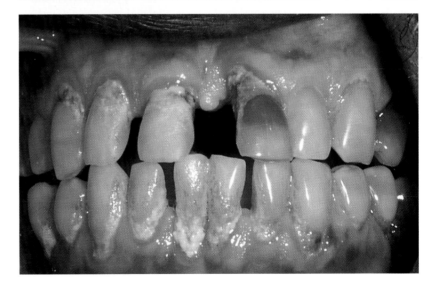

## INTERNAL RESORPTION OF TEETH

### Fig. 2.19

Internal resorption of teeth refers to removal of tooth structure that involves the inner dentinal walls by cells originating in the dental pulp. Most instances occur during adulthood and exhibit no significant sex predilection; prevalence is less than 1% of patients. Most commonly, initiation of the process is associated with some form of trauma or dental caries. In a few patients, the resorption is idiopathic, with no obvious predisposing factor identified. The resorption may occur in the root or crown and appears as an area of radiolucency overlying the affected area. Typically, the margins of the lucency are smooth and well defined. The walls of the canal appear to balloon out and cannot be followed through the center of the lesion. Rarely is more than one tooth involved. Root canal therapy may prove beneficial if the resorption has not perforated into the periodontal ligament and if the area of resorption can be properly instrumented.

## EXTERNAL RESORPTION OF TEETH

### Figs. 2.20 and 2.21

External resorption of the teeth begins along the root surface and is the result of activity of cells within the periodontal ligament. Radiographically, the lucency typically demonstrates symmetrical, ill-defined borders, often superimposed over an intact root canal system. This pattern of resorption has many known causes, but the most frequently encountered is periapical inflammation. Reimplanted teeth that are not able to reestablish their vascular supply exhibit significant resorption. Impacted teeth, tumors, and cysts may produce resorption of the adjacent teeth, mostly secondary to pressure. Orthodontic therapy also may be related to significant resorption, regardless of the duration, type of appliance, or degree of force. Not infrequently, impacted or embedded teeth also may exhibit external resorption. In the past, many cases of external resorption were thought, on radiographic examination, to represent anachoretic caries; but microscopically, the teeth exhibited no caries, only resorption.

In contrast to internal resorption, external resorption is almost universal, with all patients having at least a minor degree of resorption on one or more teeth. The resorption potential is inherent in each individual and is the single most important factor that determines the degree of resorption that occurs secondary to stimulus. When pretreatment radiographs reveal an abnormally high degree of external resorption, treatment that promotes resorption, such as orthodontics, should be undertaken with great hesitation.

Some cases of extensive external resorption are idiopathic and may involve numerous teeth. Without any known cause, these idiopathic examples are frustrating and often difficult to stop. When the resorption occurs in the cervical area, exposure and removal of the soft tissue within the lacuna and restoration of the defect may stop the destruction. On occasion, external resorption has been treated successfully through placement of calcium hydroxide into the pulp canals; this may have been possible because of small communications between the defect and the pulp.

### ► Figure 2.19
### INTERNAL RESORPTION OF TEETH

A right maxillary central incisor exhibiting large, centrally placed radiolucency of the middle portion of the root. Note the loss of pulp canal boundaries in the area of destruction. (Case courtesy of Dr. L. R. Bean.)

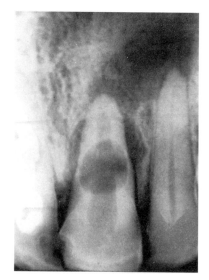

### ► Figure 2.20
### EXTERNAL RESORPTION OF TEETH

A maxillary left central incisor demonstrating extensive root destruction. The tooth was traumatically avulsed 2 years ago. At that time, root canal therapy was performed and the tooth was reimplanted.

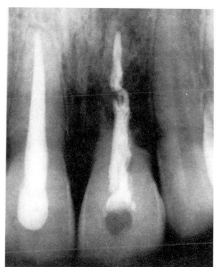

### ► Figure 2.21
### EXTERNAL RESORPTION OF TEETH

Diffuse extensive root resorption that began during orthodontic therapy.

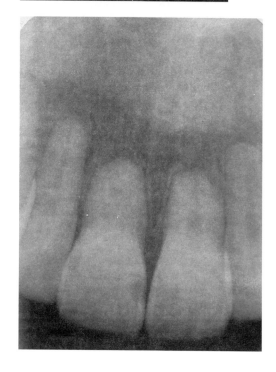

**Fig. 2.22**

Historically, natal teeth are deciduous teeth that are erupted at birth; neonatal teeth are those that erupt within the first 30 days of life. This is an artificial separation, and it seems appropriate to designate both forms as natal teeth. These prematurely erupted deciduous teeth have been termed "predeciduous dentition," but only rarely do they represent supernumerary teeth. Although other teeth may be involved, most are mandibular central incisors. Natal teeth may produce nursing difficulties because the infant may place the tongue over these teeth while nursing. This often results in the formation of a traumatic ulceration on the ventral surface of the tongue known as "Riga-Fede disease" (see page 174). In many of these cases, extraction is not necessary and resolution of the ulceration often occurs after smoothing of rough incisal edges or placement of round smooth composite over the exposed portion of the tooth.

On occasion, newly erupted natal teeth may be loose and mobile. Concern over possible aspiration seems overblown, and inhalation of a natal tooth has never been reported. Typically, natal teeth become less mobile by 1 month of age. Natal teeth should be left alone if not causing significant difficulty to the infant or mother. If removed, the soft tissue at the surgical site should be curetted to prevent further tooth development from odontogenic remnants.

## ANKYLOSIS

**Fig. 2.23 and 2.24**

Eruption is a continuous process of occlusal movement by a tooth from its developmental position to its functional position. Although the process typically continues throughout life, cessation in eruption occasionally occurs and is termed "submergence" or "infraocclusion." A tooth is considered submerged when its marginal ridges (previously in normal position) are more than 0.5 mm below the marginal ridges of the adjacent normal teeth. In rare cases, the submerged tooth may become completely encased by the growing alveolar ridge, a process termed "reimpaction." Although permanent teeth may be involved, deciduous teeth are affected most commonly.

Most cases of submerged teeth are due to ankylosis in which there is a focus of fusion between the cementum and the adjacent bone. In a few cases, the affected tooth exhibits a sharp, solid sound on percussion or radiographic absence of the periodontal ligament space in a focal area. Submergence may result in drift of adjacent teeth, super-eruption of its antagonist, plaque accumulation, gingival inflammation, and decreased alveolar bone growth.

Submerged deciduous teeth with an underlying successor usually exfoliate normally, although the process may be delayed for a few months. Appropriate therapy consists of close follow-up or, in severe cases, space maintenance or restoration to rebuild the height of the tooth. Those without successors and affected permanent teeth may be restored to proper height or extracted and replaced with a prosthesis. In addition, permanent teeth may be luxated and orthodontically moved into position.

### Figure 2.22
**NATAL TEETH**

A mandibular left central deciduous incisor that was erupted at birth. The infant developed a traumatic ulceration of the ventral tongue secondary to nursing (Riga-Fede disease). A protective shield was constructed and the tooth was retained.

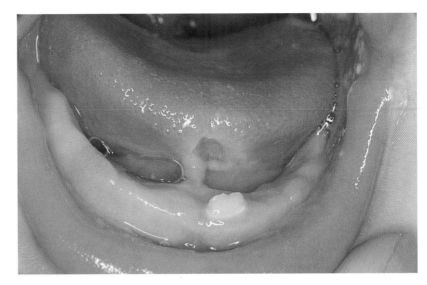

### Figure 2.23
**ANKYLOSIS**

Mirror view of a retained maxillary second deciduous molar that failed to maintain a functional level of occlusion.

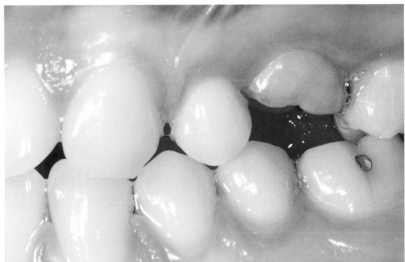

### Figure 2.24
**ANKYLOSIS**

Radiograph of dentition depicted in Figure 2.23.

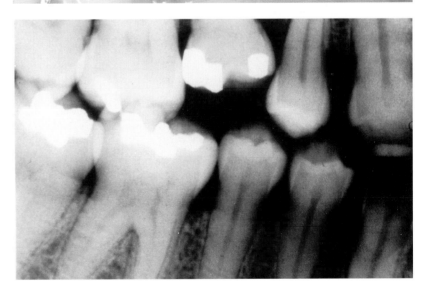

### Figs. 2.25 and 2.26

Supernumerary teeth are additional teeth present within the dental arch. These teeth are thought to arise from accessory buds of the dental lamina that develop into fully formed teeth. These extra teeth may or may not resemble the adjacent teeth.

Approximately 90% of supernumerary teeth develop in the maxilla, with the most common being the mesiodens. These supernumerary teeth occur in the anterior maxilla in the midline and may present alone or bilaterally. Since few achieve eruption, most mesiodentes are discovered secondary to lack of eruption of the adjacent maxillary incisor or on radiographic examination. Often the crowns are cone-shaped with short roots and occasionally may be inverted.

Extraction during childhood is recommended due to a significant number of possible complications related to their continued presence. Delayed eruption, dilaceration, crowding or displacement of adjacent teeth, abnormal diastema formation, tumor or cyst formation, and eruption into the nasal cavity have been associated with mesiodentes. Impacted supernumerary teeth also may create problems if they are exposed secondary to bone resorption and trauma associated with denture use. Early removal often results in spontaneous eruption and alignment of the adjacent permanent teeth within 6 months to 3 years. Removal in older adults often is difficult because of dense bone, further justifying early intervention. Heredity exerts a strong influence on the presence of supernumerary teeth, but a consistent Mendelian pattern is not evident.

## SUPERNUMERARY TEETH

### Fig. 2.27

Although the mesiodens is the most common supernumerary tooth, numerous other supernumerary teeth may occur. Fourth molars, bicuspids, maxillary lateral incisors, mandibular central incisors, and maxillary paramolars are not rare. A paramolar is a small supernumerary maxillary molar located buccal, palatal, or interproximal to a permanent maxillary molar.

In contrast to most supernumerary teeth, supernumerary bicuspids most frequently arise in the mandible rather than the maxilla. These accessory premolars typically are discovered late, with most visible initially between 12 and 14 years of age. If eruption occurs, they often produce crowding, hygiene difficulties, malalignment of teeth, and resorption of adjacent teeth.

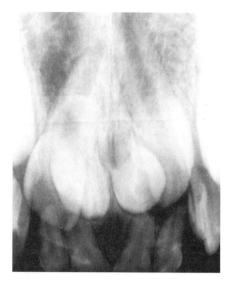

► **Figure 2.26**
**MESIODENS**
Multiple erupted supernumerary teeth of the anterior maxilla. (Courtesy of Dr. Kurt Studt.)

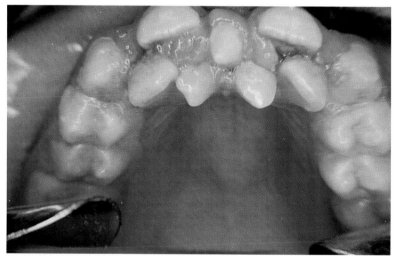

► **Figure 2.27**
**SUPERNUMERARY TEETH**
Two erupted supernumerary mandibular bicuspids.

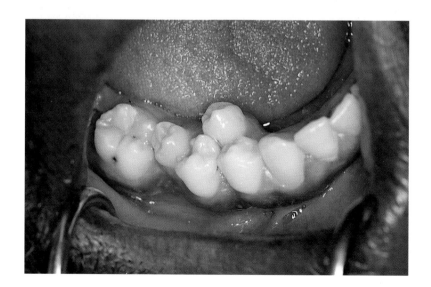

### Fig. 2.28

Although most supernumerary teeth occur in the maxilla, supernumerary mandibular teeth are not rare. Of these, accessory mandibular incisors are least common and represent less than 2% of supernumerary teeth. These teeth can be overlooked because they are not counted easily and often exhibit crowding and malalignment.

Most supernumerary teeth occur in the permanent dentition, but supernumerary deciduous teeth do occur. Typically, removal of these teeth is not recommended because most shed normally on eruption of the permanent dentition and removal may danger the underlying developing permanent tooth. Other more unusual locations for supernumerary teeth include the gingiva, soft palate, nasal cavity, incisive suture, ophthalmic conchae, sphenomaxillary fissure, maxillary tuberosity, maxillary sinus, and between the orbit and the brain.

Multiple supernumerary teeth may occur, and many are associated with one of many syndromes. More than 20 syndromes have been associated with supernumerary teeth; the most strongly correlated is cleidocranial dysplasia (see Figs. 11.4 to 11.6). Reports of impacted and supernumerary teeth associated with Gardner syndrome (see Figs. 11.11 and 11.12) are known, but many cases exhibit only permanent teeth embedded within the dense bone of the jaw osteomas.

## HYPODONTIA

### Figs. 2.29 and 2.30

Anodontia is the congenital absence of all teeth. Impaction or previous extraction of the teeth must be ruled out and is not considered true anodontia. Generalized true anodontia is rare and most often is associated with hereditary hypohidrotic ectodermal dysplasia. Absence of one or more teeth is relatively common, and is termed hypodontia. Oligodontia is a subdivision of hypodontia and refers to six or more absent teeth. Missing teeth are uncommon in the deciduous dentition, and the most commonly involved permanent teeth are the third molars, maxillary lateral incisors, and bicuspids. When present, an increased prevalence of ankylosis, disturbances of spacing, tooth eruption, and exfoliation are noted. Hypodontia is correlated positively with microdontia and exhibits a greater prevalence in females. Radiation therapy to the jaws during tooth formation can destroy the tooth buds and produce a pattern similar to hypodontia. A strong genetic influence is noted, with hypodontia demonstrating an association with close to 40 different syndromes.

▶ **Figure 2.28**
**SUPERNUMERARY TEETH**

An erupted, supernumerary left mandibular central incisor. (Courtesy of Dr. Janet Edwards.)

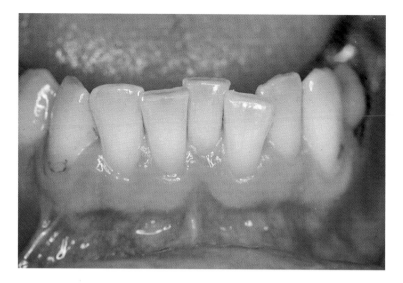

▶ **Figure 2.29**
**HYPODONTIA**

Dentition demonstrating retained deciduous teeth and the absence of numerous permanent teeth that never developed. Note the cone-shaped appearance of the posterior teeth.

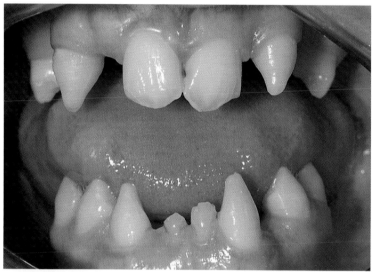

▶ **Figure 2.30**
**HYPODONTIA**

Occlusal view of the dentition described in Figure 2.29. The cuspids and the bicuspids were the only mandibular permanent teeth to develop. The patient did not exhibit any other signs or symptoms of ectodermal dysplasia.

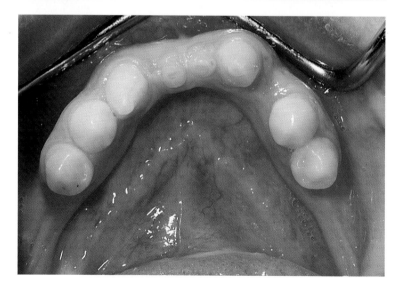

## MICRODONTIA AND MACRODONTIA

### Fig. 2.31

Microdontia refers to teeth that are smaller than normal, and macrodontia refers to teeth that are larger than normal. These disorders may be generalized to all of the teeth or they may be localized to one or more teeth. The generalized forms are rare and normally associated with pituitary dysfunction. Localized microdontia is not uncommon and most often is seen involving the maxillary lateral incisors or third molars. Affected laterals often exhibit cone-shaped crowns and are termed "peg laterals." Localized macrodontia is less common and must be separated from fusion and gemination.

Heredity exhibits a strong influence, but seems to be combined with environmental factors in many cases. Microdontia is correlated positively with hypodontia, and macrodontia is associated with an increased prevalence of hyperdontia (supernumerary teeth). Females demonstrate a higher frequency of microdontia, and males exhibit a greater degree of macrodontia.

## GEMINATION

### Figs. 2.32 and 2.33

Double teeth refers to two teeth that are totally or partially joined by dentin and maybe their pulps. These abnormal teeth are the result of gemination or fusion (see Figs. 2.34 and 2.35). Gemination is defined as a single enlarged tooth or joined (double) tooth in which the tooth count is normal when the anomalous tooth is counted as one. Classically, gemination is thought to represent the incomplete attempt of one tooth germ to divide into two. In many instances, the origin is arguable; the double tooth could have arisen from a split of a single tooth bud or fusion between a normal tooth bud and that of a supernumerary tooth. This argument is academic, and the definition of gemination need not consider this controversial aspect. Gemination is distinguished from fusion by the presence of a full complement of teeth; if no tooth is missing and an incompletely divided tooth exists, it usually is termed gemination.

Geminated teeth typically demonstrate two crowns or one large partially separated crown sharing a single root or root canal. The most commonly affected teeth are the permanent maxillary incisors and the deciduous mandibular incisors. Most examples present as isolated anomalies, but bilateral cases have been reported. Treatment is problematic and often requires extraction and prosthetic replacement of the affected teeth. Recently, investigators described sectioning and removal of the excess coronal tooth structure while retaining vitality and not performing conventional endodontics.

## Figure 2.31
### MICRODONTIA

A maxillary right lateral incisor that is smaller than normal.

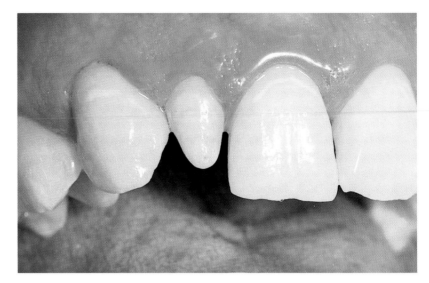

## Figure 2.32
### GEMINATION

A patient who has a full complement of teeth and demonstrates bilateral enlarged maxillary central incisors. Note the incisal groove in the left central incisor. (Case courtesy of Dr. John Mink.)

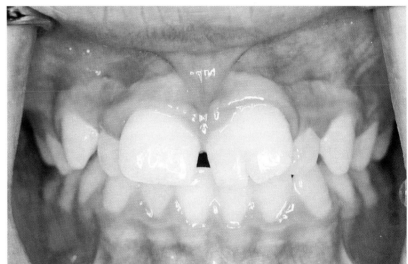

## Figure 2.33
### GEMINATION

Radiograph of a lateral incisor that has partially divided to form two incompletely separated crowns.

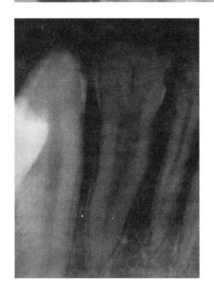

### Figs. 2.34 and 2.35

As mentioned in the discussion of gemination, double teeth may result from either fusion or gemination. Fusion is defined as a single enlarged tooth or joined (double) tooth in which the tooth count reveals a missing tooth when the anomalous tooth is counted as one. Classically, fusion is thought to arise from the union of two normally separated tooth germs. The diagnosis of fusion is best reserved for two completely or incompletely fused teeth that have arisen in the place of two normal teeth. A hereditary pattern occasionally is observed.

These teeth may appear as one large tooth, as one incompletely fused crown, or as two crowns sharing completely or incompletely fused roots. No matter what the pattern, by definition, the fusion must involve the dentin. The occurrence is seen in both deciduous and permanent teeth and has been reported more frequently in the deciduous dentition.

## CONCRESCENCE

### Fig. 2.36

Concrescence is the union of two adjacent teeth by excessive cementum production. This most commonly occurs in the molar region and may involve two normal teeth or a supernumerary tooth and a normal tooth. Concrescence normally is developmental in origin, but some cases may arise after repair of a previous inflammatory lesion. If a nonvital molar has periapical damage from inflammation, the damage may be repaired with cementum production once the inflammatory lesion resolves. Adjacent teeth may become fused after the cementum repair. This most frequently is seen with nonvital maxillary second molars and impacted third molars. Concrescence can produce extraction difficulties and problems in vitality testing.

### Figure 2.34
### FUSION

Dentition demonstrating union of the crowns of the adjacent right mandibular lateral and central incisors.

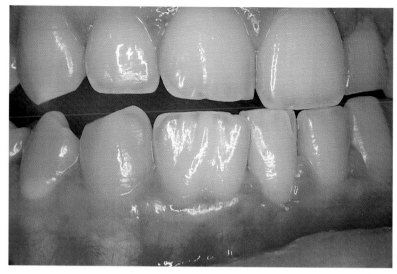

### Figure 2.35
### FUSION

Radiograph demonstrating union of the crowns of the adjacent right mandibular lateral and central incisors.

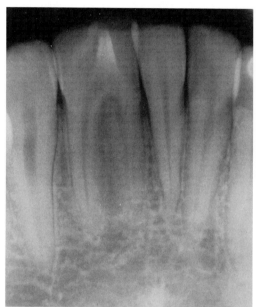

### Figure 2.36
### CONCRESCENCE

Gross photograph of maxillary third molar that is fused by cementum to the adjacent supernumerary fourth molar.

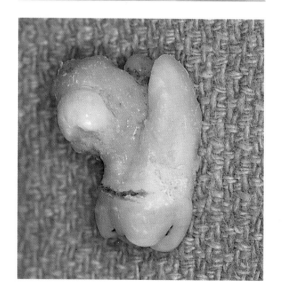

## Figs. 2.37, 2.38, and 2.39

Dens invaginatus is a deep surface invagination of the crown or, rarely, the root of a tooth that is lined by enamel and dentin; it has been termed "dens-in-dente" because it may appear to be a tooth within a tooth. The invagination may be shallow and confined to the crown of the tooth or it may extend all the way to the apex.

In the coronal variants, the defect typically is isolated but may occur in multiple teeth. Bilateral and symmetrical cases occasionally are seen. The most commonly affected tooth is the maxillary lateral incisor. The invagination normally opens at the cingulum area. Radiographically, the invagination is seen easily since it is lined by a thin but distinct layer of enamel. The invagination is constricted adjacent to the opening but often widens as it approaches the base. Occasionally, there is a bulbous enlargement of the invagination at the base that contains an abundance of dysplastic enamel.

Radicular examples of dens invaginatus are rare and arise in areas of ectopic enamel that are similar to that associated with enamel pearls (see Fig. 2.43). Rather than forming an exophytic projection, the ectopic enamel lines a surface invagination into the root. Typically, no clinical problems arise unless the radicular concavity is exposed to the oral cavity.

Coronal invaginations are prone to development of caries; without treatment, pulpal necrosis can occur rapidly. These openings should be restored prophylactically as soon as possible after eruption to prevent carious pulpal necrosis. Because of the open apex, successful endodontic therapy is difficult but has been accomplished.

Occasionally, coronal invaginations rupture out the lateral aspect of the root without communication with the associated dental pulp. Due to the direct communication between the oral cavity and the underlying bone, these teeth develop lateral radicular inflammatory lesions while often maintaining pulpal vitality. Endodontic-like restoration of the coronal invagination may result in resolution of the lateral inflammatory lesion.

**Figure 2.37**
**DENS INVAGINATUS**
Maxillary right lateral incisor demonstrating enamel-lined invagination originating in the area of the cingulum.

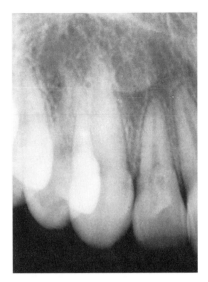

**Figure 2.38**
**DENS INVAGINATUS**
Radiograph of an extracted permanent maxillary lateral incisor that exhibits a deep surface invagination lined by enamel. The invagination originated close to the cusp tip, and the apical portion was filled with an abundance of dysplastic enamel. (Courtesy of Dr. Michael Ridley.)

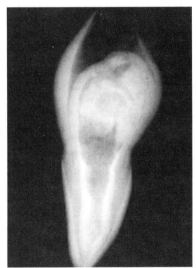

**Figure 2.39**
**DENS INVAGINATUS**
Gross photograph of a decalcified specimen demonstrating deep surface invagination that extends close to the apex.

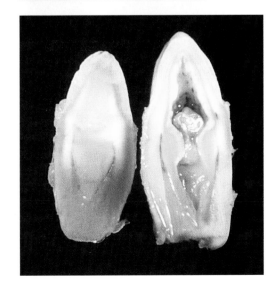

## TALON CUSP

Figs. 2.40 and 2.41

The talon cusp is an accessory cusp usually located on the lingual surface and rarely on the facial surface of permanent or deciduous incisors. The cusp arises in the cingulum area, and more than 90% affect maxillary teeth. This projection, in combination with the normal incisal edge, occasionally forms a pattern resembling an eagle's talon. The cusp often demonstrates a deep developmental groove where it joins the lingual surface of the incisor. This groove is prone to caries and should be restored prophylactically to prevent carious exposure of the pulp. Although a talon cusp may occur as an isolated finding, often additional dental abnormalities, such as shovel-shaped incisors, bifid cingula, cusps of Carabelli, and dens invaginatus, also are present.

Involvement of maxillary teeth may result in malalignment of the anterior teeth or occlusal interference with the mandibular teeth. In these instances, the cusp often must be removed to achieve normal function. It must be remembered that the cusp usually consists of enamel, dentin, and pulp; rapid removal often results in pulp exposure. To avoid exposure and the resultant endodontic therapy, the cusp can be removed a small portion at a time. Removal should cease any time the pulp is approached. The exposed dentin should be covered with calcium hydroxide or a desensitizing agent such as a fluoride varnish, and the patient told to return after the pulp has had time to recede from the surface. With time and patience, the cusp can be removed without necessitating root canal therapy. Talon cusps demonstrate a multifactorial inheritance pattern and have been seen in association with the Rubinstein-Taybi and Mohr syndromes.

## TAURODONTISM

Fig. 2.42

Taurodontism is a developmental abnormality of molar teeth in which the body of the affected tooth is very large and the associated roots are shortened, with the bifurcation near the apex. The tooth tends to be rectangular in shape, with a large pulp chamber dramatically increased in its apico-occlusal height. Variations in severity are seen. Involvement of one or more molars may be seen in one or all four of the quadrants. The permanent teeth are most commonly affected, but occurrence is seen in the deciduous dentition. The condition may occur as an isolated trait or be associated with one of close to 20 syndromes known to be associated with taurodontism. An increased prevalence of this tooth abnormality is noted in patients demonstrating oligodontia.

## ▶ Figure 2.40
### TALON CUSP

A maxillary central incisor demonstrating an accessory palatal cusp.

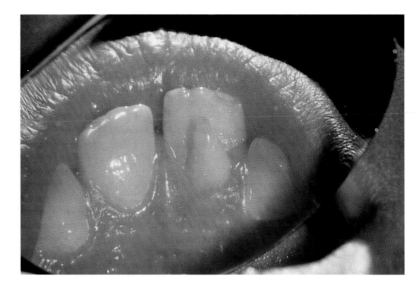

## ▶ Figure 2.41
### TALON CUSP

Radiograph of a maxillary central incisor demonstrating an accessory cusp that consists of enamel, dentin, and pulp.

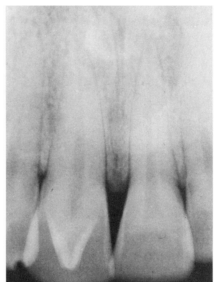

## ▶ Figure 2.42
### TAURODONTISM

A mandibular first molar exhibiting short roots, bifurcation close to the apex, and a pulp chamber that is dramatically increased in apico-occlusal height.

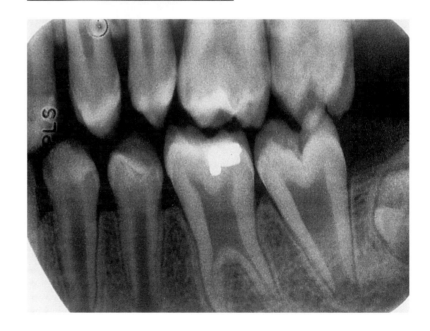

## ENAMEL PEARL

**Fig. 2.43**

The enamel pearl is an uncommon ectopic mass of enamel located near the bifurcation of molar teeth, usually in the permanent dentition. Rare cases have been documented in teeth anterior to the molars. This is thought to be a developmental abnormality that arises from a cluster of misplaced ameloblasts located in the area. The maxillary molars are affected most frequently, but mandibular cases do occur. The pearls may be seen radiographically and can be confused with calculus. Large pearls may exhibit root formation, and some believe the histogenesis is based on the ability of the carrier root to partially behave as a new tooth germ.

These globules of enamel usually do not present any clinical problems unless periodontal disease develops in the bifurcation. The ectopic enamel precludes normal periodontal attachment and may lead to hygiene problems and rapid loss of attachment. If removal is planned, it must be remembered that they may contain a fine strand of dentin and pulp. In deciduous teeth, enamel pearls may produce delayed exfoliation or deviation of the underlying permanent tooth.

## HYPERCEMENTOSIS

**Fig. 2.44**

Hypercementosis is the nonneoplastic deposition of excessive secondary cementum along the root surface of a tooth. Radiographically, no sharp dividing line can be seen between the dentin and the cementum; therefore, the diagnosis is made from the abnormal blunt shape of the enlarged root. One or more teeth may be affected, and bicuspids are involved most frequently. On occasion, excessive deposition is generalized to the entire dentition.

Typically, the process occurs in adulthood and increases in prevalence with age. Cases discovered in younger patients often demonstrate familial clustering. Hypercementosis is known to be associated with tooth repair, adjacent inflammation, and teeth that are not in occlusion (impacted, embedded, or without an antagonist). A few systemic disorders, including Paget disease, acromegaly, pituitary gigantism, thyroid goiter, rheumatic fever, arthritis, calcinosis, and possibly vitamin A deficiency, have been associated with hypercementosis. No treatment is required; however, such teeth may prove difficult to extract.

## DILACERATION

**Fig. 2.45**

Dilaceration is an abnormal bend in the root or crown of a tooth. The bend occurs much more frequently in the root but may be present anywhere along the length of the tooth. Dilaceration is thought to arise secondary to trauma during tooth formation that alters the angle between the tooth germ and the portion of the tooth already developed. On occasion, the bend is created by pressure from an adjacent cyst, tumor, or odontogenic hamartoma. The cause in some cases is difficult to ascertain.

The most frequently affected teeth are the permanent maxillary incisors, followed by the mandibular anteriors. Occasionally, deciduous teeth are affected from perinatal trauma such as laryngoscopy or intubation. The severity of the angulation seems to be related to the age of the patient and the direction and degree of the force applied. Dilaceration of the roots may produce delayed eruption or difficulties during root canal therapy or extraction; recognition on preoperative radiographs often minimizes these problems.

**Figure 2.43**
**ENAMEL PEARL**
Ectopic mass of enamel located in the bifurcation of a maxillary first molar. (Courtesy of Dr. Joseph Beard.)

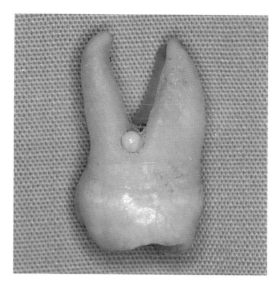

**Figure 2.44**
**HYPERCEMENTOSIS**
Radiograph of the mandibular first molar demonstrating apical enlargement and blunting of the roots secondary to excessive cementum deposition.

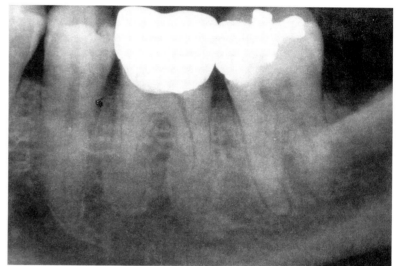

**Figure 2.45**
**DILACERATION**
Abnormal bend in the apical third of the root of the mandibular second bicuspid.

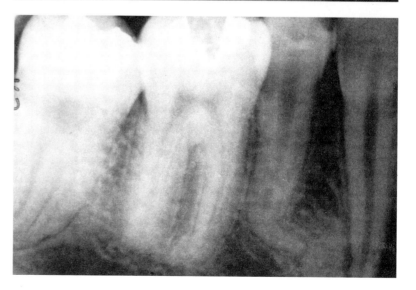

## Figs. 2.46, 2.47, and 2.48

Amelogenesis imperfecta is a complicated group of disorders that encompasses at least 15 different hereditary abnormalities of enamel formation that typically affect all of the teeth in both the deciduous and permanent dentitions in the absence of a related systemic disease. Enamel develops in three stages: first the organic matrix is laid down, then it is mineralized, and, finally, the enamel crystals mature into their final organization. Malfunction of each individual stage may be seen and be responsible for the variation of the clinical presentations. The current classification uses the inheritance pattern and clinical features to group the different forms of amelogenesis imperfecta. Several investigators have begun to formulate a more accurate classification based on the molecular biology of these hereditary enamel defects.

Hereditary defects in enamel matrix formation constitute the category of hypoplastic amelogenesis imperfecta. The affected teeth demonstrate numerous pits, vertical grooving, or a dramatically diminished thickness of enamel. Hypoplastic amelogenesis imperfecta may be inherited as an autosomal-dominant, autosomal-recessive, or X-linked–dominant disorder. When pitted, the defects may be randomly distributed over all of the teeth or localized and arranged in horizontal rows in the middle one third of the crown. In contrast to other forms of amelogenesis imperfecta, the localized pitted form may involve only scattered teeth and affect only the deciduous dentition.

Those with dramatically thin enamel may exhibit a smooth or rough surface texture; in some cases, the enamel is so thin it is termed "enamel agenesis." These patterns produce teeth that often are small and yellow with open contact points and shaped like the underlying dentin. In the X-linked–dominant pattern, affected males demonstrate diffuse involvement; females reveal vertical furrows of thin hypoplastic enamel alternating between bands of normal-thickness enamel.

Radiographically, the pitted type demonstrates numerous pits within the enamel, whereas those with thinned enamel exhibit teeth covered by a very thin shell of radiopaque enamel. To restore function and improve aesthetics, these enamel defects often are treated best with full coverage; on occasion, however, attrition reduces the crown height to such an extent that overdentures become the treatment of choice.

▶ **Figure 2.46**
**AMELOGENESIS IMPERFECTA, ROUGH HYPOPLASTIC TYPE**
Dentition demonstrating dramatic reduction in thickness of enamel that has resulted in teeth that appear smaller than normal with open contact points. The teeth are the shape and color of the underlying dentin.

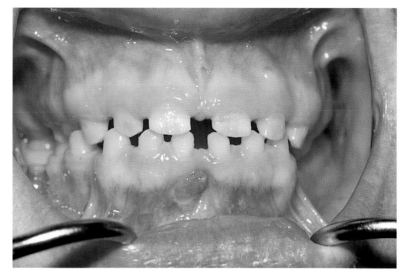

▶ **Figure 2.47**
**AMELOGENESIS IMPERFECTA, SMOOTH HYPOPLASTIC TYPE**
Shiny-surfaced dentition covered by a thin layer of hypoplastic enamel (see radiograph in Fig. 2.48). Due to crowding, the typical widely spaced dentition is lacking. Composite resin has been added to the maxillary central incisors. Note the anterior open bite. (Courtesy of Dr. John G. Stephenson.)

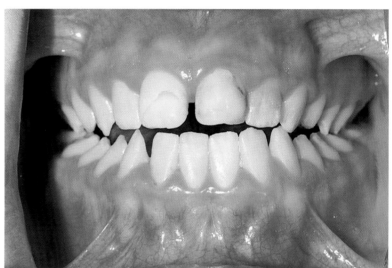

▶ **Figure 2.48**
**AMELOGENESIS IMPERFECTA, SMOOTH HYPOPLASTIC TYPE**
Radiograph of patient depicted in Figure 2.47. Note the thin radiopaque band of enamel overlying the cusps of the molars. (Courtesy of Dr. John G. Stephenson.)

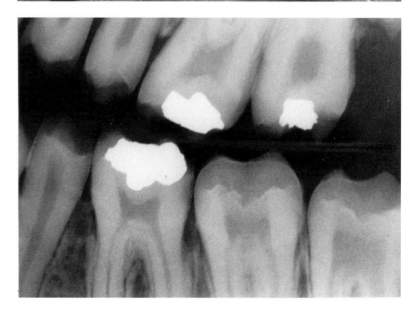

**Figs. 2.49 and 2.50**

Inheritable defects in enamel formation that prevent mineralization of the enamel matrix are termed "amelogenesis imperfecta, hypocalcified type." These teeth demonstrate white and opaque or brownish-orange enamel that can be removed easily with hand instruments and has a soft, cheesy, and crumbly texture. Before eruption, the teeth exhibit enamel of normal shape and thickness, but the radiodensity is similar to that of the underlying dentin. On eruption, the enamel can be abraded easily, and it often exhibits significant calculus accumulation. The most common form is inherited as an autosomal-dominant trait, but some cases do exhibit autosomal-recessive inheritance. Full coverage is the treatment of choice to improve aesthetics, restore function, and prevent accelerated periodontitis secondary to the significant calculus accumulation.

## AMELOGENESIS IMPERFECTA, DIFFUSE HYPOMATURATION TYPE

**Fig. 2.51**

Inheritable defects in enamel formation that prevent the final enlargement and maturation of the enamel crystals are termed "amelogenesis imperfecta, hypomaturation type." The enamel is of normal size and shape but often is lost partially by chipping. The hypomaturation may be diffuse or localized to the incisal/occlusal one third of the teeth (see Fig. 2.52).

In the typical diffuse pattern, the entire dentition is opaque yellow-white, may exhibit mottling, and is inherited as an X-linked–recessive disorder. Secondary to its mode of inheritance, males reveal uniformly diffuse involvement and affected females typically demonstrate alternating vertical bands of white opaque enamel and normal translucent enamel. The vertical pattern in females is not obvious under normal lighting conditions and is best viewed by transillumination. Clinically and radiographically, the teeth in affected males closely resemble the dental changes of fluorosis. In most instances, the dentition is not impaired functionally, and treatment centers around aesthetic improvement of the anterior teeth.

Another variant of hypomaturation amelogenesis imperfecta is termed the "pigmented pattern"; it appears diffusely agar-brown and exhibits autosomal-recessive inheritance. In this pattern, the enamel often separates from the underlying dentin and frequently is soft enough to be pierced by a dental explorer. On occasion, enamel softness similar to that seen in the hypocalcified forms is present. Treatment with full crowns in severe cases can improve aesthetics and function.

### Figure 2.49
**AMELOGENESIS IMPERFECTA, HYPOCALCIFIED TYPE**

Dentition demonstrating brown-to-orange enamel that can easily be removed with hand instruments. (Courtesy of Drs. D. S. Holbrook and S. Altman.)

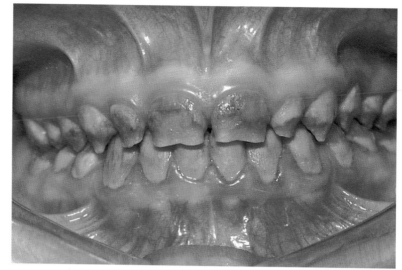

### Figure 2.50
**AMELOGENESIS IMPERFECTA, HYPOCALCIFIED TYPE**

Radiograph of the dentition depicted in Figure 2.49. Note the significant loss of enamel that has occurred from physiologic use. In addition, the radiodensity of the enamel is similar to that of the underlying dentin. (Courtesy of Drs. S. Altman and D. S. Holbrook.)

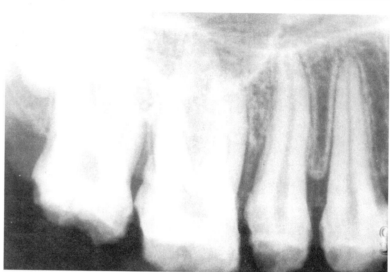

### Figure 2.51
**AMELOGENESIS IMPERFECTA, DIFFUSE HYPOMATURATION TYPE**

Dentition demonstrating enamel with diffuse white opaque and yellow discoloration.

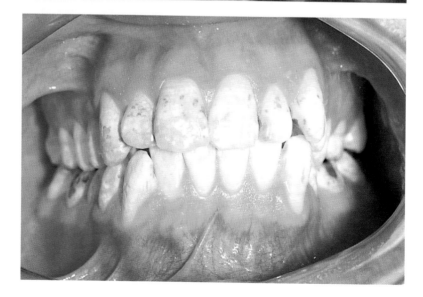

## AMELOGENESIS IMPERFECTA, SNOW-CAPPED TYPE

**Fig. 2.52**

In this pattern of amelogenesis imperfecta, areas of opaque white hypomaturation are noted in the incisal and occlusal one quarter of the teeth. The altered areas do not form a pattern consistent with environmental damage and often reveal an anterior-to-posterior distribution that has been compared with the cusp tips of a denture dipped in white paint. Both the deciduous and permanent dentitions are affected, with most cases exhibiting an X-linked pattern of inheritance. An autosomal-dominant pattern also may exist. The affected teeth typically are functionally sound and require no therapy.

## DENTIN DYSPLASIA, TYPE I

**Figs. 2.53 and 2.54**

Dentin dysplasia, type I, which also is known as "radicular dentin dysplasia," or "rootless teeth," is one of two forms of dentin dysplasia. The second, type II, is related closely to dentinogenesis imperfecta and is presented following that section (see Figs. 2.58 and 2.59). Dentin dyplasia, type I, is autosomal dominant and affects both the deciduous and the permanent dentitions.

The coronal enamel and dentin are well formed and appear normal clinically. The dentin in the roots is extremely disorganized, often resulting in short roots and total obliteration of the pulp canals. The deciduous teeth usually are affected severely and exhibit no pulp chambers. The radiographic pattern in permanent teeth varies according to the degree of dentin disorganization within the root. In some patients, the roots are extremely short with no detectable pulp; in others, the roots are slightly longer and reveal crescent or chevron-shaped pulp chambers. In mildly affected patients, the root length approaches normal, and the canals contain a centrally placed pulp stone. Frequent periapical inflammatory lesions are seen secondary to coronal exposure of superficial microscopic threads of pulpal remnants present within the defective dentin.

Early tooth loss secondary to the short roots and frequent periapical lesions may occur. A few cases have been treated endodontically, with resolution of some of the periapical lesions. The initial endodontic therapy is most difficult because the obliterated root canals have to be instrumented initially with burs. Lesions that fail to resolve are treated with apical curettage if they enlarge or become symptomatic. Otherwise, without these heroics, there is no treatment.

### ► Figure 2.52
### AMELOGENESIS IMPERFECTA, SNOW-CAPPED TYPE

Dentition demonstrating white opaque enamel in the incisal and occlusal one-quarter of the teeth.

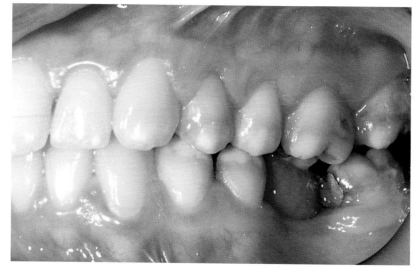

### ► Figure 2.53
### DENTIN DYSPLASIA, TYPE I

Dentition that demonstrates normal coronal structure. (Courtesy of Dr. Charles J. Cunningham.)

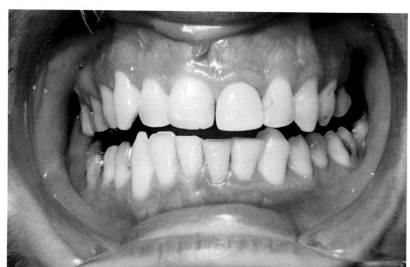

### ► Figure 2.54
### DENTIN DYSPLASIA, TYPE I

Radiograph of the posterior mandible, in which the teeth demonstrate normal coronal structure, short roots, absence of pulp canals, and only small crescents of pulp chambers. Note the numerous periapical lesions. (Courtesy of Tidwell E, Cunningham CJ. Dentinal dysplasia: endodontic treatment, with case report. J Endod 1979;5:372.)

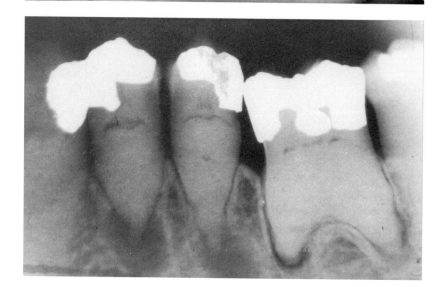

# DENTINOGENESIS IMPERFECTA (HEREDITARY OPALESCENT DENTIN, CAPDEPONT TEETH)

## Figs. 2.55, 2.56, and 2.57

Dentinogenesis imperfecta is an autosomal-dominant disturbance in dentin formation that presents with opalescent teeth in both dentitions and is not associated with a systemic disease. Similar dental findings can be seen in patients with osteogenesis imperfecta, a systemic disorder of bone exhibiting a clearly separate genetic origin. Because these two diseases are distinctly different, when altered teeth are noted in the latter disease, it should be termed "osteogenesis imperfecta with opalescent teeth" and not "dentinogenesis imperfecta."

The classic presentation involves both deciduous and permanent teeth that are clinically opalescent and radiographically exhibit premature closure of the pulp chambers and canals. Although the overlying enamel is normal, it may be lost early, with resultant severe attrition. The coloration of the teeth varies from blue-gray to yellow to brown. When large kindreds are reviewed, occasional variations in expression are noted and previously have been termed the "Brandywine isolate." In these cases, the deciduous teeth may exhibit enamel hypoplasia and multiple pulp exposures in addition to the other dentin changes. The teeth are opalescent, and although many pulps may exhibit premature closure, others are normal or greatly enlarged, forming the pattern known as "shell teeth." A similar variation in expression has been noted in patients with osteogenesis imperfecta and opalescent teeth. Although full crowns may prove beneficial in preserving the teeth, most affected individuals are candidates for full dentures or implants by age 30 years despite numerous interventions. Partial dentures are contraindicated because the roots fracture easily.

▶ **Figure 2.55**
**DENTINOGENESIS IMPERFECTA**
Dentition demonstrating translucence and grayish discoloration.

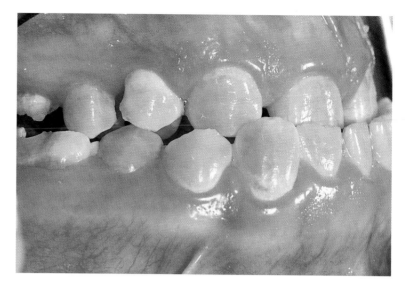

▶ **Figure 2.56**
**DENTINOGENESIS IMPERFECTA**
Occlusal view of the dentition depicted in Figure 2.55. Note the loss of enamel and the accelerated attrition.

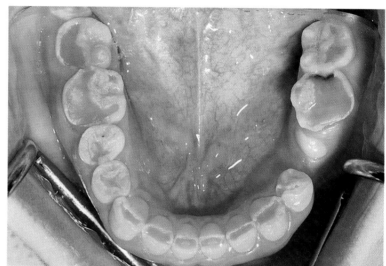

▶ **Figure 2.57**
**DENTINOGENESIS IMPERFECTA**
Radiograph of the patient depicted in Figures 2.55 and 2.56. Note the thin, pointed roots, the bulbous crowns, and the obliteration of the pulp canals.

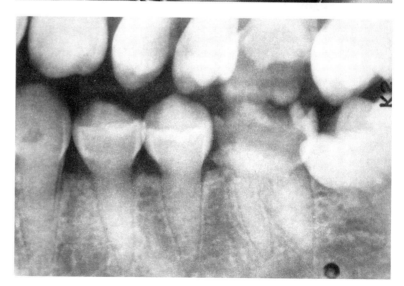

## DENTIN DYSPLASIA, TYPE II

**Figs. 2.58 and 2.59**

Dentin dysplasia, type II (coronal dentin dysplasia), is an autosomal-dominant abnormality of dentin formation that exhibits numerous features of dentinogenesis imperfecta and has been suggested to be a variant of that disorder. The deciduous teeth are opalescent and exhibit premature closure of the pulp chambers and canals. Clinically, the permanent teeth are normal without opalescence. Radiographically, they exhibit enlarged "thistle-tube" shaped pulp chambers, all of which will eventually develop pulp stones. No significant clinical problems are seen in the permanent teeth, and no treatment is required.

## REGIONAL ODONTODYSPLASIA

**Fig. 2.60**

Regional odontodysplasia or "ghost teeth" is an idiopathic developmental abnormality of enamel and dentin that is not hereditary. Although no consistent cause has been documented, many cases have been related to a variety of syndromes, growth abnormalities, neural disorders, and vascular malformations.

This condition may affect a single tooth or several contiguous teeth in a localized area. Rarely, an unaffected tooth may be interposed within a row of affected teeth. The maxilla is affected more frequently with an anterior predominance. Affected deciduous teeth typically are followed by altered permanent teeth; involvement isolated to the permanent teeth is not rare. Usually, the process is confined to a single segment, but it may be bilateral or involve two ipsilateral quadrants. Frequently, affected teeth demonstrate delayed or failed eruption. On eruption, the teeth are yellow-to-brown with a rough surface. Radiographically, a large lucent pulp is encased by a thin layer of enamel and dentin. Short roots and open apices often are present.

Frequent caries and associated periapical inflammatory disease complicate the therapeutic approach. If at all possible, the altered teeth should be retained to allow for appropriate development and preservation of the associated alveolar ridge. Frequently, persistent infection combined with poor tooth structure mandates extraction. Endodontic therapy and coronal restoration have been performed successfully on teeth with sufficient hard tissue. Retained teeth that have maintained their vitality often eventually demonstrate near-normal root formation with overlying hypoplastic crowns. Removable partial dentures can be used to cover affected embedded teeth until the skeletal growth spurt is complete.

## Figure 2.58
### DENTIN DYSPLASIA, TYPE II
Radiograph of the left posterior maxillary dentition demonstrating thistle-tube shaped pulp chambers. The clinical appearance of the teeth was within normal limits. (Case courtesy of Dr. David Besser.)

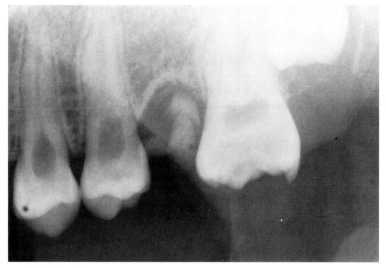

## Figure 2.59
### DENTIN DYSPLASIA, TYPE II
Radiograph of the right anterior mandibular dentition in the patient depicted in Figure 2.58. Note the thistle-tube shaped pulp canals with stones. (Case courtesy of Dr. David Besser.)

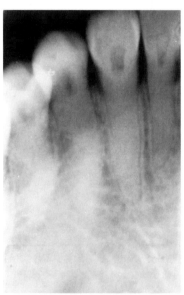

## Figure 2.60
### REGIONAL ODONTODYSPLASIA
Radiograph of the left mandible exhibiting several contiguous deciduous teeth demonstrating large pulp canals encased by a thin layer of enamel and dentin. Note that the underlying succedaneous teeth are affected similarly. Elsewhere, all other teeth are within normal limits. (Courtesy of Dr. John B. Perry.)

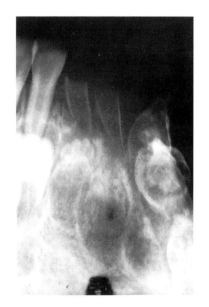

### Dental Fluorosis

Black GV, McKay FA. Mottled teeth: an endemic developmental imperfection of the enamel of teeth heretofore unknown in the literature of dentistry. Dent Cosmos 1916;58:129.

Dean HT, Arnold FA. Endemic dental fluorosis or mottled teeth. J Am Dent Assoc 1943;30:1278.

Levy SM, Kiritsy MC, Slager SL, et al. Patterns of fluoride dentifrice use among infants. Pediatr Dent 1997;19:50.

Lewis DW, Limeback H. Comparison of recommended and actual mean intakes of fluoride by Canadians. J Can Dent Assoc 1996;62:708.

Simard PL, Naccache H, Lachapelle D, et al. Ingestion of fluoride from dentifrices by children aged 12 to 24 months. Clin Pediatr 1991;30:614.

### Localized Environmental Enamel Hypoplasia

Peretz B. An unusual hypoplastic premolar: a case report. Int J Paediatr Dent 1993;3:211.

Via WF. Enamel defects induced by trauma during tooth formation. Oral Surg Oral Med Oral Pathol 1968;25:49.

von Arx T. Developmental disturbances of permanent teeth following trauma to the primary dentition. Aust Dent J 1993;38:1.

### Environmental Enamel Hypoplasia

Brook AH, Fearne JM, Smith JM. Environmental causes of enamel defects. Ciba Found Symp 1997;205:212.

El-Najjar MY, Desanti MV, Ozebek L. Prevalence and possible etiology of dental enamel hypoplasia. Am J Phys Anthropol 1978;48:185.

Needleman HL, Aldred E, Bellinger D, et al. Antecedents and correlates of hypoplastic enamel defects of primary incisors. Pediatr Dent 1992;14:158.

Norén JG, Ranggård L, Klingberg G, et al. Intubation and mineralization disturbances in the enamel of primary teeth. Acta Odontol Scand 1993;51:271.

Seow WK. Enamel hypoplasia in the primary dentition: a review. ASDC J Dent Child 1991;58:441.

Suckling GW, Herbison GP, Brown RH. Etiological factors influencing the prevalence of developmental defects of dental enamel in nine-year-old New Zealand children participating in a health and development study. J Dent Res 1987;66:1466.

### Radiation Effects on the Teeth

Dahllöf G, Rozell B, Forsberg C-M, et al. Histologic changes in dental morphology induced by high dose chemotherapy and total body radiation. Oral Surg Oral Med Oral Pathol 1994;77:56.

Kaste SC, Hopkins KP, Bowman LC. Dental abnormalities in long-term survivors of head and neck rhabdomyosarcoma. Med Pediatr Oncol 1995;25:96.

Kaste SC, Hopkins KP, Jones D, et al. Dental abnormalities in children treated for acute lymphoblastic leukemia. Leukemia 1997;11:792.

Näsman M, Björk O, Söderhäll S, et al. Disturbances in the oral cavity in pediatric long-term survivors after different forms of antineoplastic therapy. Pediatr Dent 1994;16:217.

Sonis AL, Tarbell N, Valachovic RW, et al. Dentofacial development in long-term survivors of acute lymphoblastic leukemia: a comparison of three treatment modalities. Cancer 1990;66:2645.

Takinami S, Masayuki K, Yahata H, et al. Radiation-induced hypoplasia of the teeth and mandible: a case report. Oral Surg Oral Med Oral Pathol 1994;78:382.

### Abfraction of Teeth

Grippo JO. Abfractions: a new classification of hard tissue lesions of teeth. J Esthet Dent 1991;3:14.

Grippo JO, Simring M. Dental "erosion" revisited. J Am Dent Assoc 1995;126:619.

Lee WC, Eakle WS. Possible role of tensile stress in the etiology of cervical erosive lesions of teeth. J Prosthet Dent 1984;52:374.

Lee WC, Eakle WS. Stress-induced cervical lesions: review of advances in the past 10 years. J Prosthet Dent 1996;75:487.

Owens BM, Gallien GS. Noncarious dental "abfraction" lesions in an aging population. Compend Contin Educ Dent 1995;16:552.

## Attrition of Teeth

Goldman HM. An atlas of acquired dental defects. Compend Contin Educ Dent 1982;3:275.

Johansson A, Haraldson T, Omar R, et al. An investigation of some factors associated with occlusal tooth wear in a selected high-wear sample. Scand J Dent Res 1993;101:407.

Johansson A, Kiliaridis S, Haraldson T, et al. Covariation of some factors associated with occlusal tooth wear in a selected high-wear sample. Scand J Dent Res 1993;101:398.

Mair LH. Wear in dentistry: current terminology. J Dent 1992;20:140.

Smith BGN. Toothwear: aetiology and diagnosis. Dent Update 1989;16:204.

Yaffe A, Hochman N, Ehrlich J. A functional aspect of anterior attrition or flaring and mode of treatment. Int J Prosthodont 1992;5:284.

## Abrasion of Teeth

Beckett H, Buxey-Softley G, Gilmour AG. Occupational tooth abrasion in a dental technician: loss of tooth surface resulting from exposure to porcelain powder: a case report. Quintessence Int 1995;26:217.

Bowles WH, Wilkinson MR, Wagner MJ, et al. Abrasive particle in tobacco products: a possible factor in dental attrition. J Am Dent Assoc 1995;126:327.

Eccles JD. Tooth surface loss from abrasion, attrition and erosion. Dent Update 1982;7:373.

Lussi AR, Schaffner M, Holtz P, et al. Epidemiology and risk factors of wedge-shaped defects in a Swiss population. Schweiz Montasscher Zahnmed 1993;103:276.

Nemcovsky CE, Artzi Z. Erosion-abrasion lesions revisited. Compend Contin Educ Dent 1996;17:416.

## Erosion of Teeth

Bartlett DW, Evans DF, Smith BGN. The relationship between gastro-oesophageal reflux disease and dental erosion. J Oral Rehabil 1996;23:289.

Centerwall BS, Armstrong CW, Funkhouser LS, et al. Erosion of dental enamel among competitive swimmers at a gas-chlorinated swimming pool. Am J Epidemiol 1986;123:641.

Hirschfeld Z, Stern N. Anorexia nervosa: dental manifestations and treatment. Compend Contin Educ Dent 1986;7:222.

Imfeld T. Dental erosion: definition, classification and links. Eur J Oral Sci 1996;104:151.

Järvinen VK, Rytömaa II, Heinonen OP. Risk factors in dental erosion. J Dent Res 1991;70:942.

McIntyre JM. Erosion. Aust Prosthodont J 1992;6:17-25.

Milosevic A. Sports drinks hazard to teeth. Br J Sports Med 1997;31:28.

Scheutzel P. Etiology of dental erosion: intrinsic factors. Eur J Oral Sci 1996;104:178.

Zero DT. Etiology of dental erosion: extrinsic factors. Eur J Oral Sci 1996;104:162.

## Tetracycline Staining of Teeth

Chiappinelli JA, Walton RE. Tooth discoloration resulting from long-term tetracycline therapy: a case report. Quintessence Int 1992;23:539.

Grossman ER, Walchek A, Freedman H. Tetracyclines and permanent teeth: the relation between dose and tooth color. Pediatrics 1971;47:567.

Moffitt JM, Cooley RO, Olsen NH, et al. Prediction of tetracycline induced tooth discoloration. J Am Dent Assoc 1974;88:547.

Parkins FM, Furnish G, Bernstein M. Minocycline use discolors teeth. J Am Dent Assoc 1992;123:87.

van der Bijl, Pitigoi-Aron G. Tetracyclines and calcified tissues. Ann Dent 1995;54:69.

Westbury LW, Najera A. Minocycline-induced intraoral pharmacogenic pigmentation: case reports and review of the literature. J Periodontol 1997;68:84-91.

## Extrinsic Staining of Teeth

Addy M, Moran J. Extrinsic tooth discolouration by metals and chlorhexidine: II, clinical staining produced by chlorhexidine, iron and tea. Br Dent J 1985;159:335.

Addy M, Moran J, Newcombe R, et al. The comparative tea staining potential of phenolic, chlorhexidine and anti-adhesive mouthrinses. J Clin Periodontol 1995;22:923.

Dayan D, Heifferman A, Gorski M, et al. Tooth discoloration: extrinsic and intrinsic factors. Quintessence Int 1983;14:195.

Eisenberg E, Bernick SM. Anomalies of the teeth with stains and discolorations. J Prevent Dent 1975;2:7.

Winer RA, Chauncey HH, Garcia RI. Effects of Peroxyl mouthrinse on chlorhexidine staining of teeth. J Clin Dent 1991;3:15.

## Pink Tooth of Mummery

Bakland LK. Root resorption. Dent Clin North Am 1992;36:491.
Mummery JH. The pathology of "pink spots" on teeth. Br Dent J 1920;41:301.

## Internal Resorption of Teeth

Gartner AH, Mack T, Somerlott RG, et al. Differential diagnosis of internal resorption and external root resorption. J Endod 1976;2:329.
Goldman HM. An atlas of acquired dental defects. Compend Cont Educ Dent 1982;3:275.
Gulabivala K, Searson LJ. Clinical diagnosis of internal resorption: an exception to the rule. Int Endod J 1995;28:255.
Zakhary SY. Etiology of internal resorption. Egyptian Dent J 1984;30:11.

## External Resorption of Teeth

Andreasen JO. External root resorption: its implication in dental traumatology, paedodontics, periodontics, orthodontics and endodontics. Int Endod J 1985;18:109.
Bakland LK. Root resorption. Dent Clin North Am 1992;36:491.
Moody AB, Speculand AJ, Smith AJ, et al. Multiple idiopathic external resorption of teeth. Int J Oral Maxillofac Surg 1990;19:200.
Saad AY. Calcium hydroxide in the treatment of external root resorption. J Am Dent Assoc 1989;118:579.

## Natal Teeth

Anneroth G, Isacsson G, Lindwall A, et al. Clinical, histologic, and microradiographic study of natal, neonatal, and pre-erupted teeth. Scand J Dent Res 1978;86:58.
Goho C. Neonatal sublingual traumatic ulceration (Riga-Fede disease): report of cases. J Dent Child 1996;63:362.
Kates GA, Needleman HL, Holmes LB. Natal and neonatal teeth: a clinical study. J Am Dent Assoc 1984;109:441.
Nedley MP, Stanley RT, Cohen DM. Extraction of natal and neonatal teeth can leave odontogenic remnants. Pediatr Dent 1995;17:457.
To EWH. A study of natal teeth in Hong Kong Chinese. Int J Paediatr Dent 1991;2:73.
Zhu J, King D. Natal and neonatal teeth. J Dent Child 1995;62:123.

## Ankylosis

Antoniades K, Tsodoulos S, Karakasis D. Totally submerged deciduous maxillary molars: case reports. Aust Dent J 1993;38:436.
Douglass J, Tinanoff N. The etiology, prevalence, and sequelae of infraclusion of primary molars. J Dent Child 1991;58:481.
Geiger AM, Bronsky MJ. Orthodontic management of ankylosed permanent posterior teeth: a clinical report of three cases. Am J Orthod Dentofacial Orthop 1994;106:543.
Raghoebar GM, Boering G, Vissink A. Clinical, radiographic and histological characteristics of secondary retention of permanent molars. J Dent 1991;19:164.
Williams HA, Zwemer JD, Hoyt DJ. Treating ankylosed primary teeth in adult patients: a case report. Quintessence Int 1995;26:161.

## Supernumerary Teeth

Bodin I, Julin P, Thomsson M. Hyperdontia, I: frequency and distribution of supernumerary teeth among 21,609 patients. Dentomaxillofac Radiol 1978;7:15.
Hattab FN, Yassin OM, Rawashdeh MA. Supernumerary teeth: report of three cases and review of the literature. J Dent Child 1994;61:382.
Hegde SV, Munshi AK. Late development of supernumerary teeth in the premolar region: a case report. Quintessence Int 1996;27:479.
Ida M, Nakamura T, Utsunomiya J. Osteomatous changes and tooth abnormalities in the jaws of patients with adenomatosis coli. Oral Surg Oral Med Oral Pathol 1981;52:2.
Jarvinen S, Lehtinen L. Supernumerary and congenital missing primary teeth in Finnish children: an epidemiologic study. Acta Odontol Scand 1981;39:83.

Sedano HO, Gorlin RJ. Familial occurrence of mesiodens. Oral Surg Oral Med Oral Pathol 1969;27:360.

Trimble LD, West RA, McNeill RW. Cleidocranial dysplasia: comprehensive treatment of the dentofacial abnormalities. J Am Dent Assoc 1982;105:661.

Zhu J-F, Marcushamer M, King DL, et al. Supernumerary and congenitally absent teeth: a literature review. J Clin Pediatr Dent 1996;20:87.

## Hypodontia

Aasheim B, Ögaard B. Hypodontia in 9-year-old Norwegians related to need of orthodontic treatment. Scand J Dent Res 1993;101:257.

Gorlin RJ, Pindborg JJ, Cohen MM. Syndromes of the head and neck. 2nd ed. New York: McGraw-Hill, 1976.

Graber LW. Congenital absence of teeth: a review with emphasis on inheritance patterns. J Am Dent Assoc 1978;96:266.

Jorgenson RJ. Clinician's view of hypodontia. J Am Dent Assoc 1980;101:283.

Meon R. Hypodontia of the primary and permanent dentition. J Clin Pediatr Dent 1992;16:121.

Schalk-van der Weide Y, Steen WHA, Bosman F. Distribution of missing teeth and tooth morphology in patients with oligodontia. J Dent Child 1992;59:133.

Symons AL, Stritzel F. Anomalies associated with hypodontia of the permanent lateral incisor and second molar. J Clin Pediatr Dent 1993;17:109.

## Microdontia and Macrodontia

Ooshima T, Ishida R, Mishima K, et al. The prevalence of developmental anomalies of teeth and their association with tooth size in the primary and permanent dentitions in 1650 Japanese children. Int J Paediatr Dent 1996;6:87.

Reichart PA. Macrodontia of mandibular premolar. Oral Surg Oral Med Oral Pathol 1977;44:606.

Townsend GC. Hereditability of deciduous tooth size in Australian aboriginals. Am J Phys Anthropol 1980;53:297.

Townsend GC, Brown T. Hereditability of permanent tooth size. Am J Phys Anthropol 1978;49:497.

Ufomata D. Microdontia of a mandibular second premolar. Oral Surg Oral Med Oral Pathol 1988;5:637.

## Gemination, Fusion, and Concrescence

Brook AH, Winter GB. Double teeth: a retrospective study of "geminated" and "fused" teeth in children. Br Dent J 1970;129:123.

Buenviaje TM, Rapp R. Dental anomalies in children: a clinical and radiographic survey. J Dent Child 1984;51:42.

David HT, Krakowiak PA, Pirani AB. Nonendodontic coronal resection of fused and geminated vital teeth: a new technique. Oral Surg Oral Med Oral Pathol Oral Radiol Endod 1997;83:501.

Duncan WK, Helpin ML. Bilateral fusion and gemination: a literature analysis and case report. Oral Surg Oral Med Oral Pathol 1987;64:82.

Law L, Fishelberg G, Skribner JE, et al. Endodontic treatment of mandibular molars with concrescence. J Endod 1994;20:562.

Levitas TC. Gemination, fusion, twinning, and concrescence. J Dent Child 1965;32:93.

Ruprecht A, Batniji S, El-Neweihi E. Double teeth: the incidence of gemination and fusion. J Pedod 1985;9:332.

Yuen SWH, Chan JCY, Wei SHY. Double primary teeth and their relationship with the permanent successors: a radiographic study of 376 cases. Pediatr Dent 1987;9:42.

## Dens Invaginatus

Bimstein E, Shteyer A. Dilated type of dens invaginatus in the permanent dentition: report of a case and review of the literature. J Dent Child 1976;43:410.

Oehlers FAC. Dens invaginatus (dilated composite odontome): I, variations of the invagination process and associated anterior crown forms. Oral Surg Oral Med Oral Pathol 1957;10:1204.

Oehlers FAC. Dens invaginatus (dilated composite odontome): II, associated posterior crown forms and pathogenesis. Oral Surg Oral Med Oral Pathol 1957;10:1302.

Olmez S, Uzamis M, Er N. Dens invaginatus of a mandibular central incisor: surgical endodontic treatment. J Clin Pediatr Dent 1995;20:53.

Payne M, Craig GT. A radicular dens invaginatus. Br Dent J 1990;169:94.

Rotstein I, Stabholz A, Freidman S. Endodontic therapy for dens invaginatus in a maxillary second molar. Oral Surg Oral Med Oral Pathol 1987;63:237.

Schwartz SA, Schindler WG. Management of a maxillary canine with dens invaginatus and a vital pulp. J Endod 1996;22:493.

## Talon Cusp

Chen R, Chen H. Talon cusp in primary dentition. Oral Surg Oral Med Oral Pathol 1986;62:67.

Hattab FN, Yassin OM, Al-Nimri KS. Talon cusp—clinical significance and management: case reports. Quintessence Int 1995;26:115.

Hattab FN, Yassin OM, Al-Nimri KS. Talon cusp in permanent dentition associated with other dental anomalies: review of literature and reports of seven cases. J Dent Child 1996;63:368.

Jowharji N, Noonan RG, Tylka JA. An unusual case of dental anomaly: a "facial" talon cusp. J Dent Child 1992:59:156.

Mader CL. Talon cusp. J Am Dent Assoc 1981;103:244.

Mellor JK, Ripa LW. Talon cusps: a clinically significant anomaly. Oral Surg Oral Med Oral Pathol 1970;29:225.

## Taurodontism

Durr DP, Campos CA, Ayers, CS. Clinical significance of taurodontism. J Am Dent Assoc 1980;100:378.

Ruprecht A, Batniji S, El-Neweihi E. The incidence of taurodontism in dental patients. Oral Surg Oral Med Oral Pathol 1987;63:743.

Schalk-van der Weide Y, Steen WHA, Bosman F. Taurodontism and length of teeth in patients with oligodontia. J Oral Rehabil 1993;20:401.

Shifman A, Chanannel I. Prevalence of taurodontism found in radiographic dental examination of 1,200 young adult Israeli patients. Community Dent Oral Epidemiol 1978;6:200.

## Enamel Pearl

Cavanha AO. Enamel pearls. Oral Surg Oral Med Oral Pathol 1965;19:373.

Gaspersic D. Enamel microhardness and histologic features of composite enamel pearls of different size. J Oral Pathol Med 1995;24:153.

Goldstein AR. Enamel pearls as a contributing factor in periodontal breakdown. J Am Dent Assoc 1979;99:210.

Kupietzky A, Rozenfarb N. Enamel pearls in the primary dentition: report of two cases. J Dent Child 1993;60:63.

Moskow BS, Canut PM. Studies on root enamel: (2) Enamel pearls: a review of their morphology, localization, nomenclature, occurrence, classification, histogenesis and incidence. J Clin Periodontol 1990;17:275.

Risnes S. The prevalence, location and size of enamel pearls on human molars. Scand J Dent Res 1974;82:403.

## Hypercementosis

Gardner BS, Goldstein H. The significance of hypercementosis. Dent Cosmos 1931;73:1065.

Leider AS, Garbarino VE. Generalized hypercementosis. Oral Surg Oral Med Oral Pathol 1987;63:375.

Rao VW, Karasick D. Hypercementosis: an important clue to Paget's disease of the maxilla. Skeletal Radiol 1982;9:126.

Weinberger A. The clinical significance of hypercementosis. Oral Surg Oral Med Oral Pathol 1954;7:79.

## Dilaceration

Ligh RA. Coronal dilaceration. Oral Surg Oral Med Oral Pathol 1981;51:567.

Maragakis GM. Crown dilaceration of permanent incisors following trauma to their primary predecessors. J Clin Pediatr Dent 1995;20:49.

Seow WK, Perham S, Young WG, et al. Dilaceration of a primary maxillary incisor associated with neonatal laryngoscopy. Pediatr Dent 1990;12:321.

Smith DMH, Winter GB. Root dilaceration of maxillary incisors. Br Dent J 1981;150:125.

Stewart DJ. Dilacerated unerupted maxillary central incisors. Br Dent J 1978;145:229.

van Gool AV. Injury to the permanent tooth bud after trauma to the deciduous predecessor. Oral Surg Oral Med Oral Pathol 1973;35:2.

## Amelogenesis Imperfecta

Aldred MJ, Crawford PJ. Molecular biology of hereditary enamel defects. Ciba Found Symp 1997;205:200.

Seow WK. Clinical diagnosis and management strategies of amelogenesis imperfecta variants. Pediatr Dent 1993;15:384.

Shields ED. A new classification of heritable human enamel defects and a discussion of dentin defects. Birth Defects 1983;18:107.

Sundell S, Koch G. Hereditary amelogenesis imperfecta: I, epidemiology and clinical classification in a Swedish child population. Swed Dent J 1985;9:157.

Sundell S, Valentin J. Hereditary aspects and classification of hereditary amelogenesis imperfecta. Community Dent Oral Epidemiol 1986;14:211.

Winter GB, Brook AH. Enamel hypoplasia and anomalies of the enamel. Dent Clin North Am 1975;19:3.

Witkop CJ. Amelogenesis imperfecta, dentinogenesis imperfecta and dentin dysplasia revisited: problems in classification. J Oral Pathol 1989;17:547.

Witkop CJ, Sauk JJ. Heritable defects in enamel. In: Stewart RE, Prescott GH, eds. Oral facial genetics. St. Louis: CV Mosby, 1976:151.

## Dentin Dysplasia, Type I

Bixler D. Heritable disorders affecting dentin. In: Stewart RE, Prescott GH, eds. Oral facial genetics. St. Louis: CV Mosby, 1976:227.

Dym H, Levy J, Sherman PM. Dentinal dysplasia, type I: review of the literature and report of a family. J Dent Child 1982;49:437.

O'Carroll MK, Duncan WK, Perkins TM. Dentin dysplasia: review of the literature and a proposed subclassification based on radiographic findings. Oral Surg Oral Med Oral Pathol 1991;72:119.

O'Carroll MK, Duncan WK. Dentin dysplasia type I: radiologic and genetic perspectives in a six-generation family. Oral Surg Oral Med Oral Pathol 1994;78:375.

Seow WK. Spectrum of dentin dysplasia in a family: case report and literature review. Pediatr Dent 1994;16:437.

Steidler NE, Radden BG, Reade PC. Dentinal dysplasia: a clinicopathological study of eight cases and review of the literature. Br J Oral Maxillofac Surg. 1984;22:274.

Tidwell E, Cunningham CJ. Dentinal dysplasia: endodontic treatment, with case report. J Endod 1979;5:372.

Van Dis ML, Allen CM. Dentinal dysplasia type I: a report of four cases. Dentomaxillofac Radiol 1989;18:128.

## Dentinogenesis Imperfecta

Bouvier D, Duprez J-P, Morrier J-J, et al. Strategies for rehabilitation in the treatment of dentinogenesis imperfecta in a child: a clinical report. J Prosthet Dent 1996;75:238.

Gage JP, Symons AL, Romaniuk K, et al. Hereditary opalescent dentine: variation in expression. J Dent Child 1991;58:134.

Heimler A, Sciubba J, Lieber E, et al. An unusual presentation of opalescent dentin and Brandywine isolate hereditary opalescent dentin in an Ashkenazic Jewish family. Oral Surg Oral Med Oral Pathol 1985;59:608.

Levin LS, Leaf SH, Jelmini RJ, et al. Dentinogenesis imperfecta in the Brandywine isolate (DI type III): clinical, radiologic and scanning electron microscopic studies of the dentition. Oral Surg Oral Med Oral Pathol 1983;56:267.

Lukinmaa P-L, Ranta H, Ranta K, et al. Dental findings in osteogenesis imperfecta: I, occurrence and expression of type I dentinogenesis imperfecta. J Craniofac Genet Dev Biol 1987;7:115.

Ranta H, Lukinmaa P-L, Waltimo J. Heritable dentin defects: nosology, pathology, and treatment. Am J Med Genet 1993;45:193.

Shields ED, Bixler D, El-Kafrawy AM. A proposed classification of heritable human dentine defects with a description of a new entity. Arch Oral Biol 1973;18:543.

Witkop CJ Jr. Hereditary defects of dentin. Den Clin North Am 1975;19:25.

Witkop CJ Jr. Amelogenesis imperfecta, dentinogenesis imperfecta and dentin dysplasia revisited: problems in classification. J Oral Pathol 1988;17:547.

## Dentin Dysplasia, Type II

Bixler D. Heritable disorders affecting dentin. In: Stewart RE, Prescott GH, ed. Oral facial genetics. St. Louis: CV Mosby, 1976:227.

Melnick M, Eastman JR, Goldblatt LI, et al. Dentin dysplasia, type II: a rare autosomal dominant disorder. Oral Surg Oral Med Oral Pathol 1977;44:592.

Ranta H, Lukinmaa P-L, Waltimo J. Heritable dentin defects: nosology, pathology, and treatment. Am J Med Genet 1993;45:193.

Rosenberg LR, Phelan JA. Dentinal dysplasia, type II: review of the literature and report of a family. J Dent Child 1983;50:372.

Witkop CJ Jr. Hereditary defects of dentin. Dent Clin North Am 1975;19:25.

Witkop CJ Jr. Amelogenesis imperfecta, dentinogenesis imperfecta and dentin dysplasia revisited: problems in classification. J Oral Pathol 1988;17:547.

## Regional Odontodysplasia

Gardner DG, Sapp JP. Regional odontodysplasia. Oral Surg Oral Med Oral Pathol 1973;35:351.

Guzman R, Elliot MA, Rossie KM. Odontodysplasia in a pediatric patient: literature review and case report. Pediatr Dent 1990;12:45.

Kahn MA, Hinson RL. Regional odontodysplasia: case report with etiologic and treatment considerations. Oral Surg Oral Med Oral Pathol 1991;72:462.

Lustmann J, Klein H, Ulmansky M. Odontodysplasia. Report of two cases and review of the literature. Oral Surg Oral Med Oral Pathol 1975;39:781.

Neupert EA, Wright JM. Regional odontodysplasia presenting as a soft tissue swelling. Oral Surg Oral Med Oral Pathol 1989;67:193.

Sadeghi EM, Ashrafi MH. Regional odontodysplasia: clinical, pathologic and therapeutic considerations. J Am Dent Assoc 1981;102:336.

Walton JL, Witkop CJ, Walker PO. Odontodysplasia: report of three cases with vascular nevi overlying the adjacent skin of the face. Oral Surg Oral Med Oral Pathol 1978;46:676.

Zegarelli EV, Kutscher AH, Applebaum E, et al. Odontodysplasia. Oral Surg Oral Med Oral Pathol 1963;16:187.

# chapter 3

# PULPAL, PERIAPICAL, AND PERIODONTAL PATHOLOGY

**Fig. 3.1**

Pulp stones arise predominantly in the pulp chambers and consist of either tubular dentin (true denticles) or concentric layers of dystrophic calcification (false denticles). It is thought that pulp stones begin as areas of calcification around a central nidus such as a collagen fragment, ground substance, or necrotic cell remnants. Originally, the stones are atubular; and true denticles demonstrate tubules only after being surrounded by secondary dentin. Pulp stones may be free within the pulp or attached to the inner dentinal walls. An increased prevalence of pulp stones is seen in older adults, with most teeth being affected in patients older than age 50 years. These calcifications are of little clinical significance except for occasional difficulties during root canal therapy. Although most pulp stones are not related to any disease process, pulp stones are associated with dentin dysplasia type II, pulpal dysplasia, tumoral calcinosis, calcinosis universalis, and Ehlers-Danlos syndrome, type I.

## CHRONIC HYPERPLASTIC PULPITIS (PULP POLYP)

**Fig. 3.2**

Chronic hyperplastic pulpitis is an overgrowth of chronically inflamed granulation tissue that originates from the dental pulp of a tooth with a large pulp exposure. The vast majority occur in young patients whose teeth contain large vascular pulps with high tissue reactivity. The deciduous molars and first permanent molars are involved most commonly. Bacterial contamination and mechanical irritation results in hyperplastic tissue formation that produces a pink nodule originating from the pulp chamber, often filling the coronal defect. Although the pulp is vital and often asymptomatic, the changes are irreversible; the tooth must be extracted or treated endodontically.

## CONDENSING OSTEITIS (FOCAL SCLEROSING OSTEOMYELITIS)

**Fig. 3.3**

Condensing osteitis is an inflammatory condition that results in increased radiodensity of the bone and is seen most frequently in children and young adults. Classically, it occurs around the apex of a tooth with pulpal necrosis but has been seen enveloping the apices of vital teeth that had a previous episode of significant pulpitis. Typically, the adjacent root tip is separate from the lesion; the periphery of the dense bone may blend into the surrounding normal bone or exhibit a well-defined border. Treatment consists of removal of the focus of infection either through extraction or root canal therapy. Although in approximately 85% of patients the dense bone returns to normal following elimination of the inflammatory focus, residual areas of condensing osteitis may remain and are termed "bone scars."

### Figure 3.1
**PULP STONES**

Multiple teeth with pulp chambers containing calcifications.

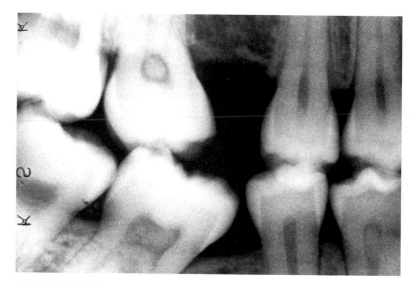

### Figure 3.2
**CHRONIC HYPERPLASTIC PULPITIS**

Hyperplastic tissue originating in pulp of maxillary first molar in an adolescent. (Courtesy of Dr. Kurt Studt.)

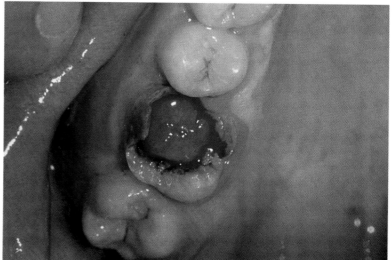

### Figure 3.3
**CONDENSING OSTEITIS**

Increased radiodensity adjacent to apex of nonvital first molar in an adolescent. Note intact periodontal ligament space.

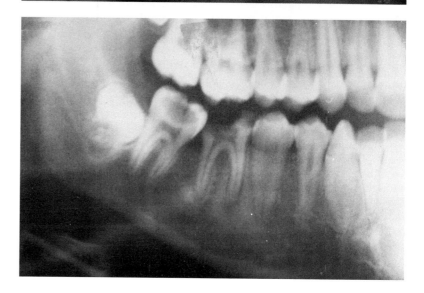

## PERIAPICAL INFLAMMATORY DISEASE

**Fig. 3.4**

Inflammatory lesions of the pulp and periapical areas are among the most common pathologic conditions involving the teeth. Once inflammation has spread from the dental pulp, it can produce a variety of pathologic alterations, the most common of which are periapical granuloma, periapical cyst, and periapical abscess (see Figures 3.5 to 3.9). The two former lesions are closely related entities that cannot be separated radiographically or clinically, and one type may transform into the other. Histopathologic examination is required for a definitive diagnosis.

Appropriate therapy is directed toward elimination of the source of the pathosis, bacterial contamination, and degenerated pulpal by-products released through the root canal. Tooth extraction or thorough removal of the diseased pulp tissue and obturation of the canal with a well-condensed filling material such as gutta-percha and root canal sealer is essential. Properly performed nonsurgical endodontic treatment can resolve most cases of periapical inflammatory disease, including both granulomas and cysts.

Lesions nonresponsive to seemingly appropriate conventional endodontic therapy should receive surgical periradicular curettage and sealing of the associated apices. The primary goal of periradicular curettage is control of the source of the irritants escaping from the root canal; once achieved, resolution is typical. Although controversial, removal of surrounding periradicular soft tissue during surgical endodontic procedures is recommended to remove minute antigenic foreign material impacted during earlier endodontic procedures, to disrupt any organized cystic structure, and to confirm the inflammatory nature of the process (and rule out pathoses such as Langerhans cell disease, giant cell granuloma, etc.).

## PERIAPICAL ABSCESS

**Fig. 3.5**

The periapical abscess is a suppurative periapical process that occurs secondary to necrosis of the dental pulp. The affected tooth does not respond to cold or electric pulp testing. The process may arise de novo or from an acute exacerbation of a periapical granuloma or cyst. Initially, the affected tooth exhibits tenderness that often is relieved by applying direct pressure. With progression, the intensity of the pain increases and typically is associated with extrusion of the tooth and sensitivity to percussion. On occasion, systemic signs of infection, such as headache, malaise, fever, and chills, arise. Without drainage through the tooth, the abscess may perforate the cortical plate and lead to parulis formation (see Figure 3.11), an overlying soft-tissue abscess (see Figure 3.12), or cellulitis. Without drainage, development into osteomyelitis may occur.

Radiographically, early de novo lesions may show little change because the rapid clinical progression precedes any observable alterations. Abscesses secondary to periapical granulomas and cysts are similar radiographically to the original lesion. Treatment is drainage via extraction of the infected tooth or through the opened pulp chamber when endodontic therapy is appropriate. Typically, patients with focal acute inflammatory disease respond favorably to local treatment and do not exhibit demonstrable benefit from antibiotic supplementation.

## PERIAPICAL GRANULOMA (CHRONIC APICAL PERIODONTITIS)

**Fig. 3.6**

The periapical granuloma arises secondary to necrosis of the dental pulp and is a mass of inflamed granulation tissue adjacent to the root canal foramen. The size of the lesion can vary from a slight thickening of the periodontal ligament to occasional lesions more than 2 cm in diameter. The periphery of the lesion may be diffuse or well circumscribed, with or without a radiopaque rim. Clinically, the lesion may be asymptomatic or may exhibit mild pain or sensitivity to percussion. As described in the previous section, treatment consists of extraction of the affected tooth or root canal therapy that may be followed by surgical endodontic procedures if the lesion does not respond to therapy.

### Figure 3.4
**PERIAPICAL INFLAMMATORY DISEASE**
Nonvital mandibular first molar demonstrating periapical lucencies enveloping each apex. Once inflammatory origin is confirmed, appropriate endodontic therapy is intitiated, regardless of the lesions being granulomas or cysts.

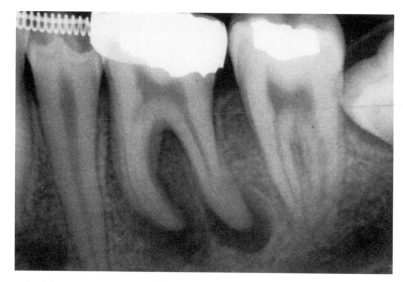

### Figure 3.5
**PERIAPICAL ABSCESS**
Radiolucency of the anterior mandible, which resolved after drainage and root canal therapy.

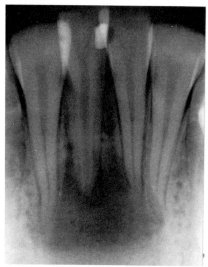

### Figure 3.6
**PERIAPICAL GRANULOMA**
Mandibular first molar exhibiting a 1.5 cm radiolucent lesion of the apices.

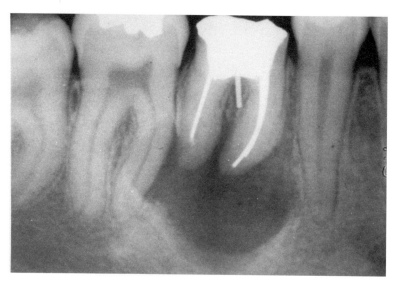

## PERIAPICAL CYST (RADICULAR CYST, APICAL PERIODONTAL CYST)

**Figs. 3.7 and 3.8**

The periapical cyst arises from a periapical granuloma containing epithelium that organizes into a true cyst. Typically, the lining is stratified squamous epithelium but can demonstrate pseudostratified columnar epithelium. The origin of the epithelium is normally the rests of Malassez, but other sources include the lining of the maxillary sinus, crevicular epithelium, or epithelium from a fistulous tract. The clinical presentation and radiographic pattern are identical to the periapical granuloma, and a definitive diagnosis is not required before initiation of appropriate therapy.

Because no reliable criteria exist for separation of granulomas from cysts, all cases of periapical inflammatory disease are approached in a similar manner. Extraction or root canal therapy is appropriate. In large lesions strongly suspected of being cystic, passage of a small file into the periapical lesion may disrupt any cystic structure and release intraluminal pressure. In addition, interim calcium hydroxide filling and decompression procedures have been used to achieve resolution without surgical endodontic procedures.

Although most patients with periapical inflammatory disease respond to nonsurgical endodontic treatment because of elimination of continued contamination through the root canal, the presence of an organized cystic structure and accumulation of tissue breakdown products within the lesion can adversely affect the healing process and lead to failure. Apicoectomy is performed if the lesion does not respond to nonsurgical root canal therapy.

## LATERAL RADICULAR CYST

**Fig. 3.9**

On occasion, odontogenic cysts of inflammatory origin present along the lateral aspect of a tooth. In most instances, these represent abnormally positioned periapical cysts that arise from the spread of inflammatory pulpal by-products through lateral foramina. In some cases, the associated tooth is vital, with the source of the inflammation being a deep periodontal pocket. Radiographically, these lesions closely resemble the pattern produced by lateral periodontal cysts. Identification and elimination of the focus of infection is the treatment of choice. Lesions that fail to respond must be removed surgically and submitted for histopathologic examination.

### Figure 3.7
**PERIAPICAL CYST**

Periapical radiolucency encircling the apex of an endodontically treated right maxillary lateral incisor.

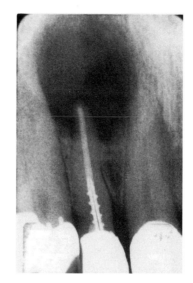

### Figure 3.8
**PERIAPICAL CYST**

Large radiolucency of the anterior mandible that extends from the right first bicuspid to the contralateral first molar.

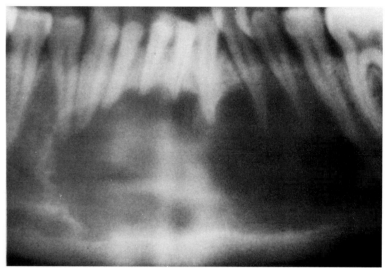

### Figure 3.9
**LATERAL RADICULAR CYST**

Radiolucency associated with the mesial aspect of the endodontically treated right maxillary lateral incisor. The cyst was inflammatory in origin and not related to periodontal disease. (Case courtesy of Dr. Larry Durand.)

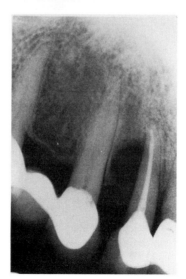

## RESIDUAL PERIAPICAL CYST

### Fig. 3.10

The residual periapical cyst arises following the extraction of an infected tooth that previously had apical inflammatory disease. Remnants of epithelium or a cyst remain in the socket after extraction and result in the residual cyst. Histopathologically, this cyst is identical to the periapical cyst.

Should curettage of the socket be performed after extraction in an attempt to prevent these cysts? The existence of the residual periapical cyst has been questioned. It has been suggested that once the inflammatory stimulus is removed, the cyst will degenerate and healing will occur. Although most cases of periapical inflammatory disease will resolve following extraction of the associated tooth, the existence of residual periapical cysts is confirmed on a regular basis in oral and maxillofacial pathology laboratories throughout the world. Although these cysts are uncommon, each clinician must weigh the chance of cyst development against the ease of simple curettage of the socket at the time of extraction.

Once established, these cysts can enlarge slowly, remain stable, or exhibit signs of degeneration, such as central dystrophic calcification. Radiographically, any number of odontogenic and nonodontogenic cysts and neoplasms can mimic the pattern presented by residual periapical cysts. Therefore, all such lesions should be surgically excised, with submission of the tissue for histopathologic examination. With complete removal, the lesion does not recur.

## PARULIS (GUMBOIL)

### Fig. 3.11

Intraosseous abscesses may perforate through the cortical plate and channel through the overlying soft tissue. When drainage occurs into the oral cavity, a parulis typically develops. This refers to a mass of subacutely inflamed granulation tissue that arises on the oral mucosal surface at the distal opening of a sinus tract. As a result of the constant drainage, abscesses associated with overlying parulides often are asymptomatic and occasionally are discovered during routine soft-tissue examination. The abscess may develop from either periapical or periodontal disease (see Figures 3.25 and 3.26). Treatment consists of resolution of the underlying focus of infection. Occasionally, the parulis may remain following successful treatment of the underlying infection. When this occurs, the lesion should be excised along with any associated residual underlying contaminated sinus tract.

## PALATAL ABSCESS

### Fig. 3.12

Odontogenic infections may spread into the soft tissues. This usually occurs toward the buccal surface because most root apices are closer to the facial surface, and the buccal cortical plate is thinner than the lingual or palatal cortical bone. In contrast, maxillary lateral incisors, the palatal roots of the maxillary molars, and mandibular second and third molars usually achieve drainage through the lingual plate. When palatal perforation does occur, significant enlargement may occur because the thick mucoperiosteum of the palate impedes drainage and promotes accumulation of the purulent exudate. Treatment involves drainage and resolution of the focus of infection.

### Figure 3.10
**RESIDUAL PERIAPICAL CYST**
Radiolucency present in the area of previously extracted mandibular first molar. (Courtesy of Dr. Brent Klinger.)

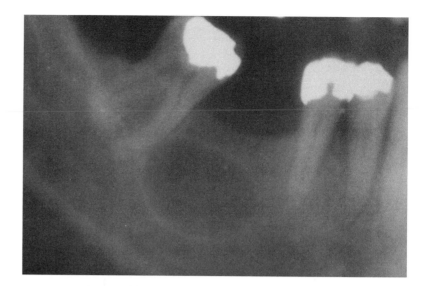

### Figure 3.11
**PARULIS**
Enlargements of the mandibular facial gingiva secondary to underlying foci of infection.

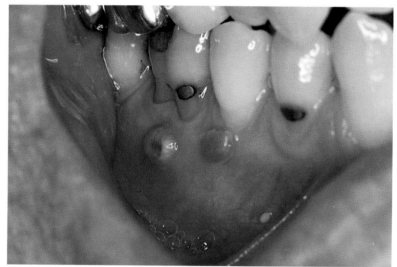

### Figure 3.12
**PALATAL ABSCESS**
Soft-tissue enlargement of the palate that arose from spread of infection from a nonvital lateral incisor.

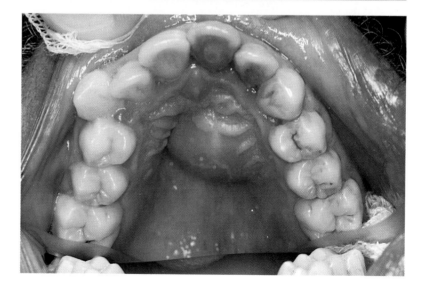

## INTRABONY FIBROUS SCAR

### Figs. 3.13 and 3.14

Intrabony fibrous scars usually arise after extraction or root canal therapy in which the site is filled with dense collagen instead of bone. The lesion usually occurs when one or both of the adjacent cortical plates are lost secondary to the primary pathologic process or from the surgical therapy. These scars often are mistaken radiographically for a periapical cyst or granuloma or may demonstrate an irregular outline and an asymmetrical pattern. In some cases, the lucency is separate from the associated apex, which may demonstrate an intact lamina dura. Occasionally, healing with bone occurs after diagnostic removal. Because radiographic resolution typically does not occur, further surgical intervention should not be performed once the definitive diagnosis has been established.

## EPULIS GRANULOMATOSUM

### Fig. 3.15

Epulis granulomatosum is the term coined to describe the overgrowth of hyperplastic tissue that arises out of a recent extraction socket. This mass of exuberant, subacutely inflamed granulation tissue often reveals fragments of nonvital bone or tooth structure; these fragments are thought to be the inciting agent responsible for the tissue overgrowth. Treatment consists of thorough removal of all of the soft tissue within the socket followed by irrigation to completely eliminate any loose fragments of tooth or bone. Histopathologic examination of the removed material is required because metastatic carcinomas occasionally masquerade as an epulis granulomatosum.

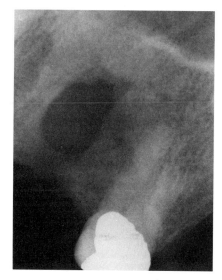

▶ **Figure 3.13**
**INTRABONY FIBROUS SCAR**
Radiolucency of the maxilla present in a previous extraction site where both cortical plates were lost. (Courtesy of Dr. C. R. Adams.)

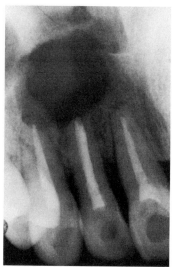

▶ **Figure 3.14**
**INTRABONY FIBROUS SCAR**
Irregular radiolucency apical to several endodontically treated teeth in the anterior maxilla on the right side. (Courtesy of Dr. Craig Little.)

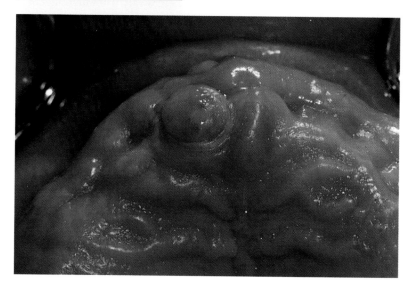

▶ **Figure 3.15**
**EPULIS GRANULOMATOSUM**
Hyperplastic tissue at site of recent extraction. Necrotic bone was found histologically within the granulation tissue.

## CHRONIC GINGIVITIS

**Fig. 3.16**    Chronic gingivitis is an inflammation of the soft tissue surrounding the teeth. Most cases are secondary to substances being released from plaque and accumulating in the gingival sulcus. In addition to the plaque-related form, other less common types include those related to allergies, medications, specific infections and certain dermatoses. Gingivitis affects most of the population, begins in childhood, and increases with age. An increased prevalence of gingivitis is noted during periods of hormonal elevation (puberty, pregnancy) and in association with diabetes mellitus, metal poisoning, trauma, mouth-breathing, smoking, or malnutrition.

Typically, the inflammation begins in the interdental papillae and presents with redness, slight enlargement, and loss of normal stippling. Bleeding may occur on manipulation. As the gingivitis progresses, the redness intensifies and spreads over the marginal gingiva, which may become blunted, receded, or enlarged. Therapy consists of elimination of the underlying cause, usually mechanical removal of dental plaque with initiation and maintenance of a system of good oral hygiene (daily home brushing and flossing combined with periodic professional care). Although effective anti-inflammatory drugs and systemic or local antimicrobials are available, these agents typically are reserved for patients with rapid or refractory disease. Gingivitis may revert to normal, stabilize, or progress on to periodontitis.

## HORMONAL GINGIVITIS

**Fig. 3.17**    The severity of gingivitis is affected by the systemic levels of sex hormones, especially progesterone, which seems to increase the permeability of gingival blood vessels and sensitize the site to irritants. Despite this, females typically exhibit less gingivitis, most likely because of better oral hygiene. The peak prevalence of gingivitis occurs around 11 years of age and seems to be related to elevated hormones present during this period. Because of this increased susceptibility, adolescents often develop significant clinical changes, termed "pubertal gingivitis," that often are present in association with minimal local factors. Following this brief period of high prevalence, the frequency of gingivitis declines for several years, then slowly increases in adulthood.

Pregnancy gingivitis arises secondary to the hormonal changes associated with pregnancy and also occurs in the presence of minimal local factors. Almost half of pregnant women exhibit increased gingival inflammation beginning near the end of the first trimester and continuing to parturition. The changes vary from mild incipient gingivitis to diffuse hyperplastic gingivitis. Occasional tumor-like masses arise in the interdental area. Each isolated enlargement is identical histopathologically to a pyogenic granuloma (see Fig. 9.14) and often is termed a "pregnancy tumor" or "granuloma gravidarum."

## ACUTE NECROTIZING ULCERATIVE GINGIVITIS (ANUG)

**Fig. 3.18**    Acute necrotizing ulcerative gingivitis is believed to be an infectious disease related to elevated levels of *Prevotella intermedia* and pathogen-related oral spirochetes. Poor hygiene, general debilitation, psychologic stress, immunosuppression, smoking, local trauma, and malnutrition promote the infection. The process was nicknamed "trench mouth" secondary to a high prevalence seen in the battlefield trenches during World War I. Acute necrotizing ulcerative gingivitis represents one of the more common symptomatic oral manifestations of acquired immunodeficiency syndrome (see Fig. 4.55).

Although the disease may occur at any age, it is seen predominantly in young and middle-aged adults. Classically, the interdental papillae demonstrate ulceration, necrosis, and loss of vertical height. Affected papillae typically are blunted and exhibit a crater-like area of necrosis. Bleeding, pain, and foul odor are present. Treatment consists of debridement followed by frequent, thorough lavage with warm water. Antibiotics may be used, although most cases resolve without medication. Without treatment, the process may lead to loss of osseous attachment (necrotizing ulcerative periodontitis) or spread to the adjacent soft tissues (necrotizing ulcerative stomatitis).

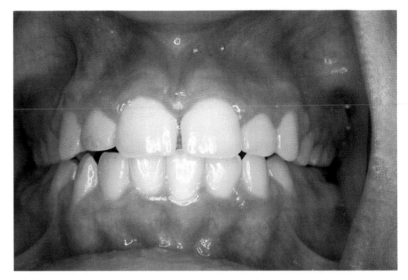

► **Figure 3.16**
**CHRONIC GINGIVITIS**
Mild redness, blunting of the interdental papillae, and rolled gingival margins. (Courtesy of Dr. Herbert Abrams)

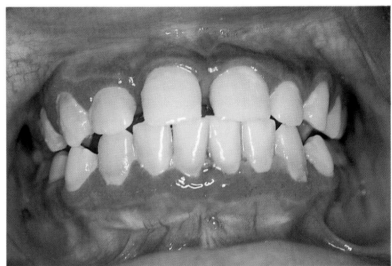

► **Figure 3.17**
**HORMONAL GINGIVITIS**
Diffuse hyperplastic and erythematous gingiva in a pregnant patient who also had a pyogenic granuloma distal to the right maxillary premolar.

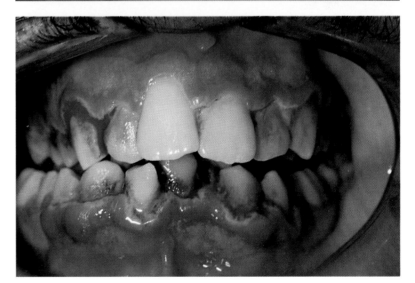

► **Figure 3.18**
**ACUTE NECROTIZING ULCERATIVE GINGIVITIS**
Ulceration of the interdental papillae with bleeding.

## Figs. 3.19, 3.20, and 3.21

Various drugs have been associated with an increased prevalence of gingival hyperplasia. The oldest and most common of these is phenytoin (Dilantin), an anticonvulsant drug commonly used in the treatment of epilepsy. Recently, the number of offending drugs is increasing, with numerous calcium channels blockers, another antiepileptic agent, sodium valproate, and the immunosuppressant drug cyclosporine joining the list. Oral contraceptives have been implicated rarely in patients, but the association is not strong. Of all the calcium channel blockers, nifedipine is correlated with increased gingival hyperplasia most frequently, but an association with diltiazem, felodipine, nitrendipine, and verapamil also has been shown. Many other calcium channel blockers exist and possibly may produce similar changes. When two offending medications are used concurrently, the degree of hyperplasia often is increased. Rather than trying to memorize the enlarging list of medications related to gingival hyperplasia, the patient's medical history must be reviewed for any possible association to a medication in all cases of unusual gingival hyperplasia.

The severity of the hyperplasia is correlated directly to the individual patient's susceptibility and the level of oral hygiene. With excellent oral hygiene, gingival hyperplasia is reduced dramatically or is not present. Despite this, occasional susceptible patients demonstrate gingival hyperplasia in the presence of good oral hygiene. Of all the medications correlated to increased gingival hyperplasia, cyclosporine is the least responsive to a rigorous program of oral hygiene.

The hyperplasia typically is generalized throughout the gingiva, beginning with enlargement of the interdental papillae after about 1 to 3 months of drug use. As the hyperplasia continues, the gingiva may grow down over the teeth and cover them. Usually only dentulous areas are involved, but rare cases show involvement of the edentulous ridge and palate if irritated by an overlying denture. Although many cases of drug-related hyperplasia may be partially or totally reversible with cessation of the medication, treatment usually consists of surgical removal of the excess tissues; this is often preferable to discontinuation of the drug. Recurrence is not rare.

Many renal transplant patients must use both cyclosporine and nifedipine. These patients demonstrate a significantly increased risk of gingival hyperplasia. In many, use of the antibiotic azithromycin has been shown to reduce the degree of gingival hyperplasia to insignificant levels.

### Figure 3.19
**DILANTIN HYPERPLASIA**
Marked enlargement of the facial and lingual gingiva. (Case courtesy of Drs. Ann Drummond and Timothy M. Johnson.)

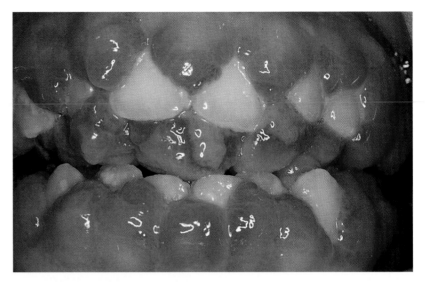

### Figure 3.20
**CYCLOSPORINE HYPERPLASIA**
Marked gingival hyperplasia in a renal transplant patient receiving cyclosporine.

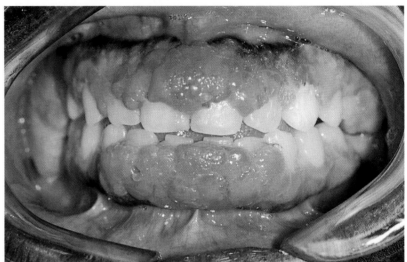

### Figure 3.21
**CYCLOSPORINE/NIFEDIPINE HYPERPLASIA**
Marked gingival hyperplasia in a patient receiving both cyclosporine and nifedipine.

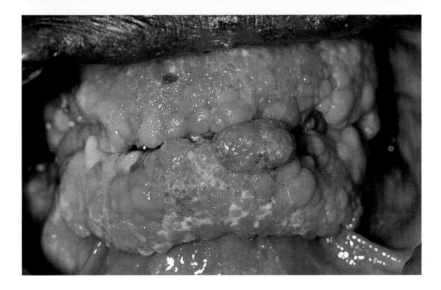

## GINGIVAL FIBROMATOSIS

**Fig. 3.22**

Gingival fibromatosis is a rare condition characterized by a generalized firm, collagenous overgrowth of the gingival tissues. Although its name suggests otherwise, gingival fibromatosis bears no relationship to the neoplastic fibromatoses. Many cases are inherited as an autosomal-dominant trait, either as an isolated entity or as a component of a variety of genetic syndromes. The most commonly associated clinical features are hypertrichosis, epilepsy, and mental retardation. The condition usually has its onset in childhood. Often, the overgrowth is correlated with eruption of teeth, and the presence of teeth is thought to be necessary for initiation of the process.

The hyperplastic gingiva typically is firm, normal colored, and smooth surfaced or finely stippled. Once initiated, the collagenous hyperplasia may delay eruption or extend to cover the crowns of the teeth. The changes may be generalized or localized to one or more quadrants, with the palatal surfaces often exhibiting more extensive involvement. Treatment consists of surgical removal of the hyperplastic tissue, but recurrence is common. Extraction of the teeth usually is accompanied by shrinkage of the tissues and cessation of recurrence.

## ALLERGIC GINGIVOSTOMATITIS (PLASMA CELL GINGIVITIS)

**Fig. 3.23**

Allergic gingivostomatitis is a characteristic pattern of mucositis that occasionally was seen for a short period between 1966 and 1971. At that time, the process was termed "plasma cell gingivitis" because of a characteristic dense infiltration of the gingival tissues by plasma cells. Investigation suggested that an agent in chewing gum may have been responsible for the mucosal reaction noted in the late 1960s. Similar, but usually not identical, cases still may be seen rarely. The list of allergens is variable and includes numerous products such as toothpaste, candy, and food additives. Occasional cases are idiopathic, and rare examples represent plasma cell dyscrasias.

Patients affected with allergic gingivostomatitis present with intense hyperemia and enlargement of the gingiva. Most current examples reveal only gingival involvement, whereas the earlier cases also demonstrated tongue and lip changes. When involved, the tongue exhibited loss of the filiform papillae, and the lips were dry, scaly, and atrophic. With severe involvement, cracking of the lips and angular cheilitis occurred. In such cases, all affected individuals complained of sore, burning tongue and gingiva. In all cases of plasma cell gingivitis, a thorough search for the offending antigen should be performed. If an association can be found, elimination of the offending agent typically results in rapid resolution. In idiopathic examples, corticosteroids may be used with variable results.

## ADULT PERIODONTITIS

**Fig. 3.24**

Periodontitis is an inflammatory disease of the periodontal structures that is preceded by gingivitis, results in resorption of crestal bone with secondary apical migration of the gingival attachment, and arises from damage mediated by bacteria in dental plaque. Periodontitis is the leading cause of tooth loss in patients older than age 35 years, with an increased prevalence noted with advancing age, high levels of dental plaque, smoking, diabetes mellitus, lower socioeconomic status, and decreased use of professional care.

The classic clinical presentation is erythematous and edematous gingiva with bleeding and exudation. The gingival margins often are blunted and apically positioned. In the absence of gingival hyperplasia, pockets greater than 4 mm indicate loss of attachment and active periodontal disease.

Treatment is directed toward plaque control and elimination of anatomic abnormalities that could harbor these microbes. Use of systemic antibiotics and nonsteroidal anti-inflammatory medications slows the progression of the disease but typically is reserved for patients who do not respond to conventional therapy. In refractory cases, microbial identification of disease sites coupled with evaluation of antibiotic sensitivity and institution of appropriate antimicrobial therapy has led to a dramatic remission of the disease progression.

**GINGIVAL FIBROMATOSIS**
Generalized firm, collagenous overgrowth
of the gingival tissues.

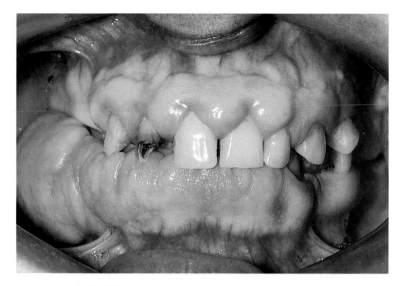

▶ **Figure 3.23**
**ALLERGIC GINGIVOSTOMATITIS**
Hyperplastic and erythematous gingivitis
and cheilitis secondary to chewing gum.

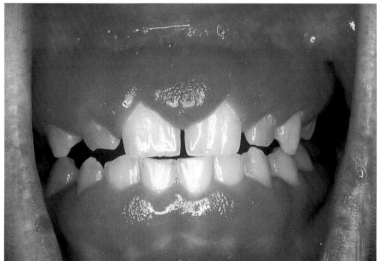

▶ **Figure 3.24**
**ADULT PERIODONTITIS**
Erythematous gingiva exhibiting blunted
gingival margins that are apically
positioned. (Courtesy of Dr. Lynn Wallace.)

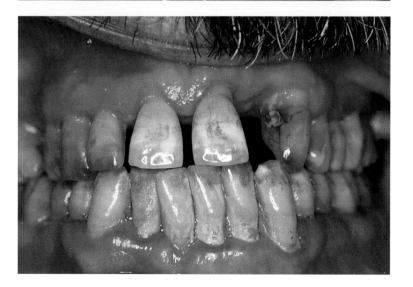

**Figs. 3.25 and 3.26**

Soft-tissue abscesses may arise from periodontal disease. The lateral periodontal abscess normally is associated with a deep, narrow periodontal pocket in which the coronal opening has become sealed and the contaminated contents produce an acute inflammatory reaction that accumulates because of the sealed pocket opening. Rarely, periodontal abscesses result from the impaction of foreign material, often food debris, into the gingival crevice. Eventual drainage may occur through the opening of the original pocket or secondary to development of an overlying sinus tract. The involved gingiva typically is erythematous and edematous, often demonstrating extreme sensitivity to palpation. A foul taste, lymphadenopathy, fever, leukocytosis, or malaise also may be present.

Treatment involves drainage of the abscess with eventual removal of the inciting cause. Typically, flap surgery provides access for removal of all of the diseased tissue and thorough cleansing of the involved teeth. In addition, any anatomic abnormalities thought to predispose the site to infection should be recontoured. In refractory cases, surgical therapy is combined with appropriate antibiotics, often guided by microbial culture and sensitivity testing. Extraction is indicated in cases not responsive to or suitable for periodontal therapy. Patients with recurrent periodontal abscesses in the absence of significant disease should be evaluated for proper immune function and systemic debilitating diseases. Cortisone therapy and diabetes have been associated with an increased prevalence of periodontal abscess formation.

## EARLY-ONSET PERIODONTITIS

**Fig. 3.27**

Although periodontitis typically is a disease of adulthood, significant disease can occur in children and young adults. Affected patients may exhibit localized or generalized involvement. In these patterns of premature periodontitis, the disease often seems to be the result of a complex interaction between genetic alterations of the immune system (leukocyte dysfunction) combined with a specific bacterial challenge. In contrast to adult periodontitis, some, but not all, cases exhibit minimal coronal plaque and gingivitis; however, subgingival plaque typically is present in sites of destruction. Culture usually reveals *Actinobacillus actinomycetemcomitans*, *Porphyromonas gingivalis*, or other periodontal pathogens also noted in adult periodontitis. These uncommon types of periodontitis arise in otherwise healthy adolescents, and the diagnosis should be reserved for cases that arise in the absence of clinical signs or symptoms of systemic disease known to produce premature periodontitis.

Unlike the treatment used for patients with adult periodontitis, mechanical removal of dental plaque and elimination of anatomic irregularities do not stop the progression of early-onset periodontitis. Antibiotics typically are combined with professional prophylaxis once a month for 6 months then every 3 months thereafter. Long-term follow-up is mandatory. Affected individuals must be informed of the possible genetic transmission of the disease process.

## Figure 3.25
### LATERAL PERIODONTAL ABSCESS
Sensitive and slightly yellow enlargement of alveolar mucosa adjacent to the medial aspect of the canine root surface.

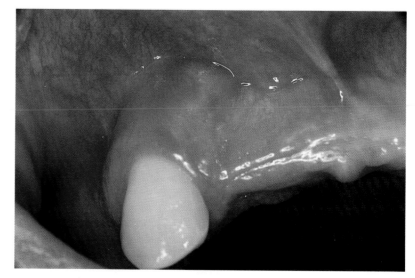

## Figure 3.26
### LATERAL PERIODONTAL ABSCESS
Radiograph of Figure 3.25 that demonstrates a deep periodontal pocket with a narrow incisal opening.

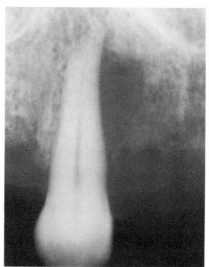

## Figure 3.27
### EARLY-ONSET PERIODONTITIS
Vertical bone loss localized to the first molar areas in a 19-year-old female. (Courtesy of Dr. Michael Gorday.)

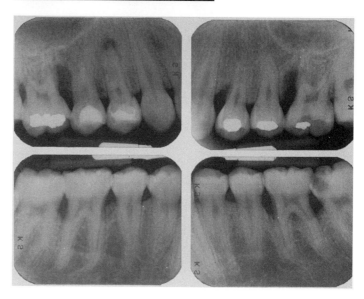

## Figs. 3.28, 3.29, and 3.30

Papillon-Lefèvre syndrome is a rare, autosomal-recessive, inherited condition characterized by palmar and plantar hyperkeratosis and early periodontal bone destruction that most likely is related to leukocyte dysfunction. Hyperkeratosis of the palms and soles usually appears during the first few years of life, presenting as red, scaly plaques. During winter, the hyperkeratotic lesions may become dry and fissured. The lesions reportedly are most severe during times of acute periodontal involvement. Fetid hyperhidrosis, especially of the feet, also may occur.

Simultaneous with the development of palmar and plantar hyperkeratosis, the gingiva becomes red, swollen, and hemorrhagic, often with a foul odor. Deep periodontal pockets develop, with associated purulence and alveolar bone destruction. The primary teeth become mobile and are exfoliated by 4 or 5 years of age. At this point, the gingival tissues revert to their normal appearance. As the permanent teeth erupt, the gingival inflammation returns, along with the severe alveolar bone destruction. By age 16 years, the patient often is nearly edentulous, except for the third molars, which have not yet erupted and may be spared. Once the permanent teeth have been lost, the alveolar tissues again return to normal and tolerate dentures well.

Treatment has been problematic, with common failures. Mechanical plaque removal alone is unsuccessful. Antibiotics often have not been useful once infected sites are present. One successful approach involves extraction of the deciduous teeth followed by antibiotic coverage during and after the eruption of the permanent teeth. In another approach, the infected sites are cultured and the offending organism (often *Actinobacillus actinomycetemcomitans*) attacked directly with antibiotics known to be effective. Through life-long combined mechanical plaque control and medical therapy, the course of the disease may be altered. In most affected patients, the skin lesions can be cleared or significantly improved through use of systemic retinoids such as etretinate.

▶ **Figure 3.28**
**PAPILLON-LEFÈVRE SYNDROME**
Hyperkeratosis of the soles. (Courtesy of Giansanti JS, Hrabak RP, Waldron CA. Palmar-plantar hyperkeratosis and concomitant periodontal destruction [Papillon-Lefèvre syndrome]. Oral Surg Oral Med Oral Pathol 1973;36:40.)

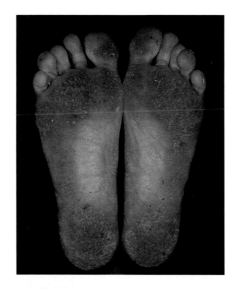

▶ **Figure 3.29**
**PAPILLON-LEFÈVRE SYNDROME**
Marked gingival inflammation.

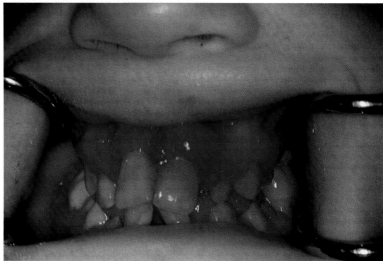

▶ **Figure 3.30**
**PAPILLON-LEFÈVRE SYNDROME**
Widespread severe periodontal bone destruction. (Courtesy of Giansanti JS, Hrabak RP, Waldron CA. Palmar-plantar hyperkeratosis and concomitant periodontal destruction [Papillon-Lefèvre syndrome]. Oral Surg Oral Med Oral Pathol 1973;36:40.)

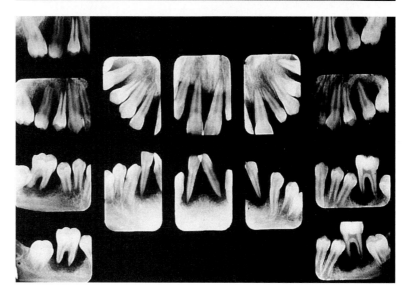

### Pulp Stones

Hillmann G, Geurtsen W. Light-microscopical investigation of the distribution of extracellular matrix molecules and calcifications in human dental pulps of various ages. Cell Tissue Res 1997;289:145.

Johnson PL, Bevelander G. Histogenesis and histochemistry of pulpal calcification. J Dent Res 1956;35:714.

Morse DR. Age-related changes of the dental pulp complex and their relationship to systemic aging. Oral Surg Oral Med Oral Pathol 1991;72:721.

Moss-Salentijn L, Hendricks-Klyvert M. Calcified structures in human dental pulps. J Endod 1988;14:184.

Sayegh FS, Reed AJ. Calcification in the dental pulp. Oral Surg Oral Med Oral Pathol 1968;25:873.

### Chronic Hyperplastic Pulpitis

Cohen S, Burns RC. Pathways of the pulp. 4th ed. St. Louis: CV Mosby, 1987.

Garfunkel A, Sela J, Ulmansky M. Dental pulp pathosis: clinicopathologic correlations based on 109 cases. Oral Surg Oral Med Oral Pathol 1973;35:110.

Ingle JI, Taintor JF. Endodontics. 3rd ed. Philadelphia: Lea & Febiger, 1985.

### Condensing Osteitis

Eliasson S, Halvarsson C, Ljungheimer C. Periapical condensing osteitis and endodontic treatment. Oral Surg Oral Med Oral Pathol 1984;57:195.

Eversole LR, Stone CE, Strub D. Focal sclerosing osteomyelitis/focal periapical osteopetrosis: radiographic patterns. Oral Surg Oral Med Oral Pathol 1984;58:456.

Hedin M, Polhagen L. Follow-up study of periradicular bone condensation. Scand J Dent Res 1979;79:436.

Panders AK, Hadders HN. Chronic sclerosing inflammation of the jaws: osteomyelitis sicca (Garre), chronic sclerosing osteomyelitis with fine-meshed trabecular structure, and very fine dense sclerosing osteomyelitis. Oral Surg Oral Med Oral Pathol 1970;30:396.

### Periapical Inflammatory Disease

Bhaskar SN. Periapical lesions—types, incidence, and clinical features. Oral Surg Oral Med Oral Pathol 1966;21:657.

Lin LM, Gaengler P, Langeland K. Periradicular curettage. Int Endod J 1996;29:220.

Maalouf EM, Gutmann JL. Biological perspective on the non-surgical endodontic management of periradicular pathosis. Int Endod J 1994;27:154.

Morse DR, Bhambhani SM. A dentist's dilemma: nonsurgical endodontic therapy or periapical surgery for teeth with apparent pulpal pathosis and an associated periapical radiolucent lesion. Oral Surg Oral Med Oral Pathol 1990;70:333.

Nair PNR, Sjögren U, Schumacher E, et al. Radicular cyst affecting a root-filled human tooth: a long-term post-treatment follow-up. Int Endod J 1993;26:225.

Stockdale CR, Chandler NP. The nature of the periapical lesion: a review of 1108 cases. J Dent 1988;16:123.

Tronstad L. Recent development in endodontic research. Scand J Dent Res 1992;100:52.

Tsurumachi T, Saito T. Treatment of large periapical lesions by inserting a drainage tube into the root canal. Endod Dent Traumatol 1995;11:41.

### Periapical Abscess

Bhaskar SN. Periapical lesions—types, incidence, and clinical features. Oral Surg Oral Med Oral Pathol 1966;21:657.

Fouad AF, Rivera EM, Walton RE. Penicillin as a supplement in resolving the localized acute apical abscess. Oral Surg Oral Med Oral Pathol 1996;81:590.

Nobuhara WK, del Rio CE. Incidence of periradicular pathoses in endodontic treatment failures. J Endod 1993;19:315.

Spatafore CM, Griffin JA, Keyes GG, et al. Periapical biopsy report: an analysis over a 10-year period. J Endod 1990;16:239.

Stockdale CR, Chandler NP. The nature of the periapical lesion: a review of 1108 cases. J Dent 1988;16:123.

### Lateral Radicular Cyst

Neville BW, Damm DD, Bouquot JE. Oral & maxillofacial pathology. Philadelphia: WB Saunders, 1995:105.

### Residual Periapical Cyst

High AS, Hirschmann PN. Age changes in residual cysts. J Oral Pathol 1986;15:524.

Lin LM, Gaengler P, Langeland K. Periradicular curettage. Int Endod J 1996;29:220.

Nair PNR, Sjögren U, Schumacher E, et al. Radicular cyst affecting a root-filled human tooth: a long term post-treatment follow-up. Int Endod J 1993;26:225.

Schaffer AB. Residual cyst? (letter). Oral Surg Oral Med Oral Pathol Oral Radiol Endod 1997;83:640.

Walton RE. The residual radicular cyst: does it exist? (editorial). Oral Surg Oral Med Oral Pathol Oral Radiol Endod 82:471, 1996.

### Parulis and Palatal Abscess

Birn H. Spread of dental infections. Dent Pract Dent Rec 1972;22:347.

Neville BW, Damm DD, Allen CM, Bouquot JE. Oral & maxillofacial pathology. Philadelphia: WB Saunders, 1995:109.

### Intrabony Fibrous Scar

Molven O, Halse A, Grung B. Incomplete healing (scar tissue) after periapical surgery: radiographic findings 8 to 12 years after treatment. J Endod 1996;22:264.

Neville BW, Damm DD, Allen CM, Bouquot JE. Oral & maxillofacial pathology. Philadelphia: WB Saunders, 1995:104.

Nobuhara WK, del Rio CE. Incidence of periradicular pathoses in endodontic treatment failures. J Endod 1993;19:315.

Spatafore CM, Griffin JA, Keyes GG, et al. Periapical biopsy report: an analysis over a 10-year period. J Endod 1990;16:239.

### Epulis Granulomatosum

Kanas RJ, Jensen JL, DeBoom GW. Painful, nonhealing tooth extraction socket. J Am Dent Assoc 1986;113:441.

Wood NK, Goaz PW. Differential diagnosis of oral lesions. 4th ed. St. Louis: CV Mosby, 1991:171.

### Chronic Gingivitis

Addy M, Renton-Harper P. Local and systemic chemotherapy in the management of periodontal disease: an opinion and review of the concept. J Oral Rehabil 1996;23:219.

Ciancio SG. Agents for the management of plaque and gingivitis. J Dent Res 1992;71:1450.

Hugoson A, Koch G, Bergendal T, et al. Oral health of individuals aged 3-80 years in Jönköping, Sweden in 1973, 1983, and 1993: II, review of clinical and radiographic findings. Swed Dent J 1995;19:243.

Orban BJ. Gingivitis. J Periodontol 1955;26:173.

Stamm JW. Epidemiology of gingivitis. J Clin Periodontol 1986;13:360.

### Hormonal Gingivitis

Addy M, Hunter ML, Kingdon A, et al. An 8-year study of changes in oral hygiene and periodontal health during adolsecence. Int J Paediatr Dent 1994;4:75.

Loe H, Silness J. Periodontal disease in pregnancy: I, prevalence and severity. Acta Odontol Scand 1964;21:533.

Muramatsu Y, Takaesu Y. Oral health status related to subgingival bacterial flora and sex hormones in saliva during pregnancy. Bull Tokyo Dent Coll 1994;35:139.

Nakagawa S, Fujii H, Machida Y, et al. A longitudinal study from prepuberty to puberty of gingivitis: correlation between the occurrence of *Prevotella intermedia* and sex hormones. J Clin Periodontol 1994;21:658.

Raber-Durlacher JE, van Steenbergen TJM, van der Velden U, et al. Experimental gingivitis during pregnancy and post-partum: clinical, endocrinological, and microbiological aspects. J Clin Periodontol 1994;21:549.

Silness J, Loe H. Periodontal disease in pregnancy: II, correlation between oral hygiene and periodontal disease. Acta Odontol Scand 1964;22:121.

## Acute Necrotizing Ulcerative Gingivitis

Hartnett AC, Shiloah J. The treatment of acute necrotizing ulcerative gingivitis. Quintessence Int 1991;22:95.

Horning GM, Cohen ME. Necrotizing ulcerative gingivitis, periodontitis, and stomatitis: clinical staging and predisposing factors. J Periodontol 1995;66:990.

Jimenez LM, Baer PN. Necrotizing ulcerative gingivitis in children: a 9 year clinical study. J Periodontol 1975;56:457.

Johnson BD, Engel D. Acute necrotizing ulcerative gingivitis: a review of diagnosis, etiology and treatment. J Periodontol 1986;57:141.

Riviere GR, Wagoner MA, Baker-Zander SA, et al. Identification of spirochetes related to *Treponema pallidum* in necrotizing ulcerative gingivitis and chronic periodontitis. N Engl J Med 1991;325:539.

Riviere GR, Weisz KS, Simonson LG, et al. Pathogen-related spirochetes identified within gingival tissues from patients with acute necrotizing ulcerative gingivitis. Infect Immun 1991;59:2653.

Uohara GI, Knapp MJ. Oral fusospirochetosis and associated lesions. Oral Surg Oral Med Oral Pathol 1967;24:113.

## Drug-Induced Gingival Hyperplasia

Boran M, Güne Z, Doruk E, et al. Improvement in cyclosporine A associated gingival hyperplasia with Azithromycin therapy. Trans Proc 1996;28:2316.

Brunet L, Miranda J, Farré M, et al. Gingival enlargement induced by drugs. Drug Safe 1996;15:219.

Butler RT, Kalkwarf KL, Kaldahl WB. Drug-induced gingival hyperplasia: phenytoin, cyclosporine, and nifedipine. J Am Dent Assoc 1987;114:56.

Hassell TM, Hefti AF. Drug-induced gingival overgrowth: old problem, new problem. Crit Rev Oral Biol Med 1991;2:103.

Lungergan WP. Drug-induced gingival enlargements. Dilantin® hyperplasia and beyond. Calif Dent Assoc J 1989;17:48.

Seymour RA. Calcium channel blockers and gingival overgrowth. Br Dent J 1991;170:376.

Seymour RA, Thomason JM, Ellis JS. The pathogenesis of drug-induced gingival overgrowth. J Clin Periodontol 1996;23:165.

Thomason JM, Seymour RA, Rice N. The prevalence and severity of cyclosporin and nifedipine-induced gingival overgrowth. J Clin Periodontol 1993;20:37.

## Gingival Fibromatosis

Bozzo L, paes de Almeida O, Scully C, et al. Hereditary gingival fibromatosis: report of an extensive four-generation pedigree. Oral Surg Oral Med Oral Pathol 1994;78:452.

Jorgenson RJ, Cocker ME. Variation in the inheritance and expression of gingival fibromatosis. J Periodontol 1974;45:472.

Rushton MA. Hereditary or idiopathic hyperplasia of the gums. Dent Pract Dent Rec 1957;7:136.

Takagi M, Yamamoto H, Mega H, et al. Heterogeneity in the gingival fibromatoses. Cancer 1991;68:2202.

## Allergic Gingivostomatitis

Kerr DA, McClatchey KD, Regezi JA. Idiopathic gingivostomatitis: cheilitis, glossitis, gingivitis syndrome: atypical gingivostomatitis, plasma-cell gingivitis, plasmacytosis of gingiva. Oral Surg Oral Med Oral Pathol 1971;32:402.

Kerr DA, McClatchey KD, Regezi JA. Allergic gingivostomatitis (due to gum chewing). J Periodontol 1971;42:709.

Serio FG, Siegel MA. Plasma cell gingivitis of unusual origin: report of a case. J Periodontol 1991;62:390.

Silverman S, Lozada F. An epilogue to plasma-cell gingivostomatitis (allergic gingivostomatitis). Oral Surg Oral Med Oral Pathol 1977;43:211.

Sollecito TP, Greenberg MS. Plasma cell gingivitis: report of two cases. Oral Surg Oral Med Oral Pathol 1992;73:690.

Timms MS, Sloan P. Association of supraglottic and gingival idiopathic plasmacytosis. Oral Surg Oral Med Oral Pathol 1991;71:451.

## Adult Periodontitis

Addy M, Renton-Harper M. Local and systemic chemotherapy in the management of periodontal disease: an opinion and review of the concept. J Oral Rehabil 1996;23:219.

Bollen CML, Quirynen M. Microbiological response to mechanical treatment in combination with adjunctive therapy: a review of the literature. J Periodontol 1996;67:1143.

Chapple ILC. Periodontal disease diagnosis: current status and future developments. J Dent 1997;25:3.

Fine DH. Microbial identification and antibiotic sensitivity testing, an aid for patients refractory to periodontal therapy: a report of 3 cases. J Clin Periodontol 1994;21:98.

Greenstein G. Periodontal response to mechanical non-surgical therapy: a review. J Periodontol 1992;63:118.

Greenwell H, Bissada NF, Wittwer JW. Periodontics in general practice: professional plaque control. J Am Dent Assoc 1990;121:642.

Leknes KN. The influence of anatomic and iatrogenic root surface characteristics on bacterial colonization and periodontal destruction: a review. J Periodontol 1997;68:507.

Newman HN. Plaque and chronic inflammatory periodontal disease: a question of ecology. J Clin Periodontol 1990;17:533.

Tanner A. Microbial etiology of periodontal disease: where are we? where are we going? Curr Opin Dent 1992;2:12.

## Periodontal and Gingival Abscesses

Fine DH. Microbial identification and antibiotic sensitivity testing, an aid for patients refractory to periodontal therapy a report of 3 cases. J Clin Periodontol 1994;21:98.

Hafström CA, Wikström MB, Renvert SN, et al. Effect of treatment on some periodontopathogens and their antibody levels in periodontal abscesses. J Periodontol 1994;65:1022.

Kareha MJ, Rosenberg ES, DeHaven H. Therapeutic considerations in the management of a periodontal abscess with an intrabony defect. J Clin Periodontol 1981;8:375.

O'Brien TJ. Diagnosis and treatment of periodontal and gingival abscesses. J Ontario Dent Assoc 1970;47:16.

Taani DSQ. An effective treatment for chronic periodontal abscesses. Quintessence Int 1996;27:697.

## Early-Onset Periodontitis

Albandar JM, Brown LJ, Brunelle JA, et al. Gingival state and dental calculus in early-onset periodontitis. J Periodontol 1996;67:953.

Albandar JM, Brown LJ, Genco RJ, et al. Clinical classification of periodontitis in adolescents and young adults. J Periodontol 1997;68:545.

Armitage GC, Van Dyke TE, et al (Committee on Research, Science and Therapy of the American Academy of Periodontology). Position Paper: periodontal disease of children and adolescents. J Periodontol 1996;67:57.

Dibart S. Children, adolescents and periodontal diseases. J Dent 1997;25:79.

Novak MJ, Novak KF. Early-onset periodontitis. Curr Opin Dent 1996;3:45.

## Papillon-Lefèvre Syndrome

Baer PN, McDonald RE. Suggested mode of periodontal therapy for patients with Papillon-Lefèvre syndrome. Periodont Case Rep 1981;3:10.

Eronat N, Ucar F, Kiline G. Papillon-Lefèvre syndrome: treatment of two cases with a clinical, microbiological and histopathological investigation. J Clin Pediatr Dent 1993;17:99.

Firatli E, Tüzü B, Efeo%glu A. Papillon-Lefèvre syndrome: analysis of neutrophil chemotaxis. J Periodontol 1996;67:617.

Hattab FN, Rawashdeh MA, Yassin OM, et al. Papillon-Lefèvre syndrome: a review of the literature and report of 4 cases. J Periodontol 1995;66:413.

Ishikawa I, Umeda M, Laosrisin N. Clinical, bacteriological, and immunological examinations and the treatment process of two Papillon-Lefèvre syndrome patients. J Periodontol 1994;65:364.

Preus HR. Treatment of rapidly destructive periodontitis in Papillon-Lefèvre syndrome: laboratory and clinical observations. J Clin Periodontol 1988;15:639.

# chapter 4
## INFECTIONS

### Fig. 4.1

Impetigo is an infection of the skin caused by *Staphylococcus aureus* and *Streptococcus pyogenes*, in combination or individually. The infection is common in children and typically arises in areas of previous trauma. The face and extremities are the most frequently involved sites, with affected areas initially displaying fragile vesicles that rapidly rupture to form honey-colored crusts. In some cases, longer-lasting bullae may be seen. Although systemic symptoms typically are not present, pruritus and regional lymphadenopathy are not rare.

Without treatment, slow enlargement and local spread often is seen. Although localized non-bullous forms often respond to topical mupirocin therapy, systemic cephalexin is the therapy of choice in patients with the bullous form or with more extensive involvement. With appropriate therapy, serious complications are rare.

## CAT SCRATCH DISEASE

### Figs. 4.2 and 4.3

Cat scratch disease is a self-limiting infectious process that normally presents in children or young adults as painful lymphadenopathy of the axilla or neck and usually follows being scratched by a cat. Often, the primary site of skin damage has resolved by the time the symptomatic lymphadenopathy becomes evident. The cause was thought to be viral, but recent evidence has shown the responsible agent to be *Bartonella henselae*, a newly described small, Gram-negative, nonacid-fast coccobacillus best viewed with the Warthin-Starry stain.

Typically, a small, inflamed papule or pustule typically develops on the skin within 3 to 10 days after a scratch that usually is trivial. In about 80% of cases, lymphadenopathy develops within 5 to 50 days (average, 2 weeks) and is the result of intranodal granulomatous inflammation with central stellate abscesses. Initially, the enlarged lymph nodes are firm and painful; with time, however, they may become soft because of abscess formation. The overlying skin can be erythematous, and fistulous tract formation may occur as the abscesses spontaneously drain.

Diagnosis often is made from the clinical presentation and history of a cat scratch. An indirect fluorescent-antibody test has been developed and is used in questionable cases. Enzyme immunoassay and polymerase chain reaction techniques also are available for diagnostic confirmation. The infection typically resolves spontaneously within 4 months, and antibiotics are not recommended in healthy patients. In severely affected patients, a variety of antibiotics, including erythromycin, doxycycline, rifampicin, ciprofloxacin, gentamycin, and trimethoprim/sulfamethoxazole, have been reported to be effective treatment. Highly symptomatic lymph nodes may require excision or incision with drainage. In patients with acquired immunodeficiency syndrome, a disseminated form termed "bacillary angiomatosis" has been documented and responds well to erythromycin treatment.

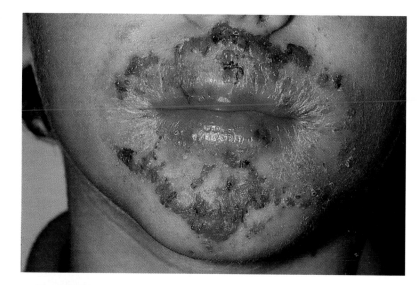

**▶ Figure 4.1**
**IMPETIGO**
Extensive amber-colored crusts of the perioral skin.

**▶ Figure 4.2**
**CAT SCRATCH DISEASE**
Male child presenting with painful right submandibular soft-tissue enlargement. (Courtesy of Dr. Robert Morris.)

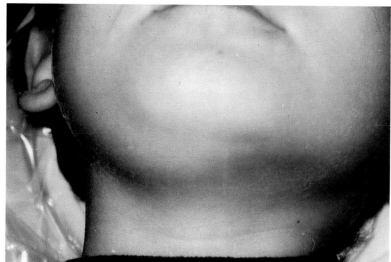

**▶ Figure 4.3**
**CAT SCRATCH DISEASE**
Small scratches caused by family cat on the right hand of the child depicted in Figure 4.2. Similar, but less prominent, scratches were noted on the right cheek. (Courtesy of Dr. Robert Morris.)

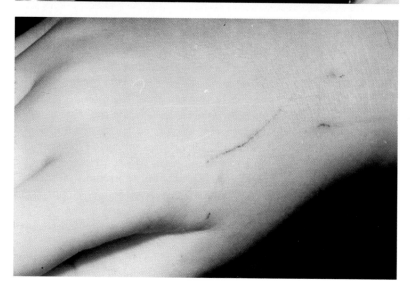

**Figs. 4.4 and 4.5**

Tuberculosis is an infectious disease produced by an acid-fast organism, usually *Mycobacterium tuberculosis,* that typically is spread through airborne droplets from patients with active disease. A variety of mycobacteria are potentially pathogenic in humans, but infection with other strains is rare. Less than 5% of patients exposed to tuberculosis progress from infection to active disease, and most progressive cases arise from reactivation of a previous infection in an immunocompromised host.

Active tuberculosis is primarily a disease of the pulmonary system, but rare secondary intraoral manifestations are seen. It is thought that most of these lesions arise from infected sputum that contacts areas of minor trauma. The most common intraoral location is the posterior tongue, but lesions also have been seen on the gingiva, palate, lips, buccal mucosa, frenulum and in the jaw bones. The classic presentation is an irregular ulceration of the dorsal tongue that slowly increases in size. Primary oral tuberculosis without pulmonary lesions is rare. On occasion, pulmonary involvement initially is discovered during the evaluation following diagnosis of associated oral lesions.

Tuberculosis infection may also occur in the cervical or submandibular lymph nodes, and this specific form of tuberculosis is known as "scrofula." These patients present with enlarged lymph nodes that are painful and may form abscesses that drain through the overlying skin. It has been suggested that this pattern develops from a primary infection in the tonsils that spreads to the nodes, but this has not been confirmed. This pattern often is produced by atypical mycobacteria rather than classic tuberculosis organisms.

Two to four weeks after initial exposure, cell-mediated immunity develops and is the basis for the tuberculin (Mantoux or PPD) skin test. A positive skin test confirms previous exposure, but diagnosis of active disease requires documentation of the organism by special stains or culture. Histopathologically, tuberculosis presents as caseating granulomatous inflammation that reveals the mycobacteria only on acid-fast staining.

*Mycobacterium tuberculosis* has shown the ability to develop resistance to single-agent therapies. Therefore, multiagent regimens form the treatment of choice and typically include isoniazid plus rifampin, ethambutol, or pyrazinamide. With appropriate therapy, relapse rates are less than 2%.

## NOMA

**Fig. 4.6**

Noma (from the Greek verb "to devour"), which also is known as "cancrum oris" or "gangrenous stomatitis," is an infection that occurs in severely debilitated individuals and is caused by components of the normal oral flora. Although the microbiologic origin is variable, it seems that species of *Fusobacterium* (*necrophorum* or *nucleatum*) initiate a polymicrobial infection with one or more bacteria, often *Prevotella intermedia, Borrelia vincentii, Staphylococcus aureus, Pseudomonas aeruginosa, Escherichia coli, Corynebacterium pyogenes,* or nonhemolytic species of streptococcus. In some instances, organisms seen in acute necrotizing ulcerative gingivitis are present, and the necrosis seems to represent the spread of acute necrotizing ulcerative gingivitis into adjacent soft tissues. Despite this, many cases develop independently of gingival involvement, often in areas of previous mucosal trauma. Poor oral hygiene, malnutrition, dehydration, blood dyscrasia, malignancy, immunosuppression, or infection with one of the exanthematous fevers often precede noma's development.

Although rare cases occur in adulthood (especially in the immunocompromised), children between the ages of 2 and 10 years are affected most frequently, with the disease presenting as a zone of blackened skin overlying an area of spreading mucosal necrosis and ulceration. Large zones of yellow necrosis replace the initial areas of discoloration and often spread into the adjacent soft tissues or bone. Malodor, pain, fever, malaise, and regional lymphadenopathy are common. Conservative debridement of the grossly necrotic areas typically is combined with antibiotics such as penicillin and metronidazole. In addition to these local factors, attention must be directed toward elimination of the predisposing factors, correcting electrolyte imbalances and providing adequate nutrition and hydration.

▶ **Figure 4.4**
**TUBERCULOSIS**

Granular-appearing mucosa of the anterior mandibular alveolar ridge. (Courtesy of Dr. Brian Blocher.)

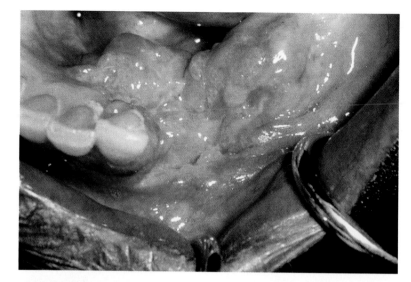

▶ **Figure 4.5**
**TUBERCULOSIS**

Multiple fistulous tracts secondary to necrosis in involved lymph nodes in a patient with scrofula. (Courtesy of Dr. Irwin Small.)

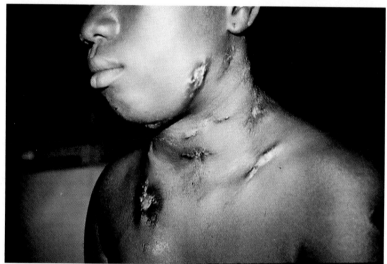

▶ **Figure 4.6**
**NOMA**

Large area of gangrenous necrosis of the buccal mucosa in a debilitated patient. (Courtesy of Budnick SD. Handbook of pediatric oral pathology. Chicago: Year Book, 1981.)

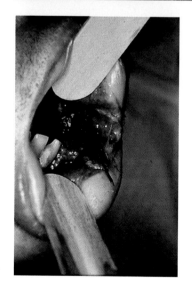

Syphilis, or lues, is an insidious infection caused by a spirochete, *Treponema pallidum*, and usually is acquired through sexual intercourse. If untreated, the disease classically progresses through three stages. The first two stages may be mild and often are ignored, but the third may result in physical disability or death. The primary stage is marked by the development of an ulceration at the site of entry, with associated nontender regional lymphadenopathy. This ulceration is known as a "chancre" and normally arises 2 to 3 weeks after inoculation. Most chancres occur in the genital areas, but oral lesions do occur. Chancres have been reported on the lips, tongue, gingiva, palate, and tonsils. Dissemination of the organism occurs during this stage, and the chancre heals in 3 to 8 weeks with or without treatment.

The secondary stage typically arises 4 to 10 weeks after the initial infection and is characterized by a generalized, reddish brown, macular skin eruption. On occasion, the rash may be subtle and ignored by the patient. Oral lesions known as "mucous patches" do occur and appear as grayish white areas of ulceration usually on the lips, buccal mucosa, gingiva, and tongue. Erythematous nodules or papules also may be seen. Ulcerated lesions, known as "split papules," may occur at the oral commissures and clinically resemble angular cheilitis. These manifestations resolve spontaneously in 3 to 12 weeks. Only during these initial two stages is the patient highly infectious.

Following the secondary stage, the disease enters a period of latency that may last for years, decades, or life. Approximately 30% of patients proceed to the tertiary stage. During this final stage, the disease can produce significant irreversible cardiovascular and central nervous system damage. In addition, localized destructive lesions known as "gummas" can occur almost anywhere in the body and present as areas of rubbery necrosis and ulceration. The tongue and palate are the most frequent locations of intraoral gummas; on occasion, perforation of the palate occurs.

For patients suspected of being initially infected, several nonspecific but relatively inexpensive screening tests are available. These include the Venereal Disease Research Laboratory and the rapid plasma reagin test, which, when results are positive, must be followed by more expensive, specific, and highly sensitive serologic tests, typically the fluorescent treponemal antibody absorption or the *Treponema pallidum* hemagglutination assays. Results of the initial screening tests become positive after the first 3 weeks of infection and continue so throughout the remainder of the first two stages. Once latency occurs, the positivity slowly fades. In contrast, the more specific assays remain positive for life. Diagnosis of a second incidence of infection is difficult because the screening tests are nonspecific and the specific assays are positive permanently. In these cases, demonstration of the organisms in tissue or exudates is required. Several recent publications continue to suggest an increased prevalence of oral cancer (especially of the tongue) in patients with a previous history of syphilis. These studies propose routine screening for the infection in patients diagnosed with oral carcinoma and increased cancer surveillance among patients with syphilis.

The treatment of choice is antibiotics, typically penicillin. Most patients obtain a clinical cure, but it must be remembered that the organism can escape the lethal effects of the therapy within the confines of lymph nodes or the central nervous system. Therefore, appropriate antibiotics only arrest the clinical manifestations, and recurrence of active infection is possible, especially if future immunosuppression develops.

### Figure 4.7
### SYPHILIS, CHANCRE

Large ulceration of dorsolateral tongue infected with treponema in patient with primary syphilis.

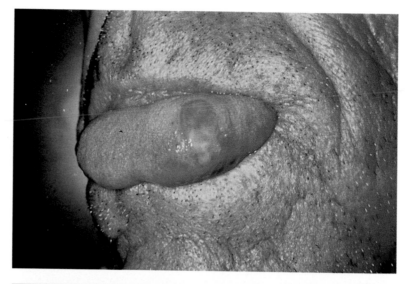

### Figure 4.8
### SYPHILIS, MUCOUS PATCH

White, circumscribed alteration of the lower labial mucosa. (Courtesy of Dr. Pete Edmonds.)

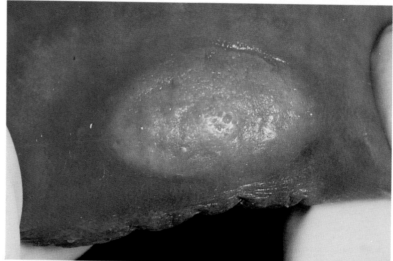

### Figure 4.9
### SYPHILIS, GUMMA

Large rubbery ulceration of the anterior dorsal tongue in a patient with tertiary syphilis. (Courtesy of Shafer WG, Hine MK, Levy BM. A textbook of oral pathology. 4th ed. Philadelphia: WB Saunders, 1983.)

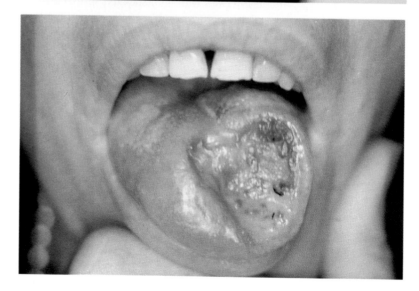

## CONGENITAL SYPHILIS

**Fig. 4.10**

Although initially the spirochete is unable to invade the placenta and infect the developing fetus, syphilis can be transmitted from an infected mother after the fifth month of gestation. The infection can spread to a developing fetus up to 5 years after the mother initially contracted the disease. This can result in abortion, stillbirth, death soon after delivery, or numerous developmental changes. The historical diagnostic features are known as the "Hutchinson Triad": enamel hypoplasia of the teeth (Hutchinson incisors and mulberry molars), eighth nerve deafness, and interstitial keratitis. In the classic case, the height of contour on all of the teeth is in the mid one-third. Screwdriver-shaped incisors and molars with occlusal anatomy similar to a mulberry are seen. Other oral findings also include short maxilla, relative mandibular prognathism, atrophic glossitis, a high-arched palate, and rhagades (premature perioral fissuring).

## ACTINOMYCOSIS

**Fig. 4.11**

Although the name implies a fungal infection, actinomycosis is an infection produced by Gram-positive filamentous bacteria, most commonly *Actinomyces israelii*. Several other species of actinomyces occasionally may be responsible, as well as a related organism, *Arachnia propionica*. Actinomyces are part of the normal flora and seem to become pathogenic only after entrance through previously created defects.

Of all cases of actinomycosis, 50% occur in the cervicofacial region. The process may present as an acute and rapidly progressing infection or as a slowly spreading chronic infection that is associated with fibrosis. In contrast to typical infections, actinomycosis does not follow fascial planes but tends to exhibit direct extension through soft tissue. The organism is associated with a purulent reaction that often is encased by dense fibrous tissue, giving the affected area a "wooden" induration. Ultimately, a central abscess develops that may reach the surface and drain yellow clusters of the bacteria that are termed "sulfur granules." Affected patients usually present with a red, elevated, firm swelling of the affected soft tissues of the neck or face that often develops multiple draining abscesses with distinctive yellow colonies. Localized actinomycotic abscesses without associated spread through adjacent tissues occasionally are seen in periapical, pericoronal, and isolated soft-tissue infections. For classic cases of cervicofacial actinomycosis, appropriate therapy requires drainage, debridement of granulation tissue, excision of any sinus tracts, and long-term antibiotic use, usually penicillin. Without initial surgical intervention the infection typically is nonresponsive to antibiotic therapy. In deep-seated infections, the antibiotic therapy may extend up to 12 months. Without prompt intervention in acute cases, cervical spread may result in life-threatening upper airway obstruction. In noninfiltrative infections, surgical debridement often is sufficient.

## CELLULITIS

**Fig. 4.12**

Cellulitis is an enlargement of soft tissue resulting from diffuse spread of an infection through the tissue spaces or fascial planes. When present in the facial tissues, it is normally the result of dental periapical infection, periodontitis, pericoronitis, or facial fractures. Cellulitis is normally present in the soft tissue adjacent to the offending tooth. Pain, fever, and lymphadenopathy usually are seen. Typically, the swollen area is diffuse, firm, red, and warm. Without appropriate therapy, spread of the infection possibly may result in cavernous sinus thrombosis, suppurative mediastinitis, airway obstruction, pleuropulmonary suppuration, or systemic bacteremia. The focus of infection should be resolved and antibiotics administered (penicillin often combined with an aminoglycoside). Warm compresses can be applied; if the infection localizes, it should be drained.

### ► Figure 4.10
### CONGENITAL SYPHILIS, HUTCHINSON INCISORS

Dentition demonstrating incisors resembling straight-edged screwdrivers secondary to constriction of the incisal one-third of the crown. (Reproduced with permission from Halstead CL, Blozis GG, Drinnan AJ, Gier RE. Physical evaluation of the dental patient. St Louis: CV Mosby, 1982.)

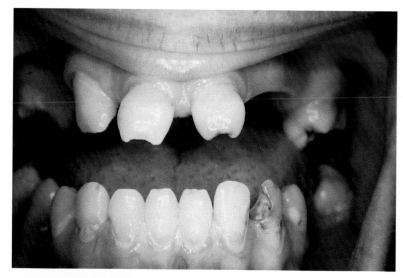

### ► Figure 4.11
### ACTINOMYCOSIS

Young adult male demonstrating erythematous and painful enlargement overlying the left mandible. Incision produced purulent exudate containing classic "sulfur granules." The focus of the infection was the adjacent mandibular first molar. (Courtesy of Dr. Richard Ziegler.)

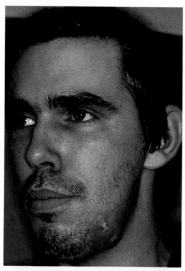

### ► Figure 4.12
### CELLULITIS

(A) Young adult female exhibiting left facial enlargement and erythema secondary to an acute periapical lesion of the left maxillary lateral incisor. An aspirin burn was present on the upper left labial mucosa. (B) Same patient following resolution of oral focus of infection.

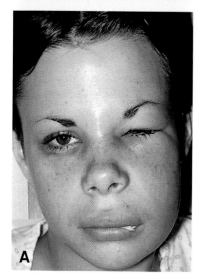
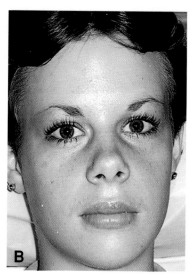

## Fig. 4.13

Ludwig's angina is a severe form of facial cellulitis in which the infection bilaterally involves all of the tissue spaces in the submandibular area: the submaxillary, sublingual, and submental spaces. In most cases, the infection is odontogenic in origin and usually arises from the area of the mandibular molars, although occasional examples arise in areas of trauma. Involvement of the sublingual space results in a boardlike swelling of the tongue, with elevation of the floor of the mouth; spread through the submandibular space creates enlargement and tenderness of the neck. Eating, swallowing, and breathing may become difficult. Fever, chills, leukocytosis, and an elevated sedimentation rate are seen occasionally. Edema of the glottis and pharyngeal spaces may require emergency tracheostomy to prevent death from suffocation. Uncontrolled spread may result in mediastinitis, subphrenic abscess formation, pneumothorax, pericardial or pleural effusion, necrotizing fasciitis, jugular venous thrombosis, rupture of the innominate artery, empyema, osteomyelitis, and systemic bacteremia. Treatment consists of maintenance of the airway, drainage, antibiotics, and elimination of the focus of infection. Penicillin often combined with an aminoglycoside is the antibiotic of choice, with metronidazole used in patients who are allergic to penicillin.

## PROLIFERATIVE PERIOSTITIS (PERIOSTITIS OSSIFICANS)

## Figs. 4.14 and 4.15

Proliferative periostitis (periostitis ossificans) is a specific pattern of chronic osteomyelitis that occurs almost exclusively in children and young adults and has been erroneously attributed to the work of Garrè and often is called "Garrè's osteomyelitis." When in the jaws, the mandible is affected more frequently than the maxilla, with most cases involving the lower border of the mandible in the premolar-molar area. This process typically arises secondary to a central low-grade chronic dental infection that has spread toward the surface of the bone. Periapical inflammatory disease and acute pericoronitis frequently represent the original focus of infection. Inflammation of the periosteum develops and results in reduplication of the cortical layers of the bone.

These patients most commonly present with symptoms related to their primary infection; on examination, a painless, hard, bony swelling is noted overlying the affected area. Occlusal radiographs classically demonstrate redundant parallel layers of cortical bone overlying the affected area of infection, but the bony enlargement will not always demonstrate this classic "onionskin" appearance. The treatment of choice is to eliminate the focus of infection, with the bone slowly reassuming its normal contour within 6 to 12 months. The presence of proliferative periostitis in the absence of infection is an indication for biopsy. Several neoplastic processes have been known to produce a similar periosteal reaction. This list includes Ewing's sarcoma, Langerhans cell histiocytosis, and metastatic disease.

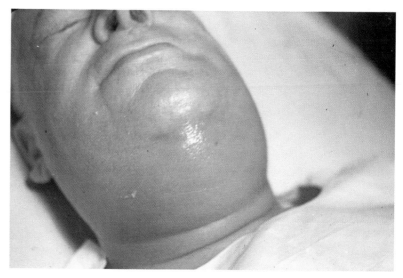

### Figure 4.13
### LUDWIG'S ANGINA
Adult male exhibiting submandibular soft tissue facial enlargement secondary to dental infection of the posterior mandible.

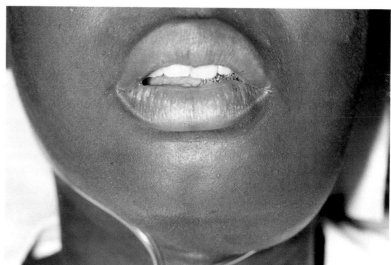

### Figure 4.14
### PROLIFERATIVE PERIOSTITIS (PERIOSTITIS OSSIFICANS)
13 year old girl with bony hard enlargement of the left mandibular body.

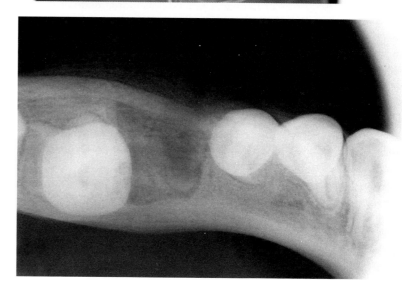

### Figure 4.15
### PROLIFERATIVE PERIOSTITIS (PERIOSTITIS OSSIFICANS)
Occlusal radiograph demonstrating reduplication of the buccal cortical bone overlying a recent extraction site. (Courtesy of Dr. Brent Klinger.)

### Fig. 4.16

Osteomyelitis is an infection within bone that spreads through the marrow spaces. In the jaws, the mandible is affected more frequently and exhibits a tendency toward greater spread of infection because of its larger marrow spaces. The most common source of the infection is odontogenic, but local trauma or hematogenous spread may be responsible. The clinical course may be acute or chronic, with the patient often presenting with fever, lymphadenopathy, and an elevated white blood cell count. The involved area is painful, and the teeth often are extruded slightly. Initially, early acute cases often demonstrate no radiographic alterations. With time, an ill-defined zone of radiolucency typically develops and may exhibit central radiopaque sequestrum formation. In many cases, computed tomographic scans and magnetic resonance images are superior to conventional radiographs in delineating the extent of the infectious process.

In acute cases, the intraosseous abscess spreads through the medullary spaces and is associated with a greater intensity of the signs and symptoms. In these cases, treatment consists of antibiotics and drainage. In chronic cases, pockets of abscess become encased in reactive fibrous connective tissue. Penetration of antibiotics into the fibrotic zones is very poor, making surgical intervention mandatory. Removal of all infected tissue down to good bleeding bone is necessary in all cases. Antibiotics also are used but often intravenously in higher dosages, with penicillin being the drug of choice and clindamycin used in those allergic to penicillin. In these chronic cases, scintigraphic techniques with technetium-99m or gallium-67 have been used to evaluate the initial spread of the infection and the subsequent response to therapy.

## OSTEORADIONECROSIS

### Figs. 4.17 and 4.18

Osteoradionecrosis of the jaws refers to osteomyelitis that has occurred subsequent to therapeutic radiation in the area. This condition usually follows radiation therapy for carcinomas of the head and neck in which elimination of the jaws from the fields of irradiation was not possible. The radiation damages the osteocytes and the microvascular system of the affected bone, thereby rendering the bone abnormally susceptible to necrosis when exposed to minor infection or trauma. The total bone dose, mode of radiation delivery, rate of delivery, and radiation fields affect the risk of future bone necrosis. Osteoradionecrosis arises from nonhealing, dead bone; although infection usually is present, it is not necessary for initiation of the process. The mandible is affected much more commonly than the more vascular maxilla.

The necrosis typically follows dental periapical infections, periodontitis, or mucosal ulcerations from denture use. Severe pain, cortical perforation, draining fistulas, and pathologic fracture are not rare. Radiographically, the affected area appears almost identical to suppurative osteomyelitis and usually presents as an ill-defined area of radiolucency that may or may not contain a central radiopaque mass of nonvital bone. Prevention is the best therapeutic approach. All necessary, foreseen oral surgical, endodontic, and periodontic procedures should be completed at least 21 days before radiation therapy. Patients who have retained all or a portion of their dentition should be taught to practice the ultimate in dental hygiene with daily application of topical fluoride. When bone necrosis develops, the sequestra should be surgically removed, with appropriate antibiotic coverage. Use of hyperbaric oxygen often improves healing and decreases the prevalence of progression and recurrence.

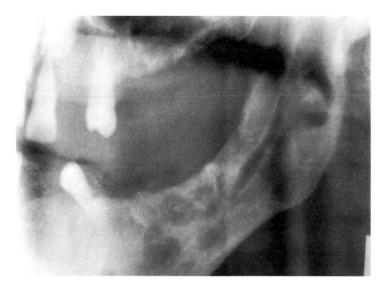

► **Figure 4.16**
**SUPPURATIVE OSTEOMYELITIS**
Mandibular body demonstrating numerous ill-defined radiolucencies. (Courtesy of Dr. Ed McGaha.)

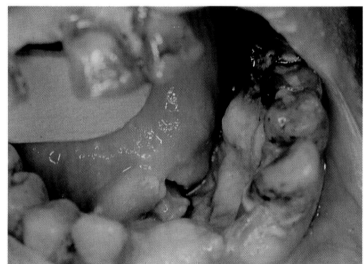

► **Figure 4.17**
**OSTEORADIONECROSIS**
Large area of ulceration and exposed bone of the left mandible that occurred as a result of a dental-related infection following radiation therapy that encompassed the area.

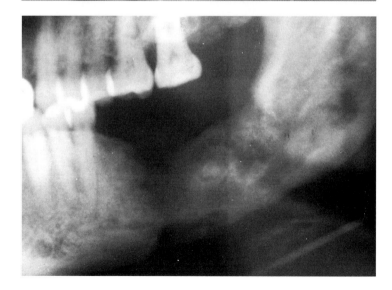

► **Figure 4.18**
**OSTEORADIONECROSIS**
Mandibular body demonstrating large, ill-defined areas of radiolucency that contain scattered radiopaque masses.

# CANDIDIASIS (CANDIDOSIS)

## Figs. 4.19, 4.20, and 4.21

Candidiasis is an opportunistic fungal infection produced most frequently by *Candida albicans* and is the most common human oral fungal infection. Although a number of additional candidal species inhabit the oral cavity, these forms rarely produce disease. Candida is present in the oral cavity of approximately 45% of healthy adults, with the percentage rising higher than 60% in denture wearers. Although clinically evident infestation may arise in otherwise healthy individuals, the infection often arises in the immunosuppressed or following antibiotic or corticosteroid therapy. Other factors associated with increased prevalence include dentures, xerostomia, epithelial damage, nutritional deficiency, hematologic pathoses, and several endocrinopathies, especially diabetes mellitus.

The classic clinical presentation is pseudomembranous candidiasis (thrush), which presents as multifocal white plaques that can be rubbed off to reveal an underlying area of mucosal erythema. The white material consists of superficial keratin intermixed with numerous fungal organisms. The plaques are rather adherent and are not removed easily with a casual scrape with a finger or mirror handle. Dry gauze should be used in any attempt to remove these plaques. Although often asymptomatic, some patients complain of mild sensitivity or an unpleasant taste. Candidiasis also may appear as numerous areas of redness or erythema that are termed "erythematous candidiasis." This pattern occurs when the affected mucosa becomes atrophic and the fungal organisms have not accumulated sufficiently to produce the typical white plaques. Affected patients frequently complain of a diffuse burning sensation of the oral mucosa that often is likened to being scalded by a hot beverage. Frequently, large zones of papillary atrophy of the tongue and angular cheilitis also are present.

Occasionally, candidiasis may be present in other white lesions that cannot be removed by scraping. Typically, the fungus represents a secondary infestation in primary oral pathoses such as keratoses with and without dysplasia, oral hairy leukoplakia, papillomas, and lichen planus. Rarely, primary candidiasis may induce epithelial hyperplasia and hyperkeratosis, termed "hyperplastic candidiasis." In many instances, these lesions cannot be separated from leukoplakia, and biopsy is mandatory.

The most common locations for oral candidiasis are the tongue, palate, and buccal mucosa, but any intraoral site may be involved. Culture is an unreliable method for diagnosis because of the high percentage of patients who harbor candida in the absence of clinical disease. Although many cases are diagnosed from the clinical presentation, exfoliative cytology represents a rapid and reliable method of diagnosis. Biopsy also is beneficial in cases resistant to therapy or thought to possibly represent secondary fungal infestation of another primary oral pathosis that is not diagnostic clinically. Life-threatening disseminated candidiasis can occur in the immunosuppressed; investigations have shown that prevention of oral lesions will dramatically lessen this possibility. Treatment of candidiasis consists of one of many antifungal medications, ranging from nystatin to fluconazole.

Multifocal white plaques of the right buccal mucosa.

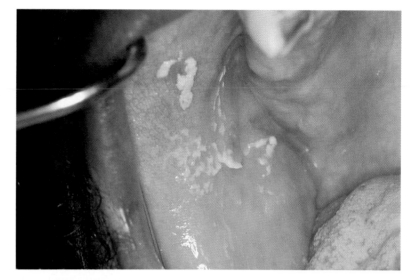

▶ **Figure 4.20**
**CANDIDIASIS**

Same patient as depicted in Figure 4.19 following removal of white plaques with dry gauze. Note the faint underlying erythema.

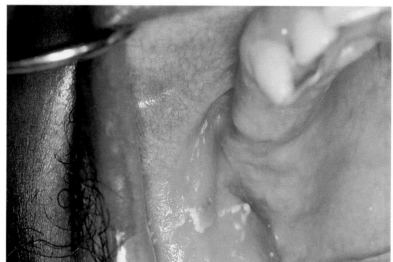

▶ **Figure 4.21**
**CANDIDIASIS**

Erythema and atrophy of the dorsal tongue mucosa.

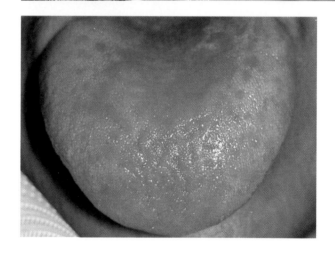

## ANGULAR CHEILITIS (PERLÈCHE)

### Fig. 4.22

Angular cheilitis is the development of symptomatic erythematous cracks or fissures at the corner of the mouth and is one of the most common oral pathologic alterations noted in the elderly. Crusts can develop at the site, and bleeding may occur if the mouth is opened wide. This disorder has been associated with nutritional deficiencies and loss of vertical dimension, but a correlation with infection by *Candida albicans* or *Staphylococcus aureus* (either organism alone or in combination) also has been made. Spontaneous remission with subsequent recurrence is not uncommon. Although most cases respond well to antifungal ointment, some examples also require topical antibiotic therapy. In all instances, any related underlying cause should be corrected to prevent recurrence. Patients must be cautioned that chronic misuse of topical antibiotics or corticosteroids often leads to the development of subsequent perioral dermatitis.

## MEDIAN RHOMBOID GLOSSITIS (CENTRAL PAPILLARY ATROPHY)

### Figs. 4.23 and 4.24

Median rhomboid glossitis is an area of erythema on the dorsal surface of the tongue in the midline, anterior to the circumvallate papillae. Total loss of the filiform papillae is seen in the affected zone. The lesion usually is smooth, although nodules or fissures may be present. Because almost all cases occur in adulthood, this entity no longer is considered developmental but to be acquired from one of several different causes.

Localized chronic candidiasis is implicated in most cases, and some resolve following antifungal therapy. Focal candidal infections of the palate have been reported in patients with median rhomboid glossitis, and inoculation from the tongue has been implicated. Biopsy samples of the area demonstrate a thick, hyalinized band of collagen between the mucosa and the underlying muscle. Some investigators have suggested that the sparse vascular supply in the area of hyalinization creates low resistance to infection and promotes candidal infestation. Others have seen abnormal pressure between the tongue and the palate during swallowing and articulation and wonder whether these factors may affect development.

### Figure 4.22
**ANGULAR CHEILITIS**
Bilateral ulceration and erythema of the oral commissures in a patient with candidiasis.

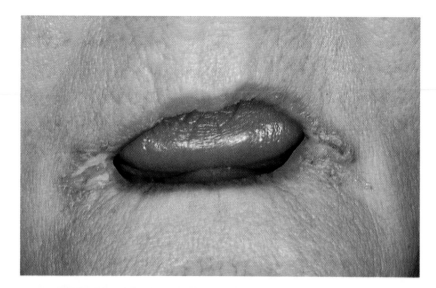

### Figure 4.23
**CANDIDIASIS IN MEDIAN RHOMBOID GLOSSITIS**
Localized erythematous mucosa of the dorsal surface of the tongue in the midline. Cytopathologic smear revealed numerous fungal organisms.

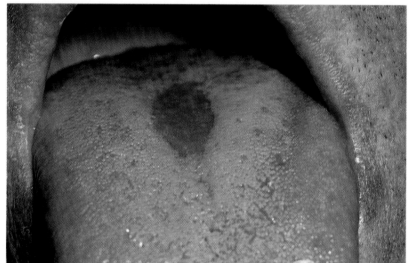

### Figure 4.24
**CANDIDIASIS**
Same patient as depicted in Figure 4.23. This localized area of mucosal erythema contacted the adjacent zone of central papillary atrophy of the tongue. Cytopathologic smear revealed numerous fungal organisms.

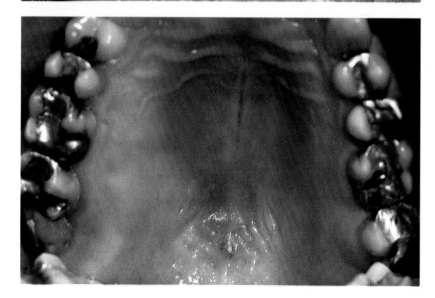

# DENTURE STOMATITIS (DENTURE SORE MOUTH)

## Figs. 4.25, 4.26, and 4.27

Denture stomatitis is a term that has been used to describe mucosal erythema present under removable dentures and is one of the most common oral pathoses in the elderly. The erythema may be multifocal, or the entire mucosa under the denture may be erythematous and delineate the exact outline of the denture. Rare cases are proven to arise from a true allergy to the denture material, and others represent pressure mucositis or mechanical trauma from the overlying prosthesis (especially related to poorly designed partial dentures). Nevertheless, a large percentage demonstrate a significant colonization of candidal organisms on the undersurface of the denture and on top of the erythematous mucosa. Because of a lack of mucosal penetration by the candidal organisms, some authors suggest the mucositis represents microbial irritation rather than a true infection.

A large percentage of these patients demonstrate poor oral hygiene and report wearing the dentures continuously. Many cases resolve when the patient cleans the prosthesis and leaves it out at night. Candidal infestation often is seen intermixed with inflammatory papillary hyperplasia and most likely is responsible for the erythematous coloration noted in that condition. A similar pattern of candidiasis also has been noted adjacent to overcontoured dentures and in the vaults of narrow, high-arched palates of dentulous patients. In most instances, denture stomatitis can be resolved by altering the defective prosthesis or by instructing the patient not to wear the appliance continuously and to follow appropriate hygiene procedures.

▶ **Figure 4.25**
**DENTURE STOMATITIS**
U-shaped denture kept in place almost
continuously for many years.

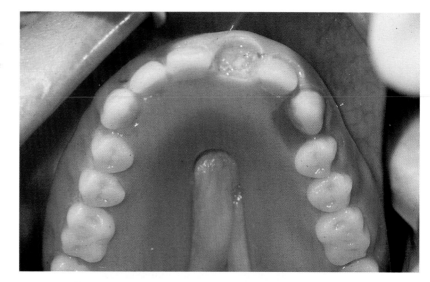

▶ **Figure 4.26**
**DENTURE STOMATITIS**
Area of erythematous palatal mucosa that
corresponds to the direct outline of the
U-shaped prosthesis depicted in Figure
4.25.

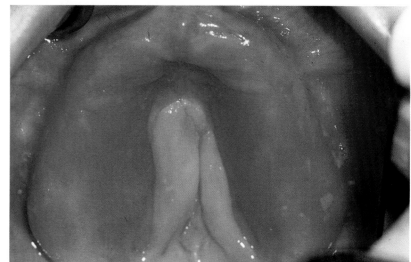

▶ **Figure 4.27**
**DENTURE STOMATITIS**
Palate of the same patient as depicted in
Figure 4.26 following cleansing and
nightly removal of the denture. Patient also
was treated with nystatin rinses.

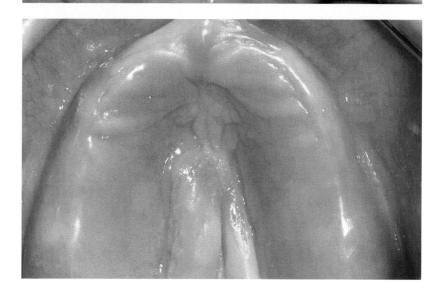

## ZYGOMYCOSIS (MUCORMYCOSIS, PHYCOMYCOSIS)

**Figs. 4.28 and 4.29** These opportunistic fungal infections are produced by the class of organisms known as the Zygomycetes whose genera include the common human pathogens *Rhizopus*, *Absidia*, and *Mucor*. Infections by all three are similar and have been grouped under the term "zygomycosis." Many of these infections are nosocomial and occur primarily in the severely and often fatally debilitated. Patients demonstrating diabetic acidosis or advanced malignancy and those receiving intensive antibiotic, steroidal, or cytotoxic medications are predisposed to contract acute and aggressive zygomycosis. The infection originates in either the nasal sinuses, lungs, or gastrointestinal tract. The pattern arising in the sinuses is seen most commonly in association with diabetic ketoacidosis. Less frequently, a more indolent chronic form is seen that occurs in patients that are not acutely or seriously ill.

The signs and symptoms include nasal obstruction, epistaxis, pain, swelling, and visual disturbances. Involvement of the maxillary sinus may result in enlargement of the maxilla with ocular displacement, movement or loosening of the maxillary dentition, or both. Sinus radiographs demonstrate opacification on the affected side. Mandibular involvement has been reported rarely. The organisms have a predilection to invade the arterial walls, which may result in areas of ischemia, infarction, and significant disfigurement. Palatal necrosis and perforation have occurred secondary to involvement of the maxillary sinus with infarction of the adjacent tissues. Unless prompt treatment is initiated, significant disfigurement can occur, along with spread into the central nervous system that may result in blindness, lethargy, seizures, hemiplegia, or death. Treatment consists of control of any underlying disease, surgical curettage of the infectious nidus, and systemic amphotericin B.

## ASPERGILLOSIS

**Fig. 4.30** *Aspergillus* is a true fungus that can produce several different forms of disease in man. *Aspergillus fumigatus* and *A. flavus* are the most common infectious species. Four main disease patterns are seen: mycetoma, allergic, invasive, and fulminant. The mycetoma (aspergilloma, fungus ball) represents a mass of fungal hyphae that fills a sinus cavity but does not demonstrate tissue invasion. Typically, this affects otherwise healthy individuals and involves one sinus, often the maxillary. Previous endodontic therapy with displacement of filling materials into the sinus seems to promote the infection. Radiographically, the involved sinus typically reveals homogeneous opacification that frequently contains radiodense foci.

Allergic fungal sinusitis usually arises in atopic young adults with a history of asthma or intranasal polyps. Radiographically, diffuse opacification and expansion are noted in multiple sinuses, occasionally with associated facial deformity. The involved sinuses are filled with laminated allergic mucin that contains numerous eosinophils, Charcot-Leyden crystals, and scattered fungal organisms.

Invasive aspergillosis normally is confined to one sinus and presents with pain, swelling, obstruction, and rhinorrhea. Radiographically, the involved sinus reveals diffuse opacification, often combined with added evidence of bone destruction. Histopathologically, tissue invasion and spread into adjacent anatomic structures is present. Late development of ocular or neurologic signs often occurs from local compression or direct invasion.

Fulminant aspergillosis is a rapidly progressing infection that typically arises in patients with diabetes mellitus, malignancy, or immunosuppressive disease. This type resembles the invasive form but demonstrates involvement of multiple sinuses. Invasion of blood vessels may lead to significant tissue necrosis and bone destruction. Rapid dissemination to the brain and lung often results in death.

Treatment of mycetoma involves surgical debridement with adequate sinus drainage, often achieved by endoscopic techniques; no antifungal therapy is necessary. Allergic fungal sinusitis requires surgical debridement of the involved sinuses with aeration of the antrum, often combined with systemic corticosteroid treatment. Invasive and fulminant disease typically is treated with surgical debridement and intravenous amphotericin B with or without flucytosine. In patients with serious infections, this initial regimen often is followed by long-term itraconazole therapy.

**Figure 4.28**
**ZYGOMYCOSIS**
Midline ulceration and necrosis of the palate. (Courtesy of Dr. E. R. Costich.)

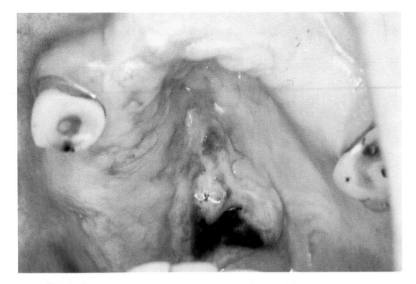

**Figure 4.29**
**ZYGOMYCOSIS**
Computed tomographic scan of the skull demonstrating a soft-tissue mass filling the maxillary sinus. (Courtesy of Dr. Jerry Bouquot.)

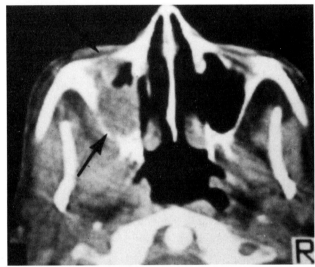

**Figure 4.30**
**ASPERGILLOSIS**
Skull radiograph demonstrating increased density of the left maxillary sinus.

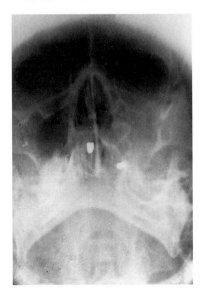

## HISTOPLASMOSIS

**Fig. 4.31**

Histoplasmosis is an infection produced by the fungal organism *Histoplasma capsulatum* and represents the most common systemic fungal infection in the United States. The disease is endemic to the Ohio and Mississippi river valleys of the United States and to other areas of the world. The organism is spread through the dust of bird and bat droppings or through contaminated soil. On exposure in healthy hosts, the organism produces no symptoms or a mild, flulike illness with fever, headache, myalgia, anorexia, or cough. Typically, the host defense system destroys or contains the organism, preventing additional clinical evidence of disease.

Chronic pulmonary involvement or disseminated disease may occur and usually is seen in the young, the old, or the immunocompromised. Common pulmonary symptoms include cough, weight loss, fever, dyspnea, hemoptysis, pain, weakness, and fatigue. With dissemination, the organism may involve the spleen, liver, lymph nodes, gastrointestinal tract, adrenals, kidneys, and central nervous system. In the United States, most oral lesions are associated with the disseminated form. In contrast, other countries occasionally demonstrate primarily extrapulmonary disease, with the oral cavity being the most frequently affected site. Although no oral mucosal site is spared, the infection most frequently involves the tongue, gingiva, palate, or buccal mucosa. Affected areas may mimic carcinoma and present as chronic ulcerations, nodular elevations, areas of slightly erythematous granularity or thickened white plaques. Severe forms of the disease require therapy with amphotericin B, whereas itraconazole may be used in the milder illnesses. In immunocompromised patients, itraconazole or fluconazole is used for maintenance therapy.

## BLASTOMYCOSIS

**Fig. 4.32**

Blastomycosis is an uncommon fungal infection produced by *Blastomyces dermatitidis*, with most cases occurring in North America. A similar disease seen in South America is produced by *Paracoccidioides brasiliensis*. The disease is prevalent in the Ohio and Mississippi river basins and the mid-Atlantic states. Like histoplasmosis, the organism's typical port of entry is the lung; following exposure, a subclinical infection, acute or chronic pulmonary disease, or disseminated disease may develop. Oral involvement may be seen and, rarely, may be the initial site of infection. These lesions typically appear as ulcerations, areas of erythema, or zones of granularity. Self-limited cases occur, and patients with chronic disease are treated with itraconazole or ketoconazole. Amphotericin B is used for seriously ill patients or infections resistant to the first-line therapies.

## MUMPS (VIRAL PAROTITIS)

**Fig. 4.33**

Mumps is an infection by a paramyxovirus usually seen in children aged 5 to 15 years. Vaccination against this virus has reduced the prevalence dramatically, but outbreaks occasionally occur. Although most outbreaks seem to be caused by lack of immunization, well-documented examples have arisen from vaccination failure. It has been suggested that a two-dose mumps vaccine may prevent similar localized epidemics. The disease normally is acquired via inhalation of infected droplets, with an incubation period ranging from 12 to 25 days. The acute illness lasts from 1 to 2 weeks with gradual improvement, although 30% of all patients are asymptomatic.

In symptomatic patients, prodromal anorexia, myalgia, fever, headache, and malaise are followed by enlargement of the salivary glands, usually the parotids. Classically, bilateral parotid involvement occurs, but sometimes the submandibular and sublingual glands also are affected. Pain exacerbated by chewing and eating is noted in the enlarged glands. The second most common pathosis is swelling, pain, and tenderness secondary to epididymo-orchitis in males. Rarely, permanent sterility occurs in severely affected patients. Other less common manifestations, including oophoritis, meningoencephalitis, pancreatitis, arthritis, carditis, hearing loss, and decreased renal function, occasionally are sufficiently severe to require hospitalization. Typical therapy is palliative and usually consists of nonaspirin analgesics and antipyretics. To minimize the orchitis, bed rest is recommended until the fever breaks in affected males.

### Figure 4.31
### HISTOPLASMOSIS

Large area of ulceration and necrosis with underlying bone loss present in the anterior maxilla. Patient was receiving heavy systemic corticosteroids for treatment of lupus erythematosus.

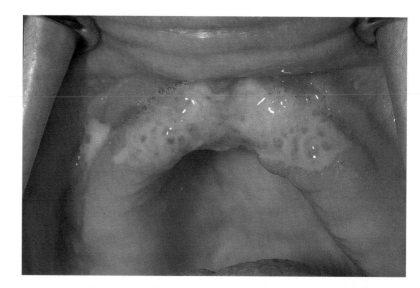

### Figure 4.32
### BLASTOMYCOSIS

Multiple areas of ulceration and granularity of the maxillary alveolar ridge and palate.

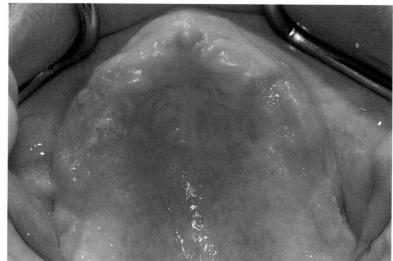

### Figure 4.33
### MUMPS (VIRAL PAROTITIS)

Young adult male demonstrating bilateral enlargement of the parotid glands.

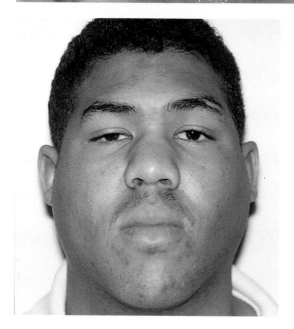

## Figs. 4.34, 4.35, and 4.36

Herpes simplex is a herpesvirus infection that classically is divided into two types. Type I usually occurs above the waist, typically in or around the mouth, and type II generally presents below the waist, classically in the genital areas. Although similar, the infections are separate and produced by different viruses. Infection by type I has occurred in close to 70% of middle-aged adults, but most of these infections are subclinical. The infection is transmitted by physical contact and typically arises in children between the ages of 6 months and 5 years but occasionally is seen in adulthood.

In patients with symptoms, the primary infection produces a distinctive intraoral ulcerative pattern known as primary herpetic gingivostomatitis. Classically, the initial symptoms are fever and lymphadenopathy, followed within a few days by diffuse involvement of the gingiva and oral mucosa. In all patients with symptoms, the gingiva demonstrates a painful and intensely erythematous alteration and often exhibits focal nicks or ulcerations of the free gingival margin. Shortly thereafter, multifocal fragile vesicles develop on any intraoral mucosal surface; these rapidly ulcerate. The individual ulcerations are usually a few millimeters in diameter, but they frequently cluster and may coalesce. On occasion, the ulcerations may resemble minor aphthous stomatitis, but the intense gingival involvement, fever, and the presence of ulcerations on bound mucosa lead away from that diagnosis.

If initiated within the first 3 days of onset, acyclovir elixir (swish and swallow) shortens the duration of symptoms and infectivity. Although acyclovir remains the treatment of choice for severe herpetic infections in both immunocompetent and immunosuppressed patients, two newer antiviral medications, famciclovir and valacyclovir, demonstrate improved bioavailability and equal efficaciousness in the immunocompetent. In addition, famciclovir may decrease the prevalence of latent infection with herpes simplex type I. Therapy to relieve the symptoms includes topical dyclonine hydrochloride or diphenhydramine elixir and ibuprofen or acetaminophen. The ulcerations typically resolve in 7 to 14 days.

▶ **Figure 4.34**
**PRIMARY HERPETIC GINGIVOSTOMATITIS**
Multifocal ulcerations present on movable
and bound mucosa. Note the intensely
erythematous gingiva without significant
plaque.

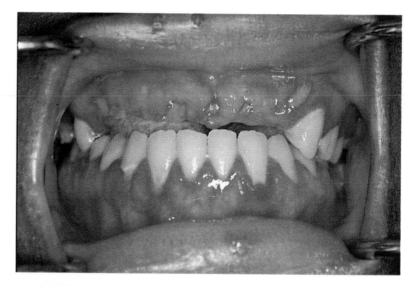

▶ **Figure 4.35**
**PRIMARY HERPETIC GINGIVOSTOMATITIS**
Palatal mucosa demonstrating numerous
small ulcerations that tend to cluster. Note
the significant erythema and ulceration of
the palatal gingiva.

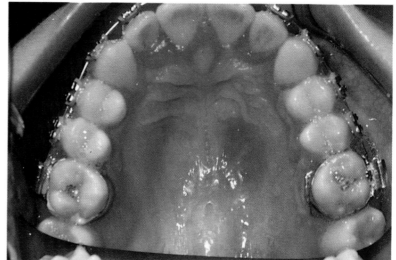

▶ **Figure 4.36**
**PRIMARY HERPETIC GINGIVOSTOMATITIS**
Multiple ulcerations of the lower labial
mucosa. The patient also demonstrated
additional lesions on both movable and
bound mucosa with the typical
erythematous and painful gingival
involvement.

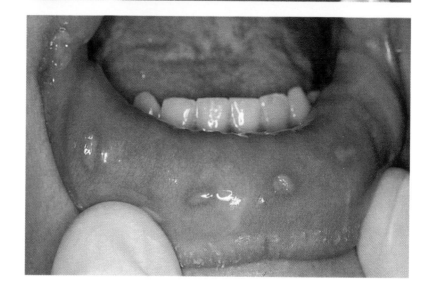

## Figs. 4.37, 4.38, and 4.39

After the initial infection, the herpes simplex virus does not remain at the site but can survive in the nerve ganglia of the area. The viral DNA is incorporated into the host DNA and is impervious to attack by the defense system or medications. The virus remains latent at this site until reactivation allows reinfection. Predisposition to reinfection may be related to minor decreases in immune function, and reports have indicated a prevalence of herpes labialis in 15 to 45% of the United States' population. Old age, trauma, extensive ultraviolet light exposure, pregnancy, allergy, respiratory illnesses, menstruation, and underlying systemic disease or malignancy have all been associated with an increased frequency of recurrence. Recurrence intervals vary widely.

Herpes simplex type I normally resides in the trigeminal ganglia; on activation, the most frequent site of involvement is the lips. Often, the lesions are preceded by prodromal symptoms that consist of burning, stinging, soreness, redness, localized warmth, and paresthesia of the affected area. The lesions appear as numerous vesicles filled with clear fluid. The vesicles are only a few millimeters in diameter but tend to cluster and coalesce. These vesicles rupture and subsequently develop a brown crust that, with movement, may crack, ooze, and bleed. Secondary infection occasionally occurs. Some patients may demonstrate significant edema associated with the presence of the lesions. Although most cases are unilateral, bilateral cases do occur; and involvement of both lips and the surrounding skin may be seen. The ulcerations usually heal in 7 to 10 days.

The effect of antiviral medications on the course of recurrent herpes labialis is controversial and most likely variable from patient to patient. If a course of acyclovir capsules is begun during the prodrome, the duration of symptoms and viral shedding is diminished in some patients. Successful prophylaxis has been achieved in severe cases with maintenance doses of acyclovir, which should be used with caution in fertile females. Although not consistently effective in immunocompetent patients, initiation of topical acyclovir or penciclovir cream during the prodrome may result in faster healing and more rapid resolution of the associated signs and symptoms. Although seen predominantly in immunocompromised patients, development of viral resistance to acyclovir has been reported and should be a warning against overuse.

### ▶ Figure 4.37
**RECURRENT HERPES LABIALIS**
Area of erythema of the right side of the lower lip that has been present for less than 1 day. The patient reports a stinging and burning sensation.

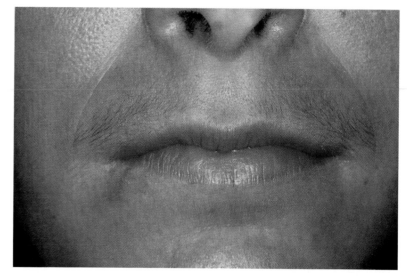

### ▶ Figure 4.38
**RECURRENT HERPES LABIALIS**
Multiple fluid-filled vesicles and erythema of the right side of the lower lip. This picture depicts the same patient 24 hours after Figure 4.37 was photographed.

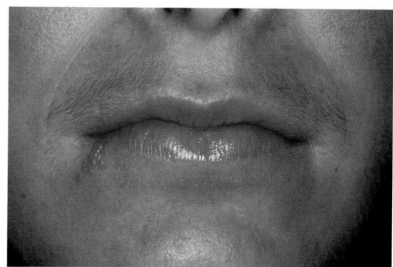

### ▶ Figure 4.39
**RECURRENT HERPES LABIALIS**
Widespread bilateral fluid-filled vesicles of both the upper and lower lips. Many of the vesicles have ruptured and formed crusts.

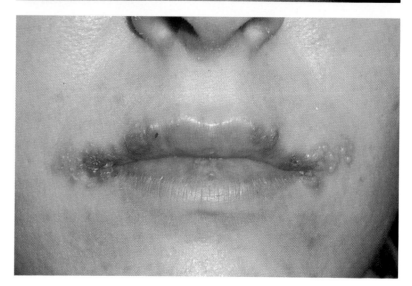

**Figs. 4.40 and 4.41**

Although recurrent herpes simplex may develop anywhere on the skin, once it crosses over the lip wetline and enters the oral cavity, the lesions occur in a specific pattern. In the immunocompetent patient, recurrent intraoral herpes simplex is seen on mucosa bound to bone as numerous pinpoint vesicles that rapidly ulcerate. Usually, they are found as small red areas only a few millimeters in diameter that commonly coalesce and, with time, develop a central zone of yellow fibrin. The palate is the usual location, but lesions do occur on the buccal gingiva. The symptoms are mild; treatment usually is not required and healing occurs in 5 to 10 days.

## HERPETIC WHITLOW (HERPETIC PARONYCHIA)

**Fig. 4.42**

Investigations have shown that approximately 50 to 60% of adults in the higher socioeconomic classes and almost 100% in poor, developing countries exhibit antibodies to herpes simplex type I. It has been shown that the virus can survive for up to 4 hours on contaminated surfaces. If barrier protection has not been maintained during both patient care and cleanup, the likelihood of contact is significant. Because a consistent barrier technique typically is used during clinical procedures today, the risk of herpetic whitlow (infection of the thumbs or fingers) has been reduced. Most examples arise from self-inoculation in children with orofacial herpes. Following the initial exposure, recurrences are possible and occasionally result in paresthesia and scarring.

**RECURRENT HERPETIC STOMATITIS**

A cluster of multiple small ulcerations of the hard palate.

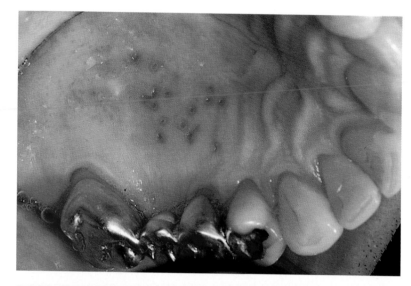

▶ Figure 4.41
**RECURRENT HERPETIC STOMATITIS**

Multiple scattered small ulcerations of the hard palate that are covered by yellowish fibrin.

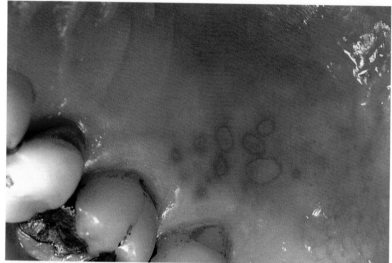

▶ Figure 4.42
**HERPETIC WHITLOW**

Multiple crusting ulcerations of the fingers. Lesions began as fluid-filled vesicles and are extremely painful.

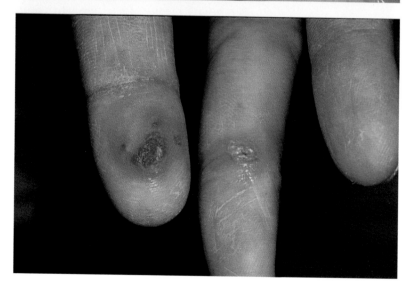

## CHRONIC HERPES SIMPLEX INFECTION

**Fig. 4.43**

Without treatment, recurrent herpetic infections require a functioning immune system for resolution. In the immunocompromised, recurrent herpes can present as chronic mucosal alterations arising in atypical oral locations. Unlike recurrent infections in healthy patients, the involved areas may occur on movable or bound mucosa and initially appear as foci of soft, elevated, and light-brown necrotic epithelium. The initial area of epithelial necrosis is replaced by a laterally spreading erosion that demonstrates a yellowish white curvilinear leading margin. The epithelial cells within the curvilinear border demonstrate the diagnostic cytopathologic effects of a herpes virus, making diagnosis from a cytologic smear simple. The presence of chronic mucosal erosion exhibiting herpetic viral cytopathologic effects strongly suggests an immunocompromised state and mandates a thorough physical evaluation. Without appropriate antiviral therapy, the lesions will continue to persist until the immune system recovers.

## CHICKENPOX (VARICELLA)

**Figs. 4.44 and 4.45**

Chickenpox is the primary infection produced by the varicella-zoster virus. Typically, it presents as an acute and highly contagious infection in children. In the immunocompetent, the disease usually is mild. The clinical phase appears after 2 to 3 weeks of viral incubation and begins with malaise, sore throat, and rhinitis. A generalized rash follows and progresses from macules to vesicles. Several crops of lesions succeed each other, beginning on the trunk and spreading to the face and extremities. The vesicles rupture, crust, and heal in about a week. Intraoral lesions may occur, may precede the skin lesions and appear as widely scattered vesicles that rupture, and may produce lesions resembling minor aphthous ulcerations.

Therapy primarily has been symptomatic, with use of nonaspirin antipyretics, warm baths with baking soda, topical calamine lotion, and either topical or systemic diphenhydramine. If initiated during the first 24 hours, systemic acyclovir has been shown in children and adults to produce rapid resolution of fever and itching, to interrupt vesicle formation, and to accelerate healing of active lesions. Valacyclovir and famciclovir also are effective against the virus, but many clinicians reserve the use of systemic antivirals for young children or infants and patients at risk for progression of the infection. Secondary and tertiary cases within a family often are more severe and represent an indication for systemic antiviral therapy. In addition, chickenpox in immunocompromised patients can be fatal, and intravenous acyclovir therapy is recommended as soon as the infection is recognized.

A vaccine that uses a live, attenuated form of the virus is available and has been shown to be 98% effective. Although used for many years elsewhere, the vaccine is just beginning to be widely used in the United States. When combined with the measles, mumps, and rubella vaccine, the resultant antibody titer to varicella was lower compared with that seen in patients who received the vaccine in a separate syringe.

▶ **Figure 4.43**
**CHRONIC HERPES SIMPLEX INFECTION**
Multiple areas of erythema, ulceration, and epithelial necrosis of the dorsal surface of the tongue. Note herpes labialis. Patient was immunocompromised.

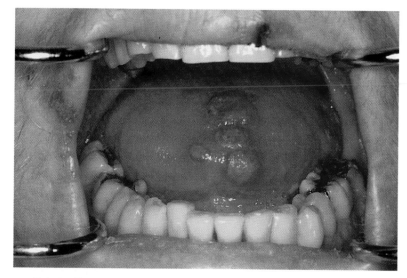

▶ **Figure 4.44**
**CHICKENPOX (VARICELLA)**
Multiple vesicles surrounded by erythematous skin on the right side of the face.

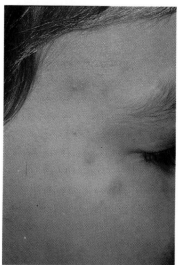

▶ **Figure 4.45**
**CHICKENPOX (VARICELLA)**
Same patient as depicted in Figure 4.44. Multiple vesicular lesions of the posterior hard palate and soft palate.

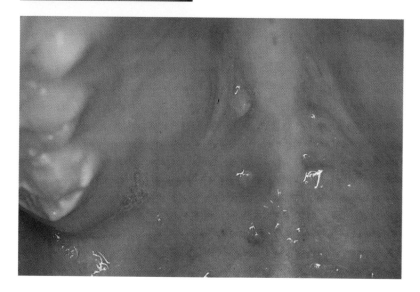

### Figs. 4.46 and 4.47

Herpes zoster represents recurrence of the virus responsible for varicella in children. This virus may become latent and reside in the sensory nerve ganglia of the infected area. Recurrence of the virus is seen during the lifetime of 10 to 20% of individuals, with the prevalence increasing with age. In contrast to herpes simplex virus, a single rather than multiple recurrences is typical. Immunosuppression, presence of malignancy, treatment with cytotoxic drugs or radiation, old age, and alcohol abuse are associated with an increased prevalence of reinfection.

On activation, a vesicular eruption of the affected skin or mucosa is seen. The eruption follows the path of the nerves and normally is unilateral, classically stopping at the midline. Bilateral involvement can be seen, however. Affected skin exhibits clusters of vesicles within areas of erythema. The vesicles ulcerate and crust within 7 to 10 days, and scarring is common. Oral lesions may involve movable or bound mucosa and usually present as 1- to 4-mm white, opaque vesicles that rupture and ulcerate. Osteonecrosis of the jaws and devitalization of teeth have occurred in areas of involvement. The lesions are extremely painful and may last for up to 5 weeks.

The major morbidity associated with herpes zoster is the development of postherpetic neuralgia. This pain lasts longer than 1 month after resolution of the infection and demonstrates an increased prevalence in patients older than age 60 years. Most cases of postherpetic neuralgia resolve within 1 year, but rare cases may last up to 20 years.

Supportive therapy includes nonaspirin antipyretics and systemic or topical diphenhydramine to decrease itching. Active skin lesions should be kept dry and clean to avoid secondary bacterial infection. Acyclovir produces cessation of the active infection, but the newer antivirals, famciclovir and valacyclovir, also seem to more rapidly speed the resolution of pain. In addition, early treatment with systemic antivirals has shown promise in reducing the prevalence and duration of postherpetic neuralgia. In many patients with neuralgia, use of topical anesthetics, such as capsaicin, is beneficial in temporarily reducing the severity. The varicella vaccine has been suggested for elderly patients in an attempt to increase the immune response to the virus and decrease the prevalence of recurrence in this population.

## HERPANGINA

### Fig. 4.48

More than 30 enteroviruses are known to be associated with patterns of infection capable of producing enanthems or exanthems in man. Within this group are a number of viruses that have been related to a distinctive clinical pattern termed "herpangina." Any 1 of 10 different strains of coxsackie A, coxsackie B, or echovirus may be responsible.

The disease begins with symptoms of sore throat, fever, malaise, and headache, occasionally with vomiting and abdominal pain. Subsequently, numerous pinhead vesicles develop, primarily on the soft palate and tonsillar pillars. The vesicles quickly rupture and develop into slightly larger areas of ulceration. Therapy is symptomatic, primarily nonaspirin antipyretics (ibuprofen or acetaminophen) and topical anesthetics (dyclonine hydrochloride or diphenhydramine elixir). The disease occurs primarily in children, is self-limiting, and produces long-lasting immunity to reinfection by the offending strain. Adults normally exhibit immunity to the numerous strains responsible for this pattern of infection.

### Figure 4.46
### HERPES ZOSTER (SHINGLES)

Adult female with an isolated zone of erythematous skin of the left hip demonstrating a cluster of fluid-filled vesicles.

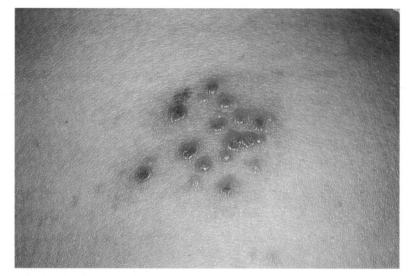

### Figure 4.47
### HERPES ZOSTER (SHINGLES)

Adult male exhibiting an acute unilateral cluster of white, opaque vesicles of the ventral surface of the tongue on the left side. Similar lesions also were noted on the left side of the hard palate. Physical evaluation revealed disseminated carcinoma of the lung.

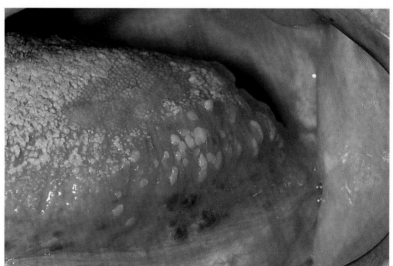

### Figure 4.48
### HERPANGINA

Multifocal areas of ulceration and erythema of the soft palate. The patient reported sore throat, fever, headache, and vomiting.

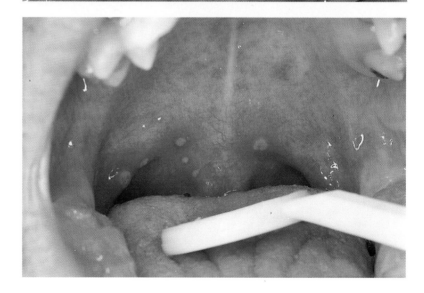

**Figs. 4.49 and 4.50**

Hand, foot, and mouth disease is another specific pattern of enterovirus infection produced by one of a number of strains of the Coxsackievirus, usually A16. The disorder arises predominantly in young children but can occur in adults. Large outbreaks of this epidemic infection have occurred in numerous cities.

Patients present with fever, malaise, and lymphadenopathy typically accompanied by lesions of the skin and oral mucosa. The skin lesions characteristically arise on the hands and feet and present as multiple vesicles surrounded by erythematous halos. A maculopapular eruption has been reported to occur occasionally on the buttocks. The skin lesions normally are asymptomatic. The oral lesions are usually on the buccal mucosa, tongue, or hard palate. These lesions begin as small vesicles that rapidly form ulcerations as large as a centimeter. Although both skin and mucosal sites are not involved consistently in all patients, almost all cases reveal some degree of skin involvement, most frequently on the hands. Most patients demonstrate oral lesions that often are responsible for the chief complaint. The severity of infection typically is associated directly with the degree of oral involvement. The infection is self-limited and normally resolves within 2 weeks. The therapy is palliative and parallels that of herpangina, with nonaspirin antipyretics and topical anesthetics used most consistently.

## ACUTE LYMPHONODULAR PHARYNGITIS

**Fig. 4.51**

Acute lymphonodular pharyngitis is another specific pattern of enterovirus infection said to be caused by the A10 strain of Coxsackievirus. The disease occurs primarily in children and young adults. These patients present with sore throat and fever associated with oral lesions. The oral lesions consist of numerous whitish yellow papules or pink nodules surrounded by obvious erythematous halos. The yellow papular lesions are similar clinically to the early lesions seen in herpangina; acute lymphonodular pharyngitis could be classified as a variation of that infection. These lesions occur primarily on the soft palate, tonsillar pillar, and oropharynx and represent hyperplastic lymphoid aggregates with overlying erythematous mucosa. The disease is self-limited, and the oral lesions usually resolve within 2 weeks. Therapy is palliative and directed toward the most severe symptoms—sore throat and fever.

▶ **Figure 4.49**
**HAND, FOOT, AND MOUTH DISEASE**
Multiple coalescing ulcers of the lateral tongue in a 3-year-old child who also had vesicular lesions of the fingers and toes. (Courtesy of Dr. Sam Jasper.)

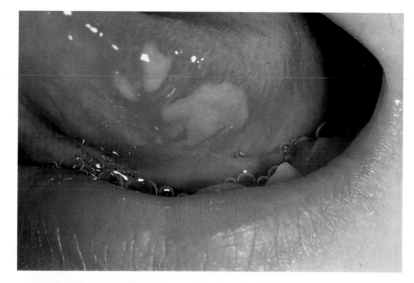

▶ **Figure 4.50**
**HAND, FOOT, AND MOUTH DISEASE**
Multiple vesicles and erythema of the fingers in the patient shown in Figure 4.49. (Courtesy of Dr. Sam Jasper.)

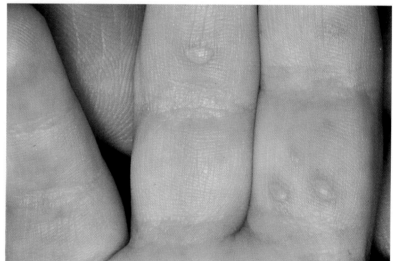

▶ **Figure 4.51**
**ACUTE LYMPHONODULAR PHARYNGITIS**
Two pink nodules immediately superior to the uvula with lateral adjacent erythema of the soft palate.

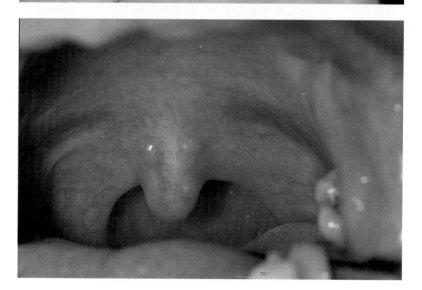

## Figs. 4.52, 4.53, and 4.54

Acquired immunodeficiency syndrome, or AIDS, is caused by an infection with the human immunodeficiency virus (HIV). This virus is capable of producing significant suppression of the immune system through its adverse effects on $CD4^+$ helper T lymphocytes. The virus is thought to be present in most bodily secretions of infected individuals and to be transmitted usually through sexual contact, exposure to infected blood, and perinatally from mother to neonate. Most cases have been diagnosed in homosexual or bisexual men and intravenous drug users.

An infected patient is considered to have AIDS when the $CD4^+$ count is less than 200 cells/$\mu$l or any of a number of "indicator" diseases are diagnosed in the absence of any other known cause of immunosuppression. The indicator diseases include a long list of opportunistic infections and cancers, which includes, but is not limited to, pneumocystis pneumonia, esophageal candidiasis, cytomegalovirus retinitis, disseminated histoplasmosis, Kaposi's sarcoma, and non-Hodgkin's lymphoma. As a result of recent advances in the treatment of patients infected with HIV and the improving prognosis, appropriate diagnosis and therapy have become increasingly more important.

Oral changes often are important clues to the definitive diagnosis. Clinically evident candidiasis of the oral cavity, in the absence of other predisposing factors, is the most common intraoral manifestation of HIV infection and often initially leads to definitive diagnosis. Up to 95% of patients with AIDS develop oropharyngeal candidiasis, and the clinical patterns are varied, including atrophic, pseudomembranous, and hyperplastic types. Angular or exfoliative cheilitis also may be indicative of a chronic candidal infestation, but it has been associated with other causes such as mixed bacterial infections.

One unique pattern of candidal infection is termed "HIV-related gingivitis" or "linear gingival erythema." Although seen most frequently in HIV-infected patients, this unusual pattern of candidiasis can occur in association with other causes of immunosuppression. Affected patients demonstrate a distinctive linear band of erythema that occurs along the gingival margin and extends 2 to 3 mm apically. The adjacent alveolar mucosa frequently exhibits scattered punctate or diffuse areas of erythema. Although typically nonresponsive to conventional oral hygiene measures, systemic fluconazole therapy usually is highly effective.

There is evidence to suggest that *Candida* species are immunosuppressive, with their presence adversely affecting the patient's ultimate prognosis. Therefore, appropriate diagnosis and therapy are mandatory. Candidiasis in patients afflicted with AIDS often does not respond typically to conventional antifungal therapies such as nystatin, clotrimazole, and amphotericin B. In many cases, these medications produce temporary resolution associated with rapid recurrence. Although resistance to multiple therapies continues to be seen, better control has been obtained with several of the newer systemic antifungal medications, such as ketoconazole, fluconazole, and itraconazole. All alterable predisposing factors, such as xerostomia, should be resolved. Despite appropriate management, maintenance therapy is required in many cases.

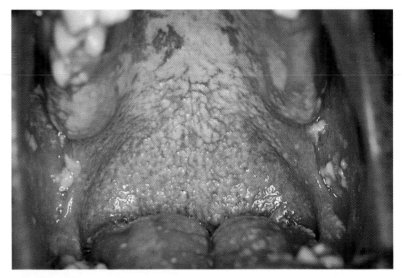

### Figure 4.52
### ACQUIRED IMMUNODEFICIENCY SYNDROME, CANDIDIASIS

Diffuse white alteration of the palate, bilateral buccal mucosa, and dorsal tongue. The surface material can be rubbed off, and smear revealed numerous fungal organisms.

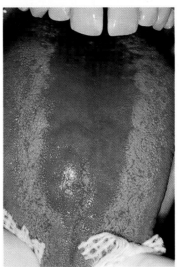

### Figure 4.53
### ACQUIRED IMMUNODEFICIENCY SYNDROME, CANDIDIASIS

Large central zone of erythema and papillary atrophy of the dorsal surface of the tongue. Cytopathologic smear revealed numerous fungal organisms.

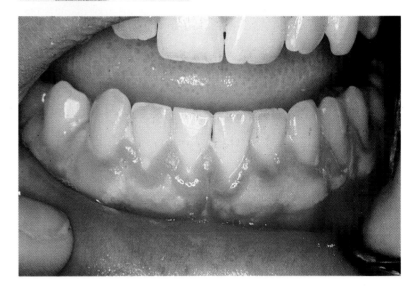

### Figure 4.54
### ACQUIRED IMMUNODEFICIENCY SYNDROME, LINEAR GINGIVAL ERYTHEMA

Distinct linear band of erythema involving the free gingival margin. Although nonresponsive to improved plaque control, the band quickly resolved following antifungal therapy. (Courtesy of Dr. Ted Raybould.)

## Figs. 4.55, 4.56, and 4.57

Although there is a greater prevalence of candidiasis in patients with AIDS, HIV-associated periodontal disease is not uncommon and occasionally is responsible for initial presentation because of associated symptoms. Unlike candidiasis, many of the periodontal pathoses are associated with significant discomfort. In addition to linear gingival erythema (see Figure 4.54), patients infected with HIV demonstrate an increased prevalence of acute necrotizing ulcerative gingivitis, advanced periodontal disease, and necrotizing stomatitis.

Acute necrotizing ulcerative gingivitis is a relatively frequent occurrence, and the related symptoms mandate appropriate care. Affected interdental papillae are blunted, highly inflamed, and edematous, with punched out areas of craterlike necrosis covered by a grayish pseudomembrane. Fetid odor, extreme pain, and spontaneous hemorrhage typically are seen. Associated lymphadenopathy, fever, and malaise are seen occasionally.

Although possessing no unique or pathognomonic characteristics, HIV-associated periodontitis occasionally reveals features that suggest the underlying cause. The resultant periodontal disease frequently is associated with severe deep pain, gingival hemorrhage, soft-tissue necrosis, and rapid loss of alveolar bone support. In some patients, up to 90% of periodontal bone support can be lost within a few weeks. Tooth mobility and necrosis of the soft tissue and bone often result in significant pain, with resultant presentation to oral health care practitioners. In contrast to conventional periodontitis, the pattern of bone loss often is irregular and associated with minimal pocketing. Surprisingly shallow periodontal pockets seem to be the result of necrosis of the gingival soft tissues that occurs in association with loss of periodontal bone support. The advanced periodontal disease may be complicated by massively destructive necrotizing lesions of the adjacent bone or soft tissue, termed "necrotizing ulcerative periodontitis." A similar pattern of infection also may be seen in soft tissue apart from bone, termed "necrotizing stomatitis," and closely resembles gangrenous stomatitis or noma.

Because of the associated destructive nature and high prevalence of significant symptoms, early appropriate management is mandatory; however, these disorders often do not respond well to conventional periodontal therapy. Treatment requires debridement (often combined with povidone-iodine lavage), local antimicrobial therapy (chlorhexidine), immediate followup care, and long-term maintenance. In patients with systemic manifestations, extensive destruction, or resistance to therapy, short-term systemic antibiotics, such as metronidazole, have been used as an adjunct to debridement and root planing. During this period of antibiotic therapy, close observation for signs of related candidal infection should be maintained.

▶ **Figure 4.55**
**ACQUIRED IMMUNODEFICIENCY SYNDROME, ACUTE NECROTIZING ULCERATIVE GINGIVITIS**
Inflamed, erythematous gingiva demonstrating necrosis of numerous interdental papillae.

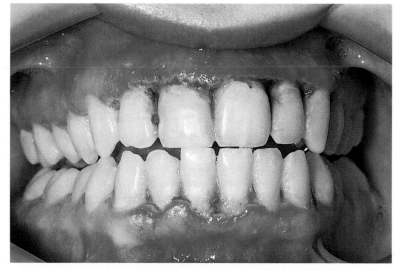

▶ **Figure 4.56**
**ACQUIRED IMMUNODEFICIENCY SYNDROME, HIV-RELATED PERIODONTITIS**
Rapidly progressing periodontal bone loss in a young adult male who is HIV positive. (Courtesy of Dr. T. L. Green.)

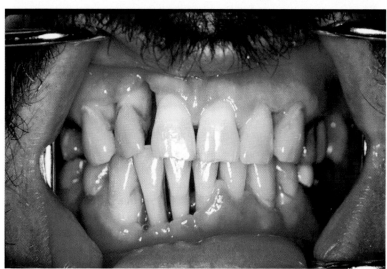

▶ **Figure 4.57**
**ACQUIRED IMMUNODEFICIENCY SYNDROME, NECROTIZING ULCERATIVE PERIODONTITIS**
Localized loss of periodontal attachment with overlying necrosis of the gingival soft tissues.

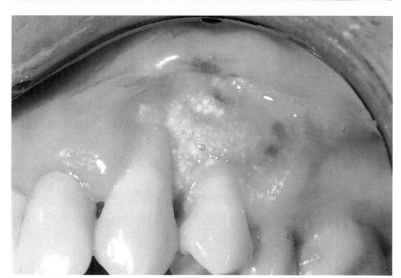

## Figs. 4.58, 4.59, and 4.60

Besides candidiasis, other fungal infections can occur from the immunosuppression seen in HIV-infected patients. Histoplasmosis, which occurs predominantly in the Ohio and Mississippi river valleys, represents the most common endemic respiratory fungal infection in the United States and is not rare in patients with AIDS. Other fungal infections that are documented less frequently include aspergillosis, zygomycosis, cryptococcosis, coccidioidomycosis and blastomycosis.

In healthy patients, exposure to histoplasmosis usually creates a subclinical and self-limited infection. Chronic disease may occur in approximately 5% of patients with AIDS residing in endemic areas. In addition, HIV-infected patients currently living outside endemic areas occasionally develop active histoplasmosis from reactivation of previous foci of infection. The oral lesions usually appear as nodular, ulcerative, or granular lesions on any mucosal surface. Although the infection may be limited to the oral cavity, physical evaluation usually demonstrates disseminated or pulmonary disease. Often, fever, weight loss, splenomegaly, and pulmonary infiltrates also are present. First-line therapy for disseminated histoplasmosis is amphotericin B, with itraconazole being the first alternative.

Not all ulcerations occurring in HIV-infected patients are related to opportunistic organisms. In this cohort, there is an increased prevalence of mucosal lesions that are indistinguishable from aphthous ulcerations. All three varieties—minor, major, and herpetiform—have been seen; and surprisingly, the most frequently detected are the usually uncommon major and herpetiform variants. The occurrence of major aphthous ulcerations in HIV-infected patients has been associated with a profound depression of the CD4$^+$ cell count and is suggestive of severe immunodepression. In most instances, minor and herpetiform aphthous ulcerations respond well to topical corticosteroid therapy; the major form occasionally requires systemic corticosteroid therapy. In nonresponsive patients, biopsy is mandatory because many infectious diseases and neoplasms may demonstrate similarities.

In immunocompromised patients, unusual oral ulcerations may arise secondary to infection by one or more viruses. In contrast to healthy patients, the pattern of virally associated oral ulcerations may be atypical and more difficult to diagnose. Classically, herpes simplex virus recurs intraorally only on mucosa bound to bone and presents as numerous small, pinhead ulcerations that tend to cluster and coalesce. In HIV-infected and other immunocompromised patients, the virus may create lesions on any mucosal surface and present as lateral spreading erosions with circinate yellow borders that reveal diagnostic cytopathologic effects of the virus (for further discussion, see Figure 4.43).

In addition, less distinctive ulcerations may be seen and require biopsy and immunohistochemical studies for appropriate diagnosis. Culture is an unreliable method because of secondary infection within a lesion that arose from another causative mechanism. Only by thorough and appropriate evaluation is the true nature of the ulceration ascertained and properly treated. Detection of causative herpes simplex virus or cytomegalovirus is not rare in chronic atypical oral ulcerations in patients with AIDS. Herpes zoster also is seen with increased frequency in HIV-infected patients. This recurrent infection is produced by the varicella-zoster virus and typically produces unilateral vesicular skin lesions that rupture and scab before resolving or intraoral white vesicles that rupture and ulcerate. Herpes simplex and zoster respond well to systemic acyclovir treatment, whereas cytomegalovirus requires the addition of systemic ganciclovir.

### Figure 4.58
### ACQUIRED IMMUNODEFICIENCY SYNDROME, HISTOPLASMOSIS

Unilateral red granular alteration of the maxillary gingiva. The facial gingiva of the involved quadrant was also affected. The lesions arose in ulcerations that were created by a recent herpes zoster infection.

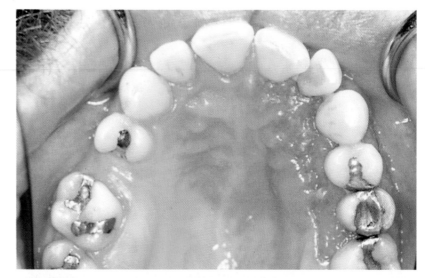

### Figure 4.59
### ACQUIRED IMMUNODEFICIENCY SYNDROME, MAJOR APHTHOUS ULCERATION

Large ulceration of the posterior soft palate on the left side. (Reproduced with permission from Neville BW, Damm DD, Allen CM, Bouquot JE. Oral & maxillofacial pathology. Philadelphia: WB Saunders, 1995.)

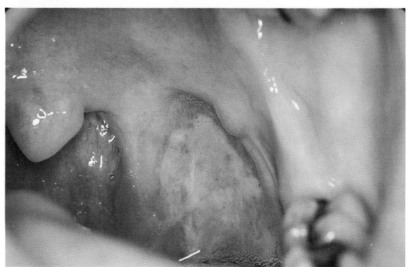

### Figure 4.60
### ACQUIRED IMMUNODEFICIENCY SYNDROME, CHRONIC HERPES SIMPLEX INFECTION

Mucosal erosion exhibiting circinate yellow periphery on the anterior dorsal surface of the tongue on the left side. (Reproduced with permission from Neville BW, Damm DD, Allen CM, Bouquot JE. Oral & maxillofacial pathology. Philadelphia: WB Saunders, 1995.)

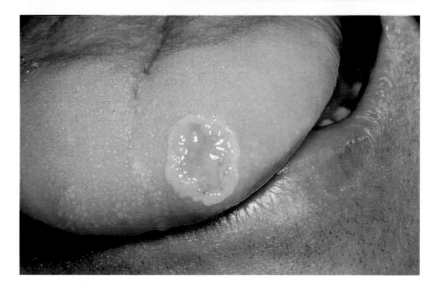

### Figs. 4.61, 4.62, and 4.63

One of the more common oral mucosal alterations related to a virus in HIV-infected patients is oral hairy leukoplakia. This somewhat distinctive lesion is associated with the Epstein-Barr virus and is characterized by thickened hyperparakeratosis and acanthosis that occur most frequently on the lateral borders of the tongue bilaterally. Although the lesion often forms vertical corrugations that strongly suggest the diagnosis, similar clinical changes have arisen from other pathoses such as cinnamon-related stomatitis and morsicatio linguarum. Oral hairy leukoplakia also histopathologically demonstrates features that are suggestive, but not pathognomonic, of the diagnosis. Demonstration of intracellular Epstein-Barr virus is required for definitive diagnosis. Although this unique pattern of mucosal pathosis is noted most frequently in association with HIV infection, cases have been documented in patients with other forms of immunosuppression and, rarely, in otherwise healthy individuals. Although treatment is not necessary, temporary resolution can be obtained with systemic acyclovir or topical podophyllum resin.

Another virus that can create mucosal alterations in HIV-infected patients is human papilloma virus (HPV). This virus induces a nonneoplastic epithelial hyperplasia that may be single or multiple. The resultant lesions present as sessile or pedunculated papules that demonstrate a pebbly surface or a highly papillary configuration. The labial mucosa, buccal mucosa, tongue, and gingiva are affected most frequently. In patients not infected with HIV, most oral HPV-related lesions are associated with types 2, 6, 11, 16, and 18. In contrast, patients with concurrent HPV and HIV infection reveal unusual types, often 7 and 32. On occasion, cytopathologic atypia is present within these HPV-related lesions and is thought to have malignant potential. Assured removal (surgery, cautery, laser, cryotherapy, etc.) is the therapy of choice, but recurrence is common as long as immunosuppression is present. One investigation suggests combined immunotherapy with interferon beta, and thymostimulin aids resolution in patients with AIDS.

## Figure 4.61
### ACQUIRED IMMUNODEFICIENCY SYNDROME, HAIRY LEUKOPLAKIA
Diffuse rough white plaque of the left lateral border of the tongue. Lesion will not rub off, and there is no history of cheek or tongue biting. (Courtesy of Dr. Carl Allen.)

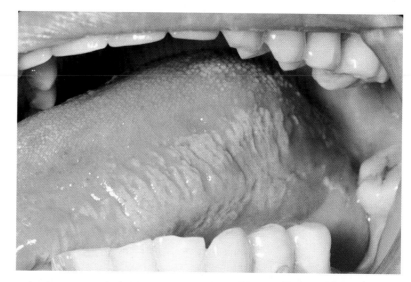

## Figure 4.62
### ACQUIRED IMMUNODEFICIENCY SYNDROME, HUMAN PAPILLOMAVIRUS INFECTION
Multiple nodules of the labial mucosa and vermilion border of the lower lip.

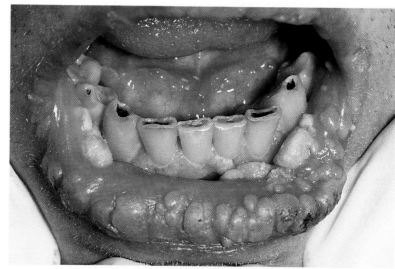

## Figure 4.63
### ACQUIRED IMMUNODEFICIENCY SYNDROME, HUMAN PAPILLOMAVIRUS INFECTION
Multiple sessile nodules of the left posterior buccal mucosa.

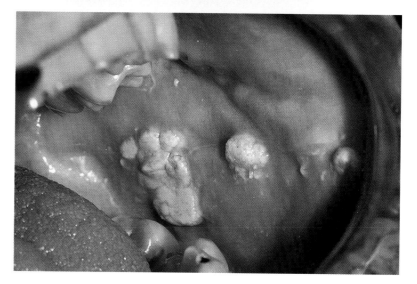

## Figs. 4.64, 4.65, and 4.66

As depicted in the preceding figures, viral infections can produce a variety of clinical presentations. Recently, investigators have discovered herpesviruslike sequences in Kaposi's sarcoma, the most commonly diagnosed malignancy in patients with AIDS. This new human herpesvirus (KSHV/HHV-8) has been detected in both AIDS- and non-AIDS–related Kaposi's sarcoma and seems to be involved in the pathogenesis of this vascular malignancy.

Kaposi's sarcoma represents 80% of all cancers that occur in patients with AIDS and exhibits a marked male predominance, with an increased prevalence in the homosexual/bisexual risk group. The neoplasm presents with oral, skin, or visceral lesions that may occur independently or synchronously. Approximately two-thirds of affected patients demonstrate oral lesions, with these being the initial presentation in greater than 20%. These tumors appear as flat or raised areas of red to purple to brown discoloration that may be confused with a hemangioma or hematoma. With enlargement, oral lesions may be associated with pain, dysphagia, bleeding, difficulty in mastication, and aesthetic concerns.

Kaposi's sarcoma is a progressive malignancy that may disseminate widely to lymph nodes and various organs. The treatment typically is palliative because systemic therapy often aggravates the associated immunosuppression. When used, systemic therapy typically consists of alternating vincristine/vinblastine or etoposide. The oral lesions frequently are a source of major morbidity and often necessitate local therapy. Intralesional injection of vinblastine or sodium tetradecyl sulfate (sclerosing agent), radiation therapy, and laser ablation have been used to minimize problematic oral lesions.

Another malignancy, lymphoma, is the second most common cancer noted in patients with AIDS. In the face of numerous chronic opportunistic infections and the resultant reaction of the remaining immune system, development of lymphoproliferative disorders in AIDS is not surprising. Although most are neoplasms of non-Hodgkin's B cells, T-cell lymphomas and Hodgkin's disease are reported less frequently. Many of these tumors appear to arise from a combination of promotion by Epstein-Barr virus, antigenic stimulation, and immunodysfunction.

In contrast to those without HIV, patients with AIDS who develop lymphoma often have tumors in nonnodal locations. Intraoral involvement is not rare and most frequently presents as a soft-tissue enlargement of the palate/maxillary region, mandible/retromolar trigone, tonsillar pillar/hypopharynx, or tongue. Treatment consists of systemic chemotherapy and radiation, with post-therapeutic survival usually less than 1 year.

### Figure 4.64
**ACQUIRED IMMUNODEFICIENCY SYNDROME, KAPOSI'S SARCOMA**
Bilateral areas of brownish discoloration of the midline of the hard palate. Also note the brown exophytic mass palatal to the maxillary third molar.

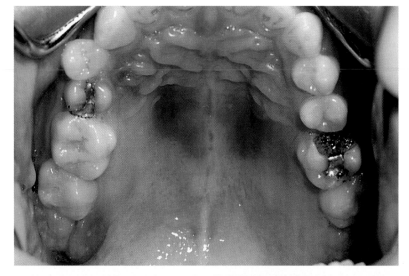

### Figure 4.65
**ACQUIRED IMMUNODEFICIENCY SYNDROME, KAPOSI'S SARCOMA**
Hemorrhagic and exophytic mass of the anterior maxillary gingiva.

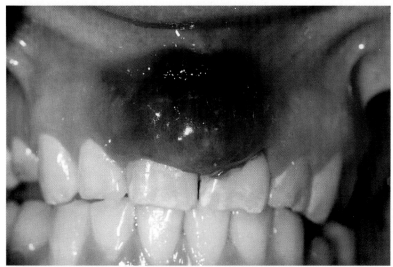

### Figure 4.66
**ACQUIRED IMMUNODEFICIENCY SYNDROME, LYMPHOMA**
Hemorrhagic and exophytic mass of the anterior gingiva.

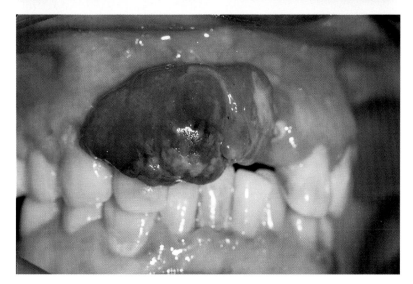

### Impetigo

Bass JW, Chan DS, Creamer KM, et al. Comparison of oral cephalexin, topical mupirocin and topical bacitracin for treatment of impetigo. Pediatr Infect Dis J 1997;16:708.

Darmstadt GL, Lane AT. Impetigo: an overview. Pediatr Dermatol 1994;11:293.

Demidovich CW, Wittler RR, Ruff ME, et al. Impetigo: current etiology and comparison of penicillin, erythromycin and cephalexin therapies. Am J Dis Child 1990;144:1313.

Macko D, Krutchkoff D, Poole A. Oral manifestations of impetigo: report of two cases. J Pedod 1977;1:318.

Shriner DL, Schwartz RA, Janniger CK. Impetigo. Cutis 1995;56:30.

### Cat Scratch Disease

Carithers HA. Cat-scratch disease: an overview based on a study of 1,200 patients. Am J Dis Child 1985;139:1124.

Chen SCA, Gilbert GL. Cat scratch disease: past and present. J Paediatr Child Health 1994;30:467.

Midani S, Ayoub EM, Anderson B. Cat-scratch disease. Adv Pediatr 1996;43:397.

Shenep JL. Cat-scratch disease and *Bartonella henselae* infections in children. Pediatr Ann 1996;25:518.

Smith DL. Cat-scratch disease and related clinical syndromes. Am Fam Physician 1997;55:1783.

Wear DJ, Margileth AM, Hadfield TL, et al. Cat scratch disease: a bacterial infection. Science 1983;221:1403.

Zachariades N, Xypolyta A. Cat scratch disease (report of a case). J Oral Med 1986;41:207.

### Tuberculosis

Eng H-L, Lu S-Y, Yang C-H, et al. Oral tuberculosis. Oral Surg Oral Med Oral Pathol Oral Radiol Endod 1996;81:415.

Fujibayshi T, Takahashi Y, Yoneda T, et al. Tuberculosis of the tongue: a case report with immunologic study. Oral Surg Oral Med Oral Pathol 1979;47:427.

Kolokotronis A, Antoniadis D, Trigonidis G, et al. Oral tuberculosis. Oral Dis 1996;2:242.

Lee KC, Schecter G. Tuberculosis infections of the head and neck. Ear Nose Throat J 1995;74:395.

Mani NJ. Tuberculosis initially diagnosed by asymptomatic oral lesions: report of three cases. J Oral Med 1985;40:39.

Penfold CN, Revington PJ. A review of 23 patients with tuberculosis of the head and neck. Br J Oral Maxillofac Surg 1996;34:508.

Talmi YP, Finkelstein Y, Tov YS, et al. Scrofula revisited. J Laryngol Otol 1988;102:387.

### Noma

Adolph HP, Yugueros P, Woods JE. Noma: a review. Ann Plast Surg 1996;37:657.

Enwonwu CO. Noma: a neglected scourge of children in sub-Saharan Africa. Bull World Health Organ 1995;73:541.

Malden N. An interesting case of adult facial gangrene (from Papua, New Guinea). Oral Surg Oral Med Oral Pathol 1985;59:279.

Uohara GI, Knapp MJ. Oral fusospirochetosis and associated lesions. Oral Surg Oral Med Oral Pathol 1967;24:113.

### Syphilis

Chapel TA. Syphilis: review and update. Compr Ther 1986;12:63.

Dickenson AJ, Currie WJR, Avery BS. Screening for syphilis in patients with carcinoma of the tongue. Br J Oral Maxillofac Surg 1995;33:319.

Fiumara NJ. Venereal diseases of the oral cavity. J Oral Med 1976;31:36.

Mani NJ. Secondary syphilis initially diagnosed from oral lesions. Oral Surg Oral Med Oral Pathol 1984;58:47.

Manton SL, Egglestone SI, Alexander I, et al. Oral presentation of secondary syphilis. Br Dent J 1986;160:237.

Michalek AM, Mahoney MC, McLaughlin CC, et al. Historical and contemporary correlates of syphilis and cancer. Int J Epidemiol 1994;23:381.

Robinson RCV. Congenital syphilis. Arch Dermatol 1969;99:599.

Seigel MA. Syphilis and gonorrhea. Dent Clin North Am 1996;40:369.

## Actinomycosis

Balatsouras DG, Kaberos AK, Eliopoulos PN, et al. Cervicofacial actinomycosis presenting as acute upper respiratory tract. J Laryngol Otol 1994;108:801.

Bennhoff DF. Actinomycosis: diagnostic and therapeutic considerations and a review of 32 cases. Laryngoscope 1984;94:1198.

Benoliel R, Asquith J. Actinomycosis of the jaws. Int J Oral Surg 1985;14:195.

Gupta DS, Gupta MK. Mandibular osteomyelitis by *Actinomyces israelii*. J Maxillofac Surg 1986;14:291.

Nagler R, Peled M, Laufer D. Cervicofacial actinomycosis: a diagnostic challenge. Oral Surg Oral Med Oral Pathol Oral Radiol Endod 1997;83:652.

Stenhouse D, MacDonald DG, MacFarland TW. Cervico-facial and intra-oral actinomycosis: a 5-year retrospective study. Br J Oral Surg 1975;13:172.

## Cellulitis and Ludwig's Angina

Bullock JD, Fleishman JA. The spread of odontogenic infections to the orbit: diagnosis and management. J Oral Maxillofac Surg 1985;43:749.

Dierks EJ, Meyerhoff WL, Schultz B, et al. Fulminant infections of odontogenic origin. Laryngoscope 1987;97:271.

Moreland LW, Corey J, McKenzie R. Ludwig's angina: report of a case and review of the literature. Arch Intern Med 1988;148:461.

Owens BM, Schuman NJ. Ludwig's angina. Gen Dent 1994;42:84.

Pynn BR, Sands T, Pharoah MJ. Odontogenic infections, I: anatomy and radiology. Oral Health 1995;85:7.

Spitalnic SJ, Sucov A. Ludwig's angina: case report and review. J Emerg Med 1994;13:499.

Zeitoun IM, Dhanarajani PJ. Cervical cellulitis and mediastinitis caused by odontogenic infections: report of two cases and review of literature. J Oral Maxillofac Surg 1995;53:203.

## Proliferative Periostitis

Eversole LR, Leider AS, Corwin JO, et al. Proliferative periostitis of Garré: its differentiation from other neoperiostoses. J Oral Surg 1979;37:725.

Kawai T, Murakami S, Sakuda M, et al. Radiographic investigation of mandibular periostitis ossificans in 55 cases. Oral Surg Oral Med Oral Pathol Oral Radiol Endod 1996;82:704.

Nortjé CJ, Wood RE, Grotepass F. Periostitis ossificans versus Garrè's osteomyelitis, II: radiologic analysis of 93 cases in the jaws. Oral Surg Oral Med Oral Pathol 1988;66:249.

Van Doorne L, Soubry R, Wackens G, et al. Periostitis ossificans. Acta Stomatologica Belgica 1995;92:131.

Wood RE, Nortjé CJ, Grotepass F, et al. Periostitis ossificans versus Garrè's osteomyelitis, I: what did Garrè really say? Oral Surg Oral Med Oral Pathol 1988;65:773.

## Osteomyelitis

Calhoun KH, Shapiro RD, Stiernberg CM. Osteomyelitis of the mandible. Arch Otolaryngol Head Neck Surg 1988;114:1157.

Kaneda T, Minami M, Ozawa K, et al. Magnetic resonance imaging of osteomyelitis in the mandible: comparative study with other radiologic modalities. Oral Surg Oral Med Oral Pathol Oral Radiol Endod 1995;79:634.

Koorbusch GF, Fotos P, Terhark K. Retrospective assessment of osteomyelitis: etiology, demographics, risk factors, and management in 35 cases. Oral Surg Oral Med Oral Pathol 1992;74:149.

Marx RE. Chronic osteomyelitis of the jaws. Oral Maxillofac Clin North Am 1991;3:367.

Rohlin M. Diagnostic value of bone scintigraphy in osteomyelitis of the mandible. Oral Surg Oral Med Oral Pathol 1993;75:650.

Schuknecht BF, Carls FR, Valavanis A, et al. Mandibular osteomyelitis: evaluation and staging in 18 patients, using magnetic resonance imaging, computed tomography and conventional radiographs. J Craniomaxillofac Surg 1997;25:24.

## Osteoradionecrosis

Carlson ER. The radiobiology, treatment, and prevention of osteoradionecrosis of the mandible. Recent Results Cancer Res 1994;134:191.

Curi MM, Dib LL. Osteoradionecrosis of the jaws: a retrospective study of the background factors and treatment in 104 cases. J Oral Maxillofac Surg 1997;55:540.

Epstein J, van der Meij E, McKenzie M, et al. Postradiation osteonecrosis of the mandible: a long-term follow-up study. Oral Surg Oral Med Oral Pathol Oral Radiol Endod 1997;83:657.

Friedman RB. Osteoradionecrosis: causes and prevention: consensus development conference on oral complications of cancer therapies: diagnosis, prevention, and treatment. NCI Monogr 1990;9:159.

Kluth EV, Jain PR, Stuchell RN, et al. A study of factors contributing to the development of osteoradionecrosis of the jaws. J Prosthet Dent 1988;59:194.

Marx RE, Johnson RP. Studies in the radiobiology of osteoradionecrosis and their clinical significance. Oral Surg Oral Med Oral Pathol 1987;64:379.

van Merkesteyn JPR, Bakker DJ, Borgmeijer-Hoelen AMMJ, et al. Hyperbaric oxygen treatment of osteoradionecrosis of the mandible: experience in 29 patients. Oral Surg Oral Med Oral Pathol Oral Radiol Endod 1995;80:12.

Wood GA, Liggins SJ. Does hyperbaric oxygen have a role in the management in osteoradio-necrosis? Br J Oral Maxillofac Surg 1996;34:424.

## Candidiasis

Allen CM. Diagnosing and managing oral candidiasis. J Am Dent Assoc 1992;123:77.

Dreizen S. Oral candidiasis. Am J Med 1984;77:28.

Ferretti GA, Ash RC, Brown AT, et al. Chlorhexidine for prophylaxis against oral infections and associated complications in bone marrow transplant patients. J Am Dent Assoc 1987;114:461.

Fotos PG, Ray TL. Oral and perioral candidosis. Semin Dermatol 1994;13:118.

Fotos PG, Vincent SD, Hellstein JW. Oral candidosis: clinical, historical and therapeutic features of 100 cases. Oral Surg Oral Med Oral Pathol 1992;74:41.

Lewis MAO, Samaranayake LP, Lamey P-J. Diagnosis and treatment of oral candidosis. J Oral Maxillofac Surg 1991;49:996.

Quintiliani R, Owens NJ, Quercia RA, et al. Treatment and prevention of oropharyngeal candidiasis. Am J Med 1984;77:44.

Scully C, El-Kabjr M, Samaranayake LP. Candida and oral candidosis: a review. Crit Rev Oral Biol Med 1994;5:125.

Shay K, Truhlar MR, Renner RP. Oropharyngeal candidosis in the older patient. J Am Geriatr Soc 1997;45:863.

## Angular Cheilitis

Dahlen G, Linde A, Moller A, et al. A retrospective study of microbiologic samples from oral mucosal lesions. Oral Surg Oral Med Oral Pathol 1982;53:250.

Dias AP, Samaranayake LP. Clinical, microbiological and ultrastructural features of angular cheilitis lesions in Southern Chinese. Oral Dis 1995;1:43.

Nevalainen MJ, Narhi TO, Ainamo A. Oral mucosal lesions and oral hygiene habits on the home-living elderly. J Oral Rehabil 1997;24:332.

Öhman S-C, Dahlen G, Moller A, et al. Angular cheilitis: a clinical and microbial study. J Oral Pathol 1986;15:213.

Samaranayake LP, Wilkieson CA, Lamey P-J, et al. Oral disease in the elderly in long-term hospital care. Oral Dis 1995;1:147.

Sweeney MP, Bagg J, Fell GS, et al. The relationship between micronutrient depletion and oral health in geriatrics. J Oral Pathol Med 1994;23:168.

## Median Rhomboid Glossitis

Baughman RA. Median rhomboid glossitis: a developmental anomaly? Oral Surg Oral Med Oral Pathol 1971;31:56.

Brown RS, Krakow AM. Median rhomboid glossitis and a "kissing" lesion of the palate. Oral Surg Oral Med Oral Pathol Oral Radiol Endod 1996;82:472.

Carter LC. Median rhomboid glossitis: review of a puzzling entity. Compend Contin Educ Dent 1990;11:446.

Kessler HP. Median rhomboid glossitis. Oral Surg Oral Med Oral Pathol Oral Radiol Endod 1996;82:360.

Pindborg JJ. Revival of "median rhomboid glossitis"? Oral Surg Oral Med Oral Pathol Oral Radiol Endod 1995;80:2.

Touyz LZG, Peters E. Candidal infection of the tongue with nonspecific inflammation of the palate. Oral Surg Oral Med Oral Pathol 1987;63:304.

van der Waal I, Beemster G, van der Kwast W. Median rhomboid glossitis caused by Candida? Oral Surg Oral Med Oral Pathol 1979;47:31.

Whitaker SB, Singh BB. Cause of median rhomboid glossitis. Oral Surg Oral Med Oral Pathol Oral Radiol Endod 1996;81:379.

## Denture Stomatitis

Arendorf TM, Walker DM. Denture stomatitis: a review. J Oral Rehabil 1987;14:217.

Budtz-Jørgensen E, Mojon P, Banon-Clément JM, et al. Oral candidosis in long-term hospital care: comparison of edentulous and dentate subjects. Oral Dis 1996;2:285.

Jeganathan S, Payne JA, Thean HPY. Denture stomatitis in an elderly edentulous Asian population. J Oral Rehabil 1997;24:468.

Jeganathan S, Thean HPY, Thong KT, et al. A clinical viable index for quantifying denture plaque. Quintessence Int 1996;27:569.

Kobayashi T, Sakuraoka K, Hasegawa Y, et al. Contact dermatitis due to an acrylic dental prosthesis. Contact Dermatitis 1996;35:370.

Morimoto K, Kihara A, Suetsugu T. Clinico-pathological study on denture stomatitis. J Oral Rehabil 1987;14:513.

Neville BW, Damm DD, Allen CM, Bouquot JE. Oral & maxillofacial pathology, Philadelphia: WB Saunders, 1995:166.

## Zygomycosis

Berger CJ, Disque FC, Topazian RG. Rhinocerebral mucormycosis: diagnosis and treatment: report of two cases. Oral Surg Oral Med Oral Pathol 1975;40:27.

Brown OE, Finn R. Mucormycosis of the mandible. J Oral Maxillofac Surg 1986;44:132.

Butugan O, Sanchez TG, Goncalez F, et al. Rhinocerebral mucormycosis: predisposing factors, diagnosis, therapy, complications and survival. Rev Laryngol Otol Rhinol (Bord) 1996;117:53.

Economopoulou P, Laskaris G, Ferekidis E, et al. Rhinocerebral mucormycosis with severe oral lesions: a case report. J Oral Maxillofac Surg 1995;53:215.

Harrill WC, Stewart MG, Lee AG, et al. Chronic rhinocerebral mucormycosis. Laryngoscope 1996;106:1292.

Hauman CHJ, Raubenheimer EJ. Orofacial mucormycosis. Oral Surg Oral Med Oral Pathol 1989;68:624.

Jones AC, Bentsen TY, Freedman PD. Mucormycosis of the oral cavity. Oral Surg Oral Med Oral Pathol 1993;75:455.

Parfey NA. Improved diagnosis and prognosis of mucormycosis: a clinicopathologic study of 33 cases. Medicine 1986;65:113.

Peterson KL, Wang M, Canalis RF, et al. Rhinocerebral mucormycosis: evolution of the disease and treatment options. Laryngoscope 1997;107:855.

Rinaldi MG. Zygomycosis. Infect Dis Clin North Am 1989;3:19.

## Aspergillosis

Falworth MS, Herold J. Aspergillosis of the paranasal sinuses: a case report and radiographic review. Oral Surg Oral Med Oral Pathol Oral Radiol Endod 1996;81:255.

Ferreiro JA, Carlson BA, Cody DT. Paranasal sinus fungus balls. Head Neck 1997;19:481.

Kobayashi A. Asymptomatic aspergillosis of the maxillary sinus associated with foreign body of endodontic origin: report of a case. Int J Oral Maxillofac Surg 1995;24:243.

Lenglinger FX, Krennmair G, Müller-Schelken H, et al. Radiodense concretions in maxillary sinus aspergillosis: pathogenesis and the role of CT densitometry. Eur Radiol 1996;6:375.

Panayiotopoulou M, Freedman PD, Weber F, et al. The synchronous occurrence of aspergillosis and myospherulosis of the maxillary sinus: report of a case with review of the literature. Oral Surg Oral Med Oral Pathol 1987;63:582.

Rowe-Jones JM, Moore-Gillon V. Destructive noninvasive paranasal sinus aspergillosis: component of a spectrum of disease. J Otolaryngol 1994;23:92.

Willinger B, Beck-Mannagetta J, Hirschl AM, et al. Influence of zinc oxide on *Aspergillus* species: a possible cause of local, non-invasive aspergillosis of the maxillary sinus. Mycoses 1996;39:361.

## Histoplasmosis

Boutros HH, van Winckle RB, Evan GA, et al. Oral histoplasmosis masquerading as an invasive carcinoma. J Oral Maxillofac Surg 1995;53:1110.

Gerber ME, Rosdeutscher JD, Seiden AM, et al. Histoplasmosis: the otolaryngologist's perspective. Laryngoscope 1995;105:919.

Ng KH, Siar CH. Review of oral histoplasmosis in Malaysians. Oral Surg Oral Med Oral Pathol Oral Radiol Endod 1996;81:303.

Padhye AA, Pathak AA, Katkar VJ, et al. Oral histoplasmosis in India: a case report and an overview of cases reported during 1968-92. J Med Vet Mycology 1994;32:93.

Toth BB, Frame RR. Oral histoplasmosis: diagnostic complication and treatment. Oral Surg Oral Med Oral Pathol 1983;55:597.

Wheat J. Histoplasmosis: recognition and treatment. Clin Infect Dis 1994;19(Suppl 1):S19.

Young LL, Dolan CT, Sheridan PJ, et al. Oral manifestations of histoplasmosis. Oral Surg Oral Med Oral Pathol 1972;33:191.

## Blastomycosis

Bell WA, Gamble J, Garrington GE. North American blastomycosis with oral lesions. Oral Surg Oral Med Oral Pathol 1969;28:914.

Bradsher RW. Blastomycosis. Clin Infect Dis 1992;14(Suppl):S82.

Kauffman CA. Role of azoles in antifungal therapy. Clin Infect Dis 1996;22 (Suppl):S148.

Page LR, Drummond JF, Daniel HT, et al. Blastomycosis with oral lesions: report of two cases. Oral Surg Oral Med Oral Pathol 1979;47:157.

Reder PA, Neel B. Blastomycosis in otolaryngology: review of a large series. Laryngoscope 1993;103:53.

Rose HD, Gingrass DJ. Localized oral blastomycosis mimicking actinomycosis. Oral Surg Oral Med Oral Pathol 1982;54:12.

## Mumps

Cheek JE, Baron R, Atlas H, et al. Mumps outbreak in a highly vaccinated school population. Arch Pediatr Adolesc Med 1995;149:774.

Cochi SL, Preblud SR, Orenstein WA. Perspectives on the relative resurgence of mumps in the United States. Am J Dis Child 1988;142, 499.

Manson AL. Mumps orchitis. Urology 1990;36:355.

McAnally T. Parotitis: clinical presentation and management. Postgrad Med 1982;71:87.

Meyer C, Cotton RT. Salivary gland disease in children: a review, I: acquired non-neoplastic disease. Clin Pediatr 1986;25:314.

Nussinovitch M, Volovitz B, Varsano I. Complications of mumps requiring hospitalization in children. Eur J Pediatr 1995;154:732.

## Herpes Simplex Infections

Acosta EP, Fletcher CV. Valacyclovir. Ann Pharmacother 1997;31:185.

Amir J, Harel L, Smetana Z, et al. Treatment of herpes simplex gingivostomatitis with aciclovir in children: a randomized double blind placebo controlled trial. BMJ 1997;314:1800.

Axéll T, Liedholm R. Occurrence of recurrent herpes labialis in an adult Swedish population. Acta Odontol Scand 1990;48:119.

Cohen SG, Greenberg MS. Chronic oral herpes simplex virus infection in immunocompromised patients. Oral Surg Oral Med Oral Pathol 1985;59:465.

Epstein JB, Scully C. Herpes simplex virus in immunocompromised patients: growing evidence of drug resistance. Oral Surg Oral Med Oral Pathol 1991;72:47.

Epstein JB, Sherlock C, Page JL, et al. Clinical study of herpes simplex virus infection in leukemia. Oral Surg Oral Med Oral Pathol 1990;70:38.

Erlich KS, Mills J, Chatis P, et al. Acyclovir-resistant herpes simplex virus infections in patients with the acquired immunodeficiency syndrome. N Engl J Med 1989;320:293.

Feder HM, Long SS. Herpetic whitlow: epidemiology, clinical characteristics, diagnosis and treatment. Am J Dis Child 1983;137:861.

Kinghorn GR. Long-term suppression with oral acyclovir of recurrent herpes simplex infections in otherwise healthy patients. Am J Med 1988;85(Suppl 2A):26.

Lamey P-J, Biagioni PA. Thermographic resolution of the prodromal phase of herpes labialis treated with acyclovir. Dentomaxillofac Radiol 1995;24:201.

Luber AD, Flaherty JF Jr. Famciclovir for treatment of herpesvirus infections. Ann Pharmacother 1996;30:978.

Macphail L, Greenspan D. Herpetic gingivostomatitis in a 70-year old man. Oral Surg Oral Med Oral Pathol Oral Radiol Endod 1995;79:50.

Main DMG. Acute herpetic stomatitis: referrals to Leeds Dental Hospital 1978-1987. Br Dent J 1989;166:14.

Mechant VA, Molinari JA, Sabes WR. Herpetic whitlow: report of a case with multiple recurrences. Oral Surg Oral Med Oral Pathol 1983;55:568.

Perna JJ, Eskinazi DP. Treatment of oro-facial herpes simplex infection with acyclovir: a review. Oral Surg Oral Med Oral Pathol 1988;65:689.

Poland JM. Current therapeutic management of recurrent herpes labialis. Gen Dent 1994;42:46.

Pottage JC Jr, Kessler HA. Herpes simplex virus resistance to acyclovir: clinical relevance. Infect Agent Dis 1995;4:115.

Raborn GW, McGaw WT, Grace M, et al. Herpes labialis treatment with acyclovir 5% modified aqueous cream: a double-blind randomized trial. Oral Surg Oral Med Oral Pathol 1989;67:676.

Raborn GW, McGaw WT, Grace M, et al. Treatment of herpes labialis with acyclovir: review of three clinical trials. Am J Med 1988;85:39.

Schwandt NW, Mjos DP, Lubow RM. Acyclovir and the treatment of herpetic whitlow. Oral Surg Oral Med Oral Pathol 1987;64:255.

Scully C. Orofacial herpes simplex virus infections: current concepts in the epidemiology, pathogenesis, and treatment, and disorders in which the virus may be implicated. Oral Surg Oral Med Oral Pathol 1989;68:701.

Spruance SL, Rea TL, Thoming C, et al. Penciclovir cream for the treatment of herpes simplex labialis: a randomized, multicenter, double-blind, placebo-controlled trial. JAMA 1997;277:1374.

Stein GE. Pharmacology of new antiherpes agents: famciclovir and valacyclovir. J Am Pharm Assoc (Wash) 1997;NS37:157–163.

Weathers DR, Griffin JW. Intraoral ulcerations of recurrent herpes simplex and recurrent aphthae: two distinct clinical entities. J Am Dent Assoc 1970;81:81.

Worrall G. Acyclovir in recurrent herpes labialis: justified as oral prophylaxis only in severely affected people. BMJ 1996;312:6.

## Varicella-Zoster Viral Infections

Arvin AM. Varicella-zoster virus: overview and clinical manifestations. Semin Dermatol 1996;15(Suppl 1):4.

Badger GR. Oral signs of chickenpox (varicella): report of two cases. J Dent Child 1980;47:349.

Balfour HH Jr. Clinical aspects of chickenpox and herpes zoster. J Int Med Res 1994;22(Suppl 1):3A.

Balfour HH Jr, Kelly JM, Suarez JM, et al. Acyclovir treatment of varicella in otherwise healthy children. J Pediatr 1990;116:633.

Chiodo F, Manfredi R, Antonelli P, et al. Varicella in immunocompetent children in the first two years of life: role of treatment with oral acyclovir: Italian Acyclovir-Chickenpox Study Group. J Chemother 1995;7:62.

Choo DCA, Chew SK, Tan EH. Oral acyclovir in the treatment of adult varicella. Ann Acad Med Singapore 1995;24:316.

Dunkle LM, Arvin AM, Whitley RJ, et al. A controlled trial of acyclovir for chickenpox in normal children. N Engl J Med 1991;325:1539.

Gershon AA. Epidemiology and management of postherpetic neuralgia. Semin Dermatol 1996;15(Suppl 1):8.

Jackson JL, Gibbons R, Meyer G, et al. The effect of treating herpes zoster with oral acyclovir in preventing postherpetic neuralgia. Arch Intern Med 1997;157:909.

Markovitis E, Gilhar A. Capsaicin–an effective topical treatment in pain. Int J Dermatol 1997;36:40.

Mostofi R, Marchmost-Robinson H, Freije S. Spontaneous tooth exfoliation and osteonecrosis following a herpes zoster infection of the fifth cranial nerve. J Oral Maxillofac Surg 1987;45:264.

Nally FF, Ross IH. Herpes zoster of the oral and facial structures. Oral Surg Oral Med Oral Pathol 1971;32:221.

Stein GE. Pharmacology of new antiherpes agents: famciclovir and valacyclovir. J Am Pharm Assoc (Wash) 1997;NS37:157.

Straus SE, Ostrove JM, Inchauspe G, et al. NIH conference: varicella-zoster virus infections: biology, natural history, treatment and prevention. Ann Intern Med 1988;108:221.

Tyring SK. Efficacy of famciclovir in the treatment of herpes zoster. Semin Dermatol 1996;15(Suppl 1):27.

White CJ, Stinson D, Staehle B, et al. Measles, mumps, rubella, and varicella combination vaccine: safety and immunogenicity alone and in combination with other vaccines given to children: Measles, Mumps, Rubella, Varicella Vaccine Study Group. Clin Infect Dis 1997;24:925.

Wood MJ, Kay R, Dworkin RH, et al. Oral acyclovir therapy accelerates pain resolution in patients with herpes zoster: a meta-analysis of placebo-controlled trials. Clin Infect Dis 1996;22:341.

## Enterovirus Infections

Bârlean L, Avram G, Pavlov E, et al. Investigation of five cases of vesicular enteroviral stomatitis with exanthema induced by Coxsackie A5 virus. Rev Roum Virol 1994;45:1.

Buchner A. Hand, foot and mouth disease. Oral Surg Oral Med Oral Pathol 1976;41:333.

Huebner RJ, Cole RM, Bell JA, et al. Herpangina: etiological studies of a specific infectious disease. JAMA 1951;145:628.

Nakayama T, Urano T, Osano M, et al. Outbreak of herpangina associated with coxsackievirus B3 infection. Pediatr Infect Dis 1989;8:495.

Robinson CR, Doane FW, Rhodes AJ. Report of an outbreak of febrile illness with pharyngeal lesions and exanthem. Can Med Assoc J 1958;79:615.

Steigman AJ, Lipton MM, Braspennickx H. Acute lymphonodular pharyngitis: a newly described condition due to Coxsackie A virus. J Pediatr 1962;61:331.

Tindall JP, Callaway JL. Hand-foot-mouth disease—it's more common than you think. Am J Dis Child 1972;124:372.

White JM, Fairley CK, Owen D, et al. Epidemiological, virological, and clinical features of an epidemic of hand, foot, and mouth disease in England and Wales. Commun Dis Rep CDR Rev 1996;6:R81.

Yamadera S, Yamashita K, Kato N, et al. Herpangina surveillance in Japan, 1982-1989. Jpn J Med Sci Biol 1991;44:29.

## Acquired Immunodeficiency Syndrome (AIDS)

Carbone A, Vaccher E, Barzan L, et al. Head and neck lymphomas associated with human immunodeficiency virus infection. Arch Otolaryngol Head Neck Surg 1995;121:210.

Castro KG, Ward JW, Slutsker L, et al. 1993 revised classification system for HIV infection and expanded surveillance case definition for AIDS among adolescents and adults. MMWR Morb Mortal Wkly Rep 1993;4(RR-17):1.

Ceballos-Salobreña A, Aguirre-Urizar JM, Bagan-Sebastian JV. Oral manifestations associated with human immunodeficiency virus infection in a Spanish population. J Oral Pathol Med 1996;25:523.

Chang Y, Cesarman E, Pessin MS, et al. Human herpesvirus-like DNA sequences in AIDS-associated Kaposi's sarcoma. Science 1994;266:1865.

Dodd CL, Greenspan D, Schiødt M, et al. Unusual oral presentation of non-Hodgkin's lymphoma in association with HIV infection. Oral Surg Oral Med Oral Pathol 1992;73:603.

EC-Clearinghouse on Oral Problems Related to HIV Infection and WHO Collaborating Centre on Oral Manifestations of the Immunodeficiency Virus. Classification and diagnostic criteria for oral lesions in HIV infection. J Oral Pathol Med 1993;22:289.

Eisenberg E, Krutchkoff D, Yamase H. Incidental oral hairy leukoplakia in immunocompetent persons: report of two cases. Oral Surg Oral Med Oral Pathol 1992;74:332.

Epstein JB, Scully C. HIV infection: clinical features and treatment of thirty-three homosexual men with Kaposi's sarcoma. Oral Surg Oral Med Oral Pathol 1991;71:38.

Epstein JB, Sherlock CH, Wolber RA. Hairy leukoplakia after bone marrow transplantation. Oral Surg Oral Med Oral Pathol 1993;75:690.

Epstein JB, Silverman S Jr. Head and neck malignancies associated with HIV infection. Oral Surg Oral Med Oral Pathol 1992;73:193.

Eversole LR. Viral infections of the head and neck among HIV-seropositive patients. Oral Surg Oral Med Oral Pathol 1992;73:155.

Ficarra G, Shillitoe EJ. HIV-related infection of the oral cavity. Crit Rev Oral Biol Med 1992;3:207.

Flaitz CM, Jin Y-T, Hicks MJ, et al. Kaposi's sarcoma-associated herpesvirus-like DNA sequences (KSHV/HHV-8) in oral AIDS-Kaposi's sarcoma: a PCR and clinicopathologic study. Oral Surg Oral Med Oral Pathol Oral Radiol Endod 1997;83:259.

Flaitz CM, Nichols CM, Hicks MJ, et al. Herpesviridae-associated persistent mucocutaneous ulcers in acquired immunodeficiency syndrome: a clinicopathologic study. Oral Surg Oral Med Oral Pathol Oral Radiol Endod 1996;81:433.

Frega A, di Renzi F, Stentella P, et al. Management of human papilloma virus vulvo-perineal infection with systemic beta-interferon and thymostimulin in HIV-positive patients. Int J Gynaecol Obstet 1994;44:255–258.

Gowdey G, Lee RK, Carpenter WM. Treatment of HIV-related hairy leukoplakia with podophyllum resin 25% solution. Oral Surg Oral Med Oral Pathol 1995;79:64.

Green TL, Eversole LR. Oral lymphomas in HIV-infected patients: association with Epstein-Barr virus DNA. Oral Surg Oral Med Oral Pathol 1989;67:437.

Greenspan D, deVilliers EM, Greenspan GS, et al. Unusual HPV types in oral warts in association with HIV infection. J Oral Pathol 1988;17:482.

Greenspan D, Greenspan JS. Significance of oral hairy leukoplakia. Oral Surg Oral Med Oral Pathol 1992;73:151.

Greenspan D, Greenspan JS, Hearst NG, et al. Relation of oral hairy leukoplakia to infection with the human immunodeficiency virus and the risk of developing AIDS. J Infect Dis 1987;155:475.

Heinic GS, Stevens DA, Greenspan D, et al. Fluconazole-resistant Candida in AIDS patients: report of two cases. Oral Surg Oral Med Oral Pathol 1993;76:711.

Lozado-Nur F, de Sanz S, Silverman S, et al. Intraoral non-Hodgkin's lymphoma in seven patients with acquired immunodeficiency syndrome. Oral Surg Oral Med Oral Pathol Oral Radiol Endod 1996;82:173.

Lucatorto FM, Sapp JP. Treatment of oral Kaposi's sarcoma with a sclerosing agent in AIDS patients: a preliminary study. Oral Surg Oral Med Oral Pathol 1993;75:192.

MacPhail LA, Greenspan D, Feigal DW, et al. Recurrent aphthous ulcers in association with HIV infection: description of ulcer types and analysis of T-lymphocyte subsets. Oral Surg Oral Med Oral Pathol 1991;71:678.

MacPhail LA, Greenspan D, Greenspan JS. Recurrent aphthous ulcers in association with HIV infection: diagnosis and treatment. Oral Surg Oral Med Oral Pathol 1992;73:283.

McCarthy GM. Host factors associated with HIV-related oral candidiasis: a review. Oral Surg Oral Med Oral Pathol 1992;73:181.

Muzyka BC, Glick M. Major aphthous ulcers in patients with HIV disease. Oral Surg Oral Med Oral Pathol 1994;77:116.

Phelan JA, Eisig S, Freedman PD, et al. Major aphthous-like ulcers in patients with AIDS. Oral Surg Oral Med Oral Pathol 1991;71:68.

Phelan JA, Saltzman BR, Friedland GH, et al. Oral findings in patients with acquired immunodeficiency syndrome. Oral Surg Oral Med Oral Pathol 1987;64:50.

Piluso S, Ficarra G, Lucatorto FM, et al. Cause of oral ulcers in HIV-infected patients: a study of 19 cases. Oral Surg Oral Med Oral Pathol Oral Radiol Endod 1996;82:166.

Regezi JA, Greenspan D, Greenspan JS, et al. HPV-associated epithelial atypia in oral warts in HIV+ patients. J Cutan Pathol 1994;21:217.

Reichart PA, Weigel D, Schmidt-Westhausen A, et al. Exfoliative cheilitis (EC) in AIDS: association with *Candida* infection. J Oral Pathol Med 1997;26:290.

Riley C, London JP, Burnmeister JA. Periodontal health in 200 HIV-positive patients. J Oral Pathol Med 1992;21:124.

Scully C, Laskaris G, Pindborg J, et al. Oral manifestations of HIV infection and their management, I: more common lesions. Oral Surg Oral Med Oral Pathol 1991;71:158.

Scully C, Laskaris G, Pindborg J, et al. Oral manifestations of HIV infection and their management, II: less common lesions. Oral Surg Oral Med Oral Pathol 1991;71:167.

Silverman S Jr. AIDS update: oral findings, diagnosis, and precautions. J Am Dent Assoc 1987;115:559.

Silverman S Jr, Migliorati CA, Lozada-Nur F, et al. Oral findings in people with or at high risk for AIDS: a study of 375 homosexual males. J Am Dent Assoc 1986;112:187.

Smith GLF, Felix DH. Current classification of HIV-associated periodontal diseases. Br Dent J 1993;174:102.

Swindells S, Durham T, Johansson SL, et al. Oral histoplasmosis in a patient infected with HIV: a case report. Oral Surg Oral Med Oral Pathol 1994;77:126.

Volter C, He Y, Delius H, et al. Novel HPV types present in oral papillomatous lesions from patients with HIV infection. Int J Cancer 1996;66:453.

Warnakulasuriya KAAS, Harrison JD, Johnson NW, et al. Localised oral histoplasmosis lesions associated with HIV infection. J Oral Pathol Med 1997;26:294.

Winkler JR, Robertson PB. Periodontal disease associated with HIV infection. Oral Surg Oral Med Oral Pathol 1992;73:145.

# chapter 5
# PHYSICAL AND CHEMICAL INJURIES

**Fig. 5.1**

Linea alba is a grayish-white line that occurs along the buccal mucosa at the level of the occlusal plane. The lesion is typically bilateral. Although few studies have been done, linea alba is common, with one investigation finding a prevalence of 13% in a sample of 256 young adults. Linea alba is probably related to frictional trauma along the occlusal plane and may be associated with negative intraoral pressure that pulls the buccal mucosa between the upper and lower teeth. It does not seem to be related to rough cusps or insufficient horizontal overlap of the teeth. The white appearance is probably created by hyperkeratosis of the epithelium. The lesion is totally benign and no treatment is necessary.

## MORSICATIO BUCCARUM (CHEEK-BITING)

**Fig. 5.2**

Morsicatio buccarum is a self-inflicted injury in which a patient habitually chews or sucks on the buccal mucosa. The habit is often a conscious one, although it may be subconscious in some individuals. The mucosa exhibits a grayish-white macerated or parchment appearance that is characterized by irregular areas of flaky desquamation and small erosions. The lesions are confined to areas that can be reached by the teeth. The condition is often bilateral and may also involve the lips (morsicatio labiorum) and lateral tongue (morsicatio linguarum). The condition is benign and usually no treatment is indicated except to try to motivate the patient to discontinue the habit. In some cases, a modified maxillary occlusal splint can be fabricated to cover the teeth and prevent the trauma.

## SUBMUCOSAL HEMORRHAGE (PETECHIA, ECCHYMOSIS, HEMATOMA)

**Fig. 5.3**

Intraoral hemorrhage is caused by rupture of blood vessels, which may occur secondary to trauma, surgery, or some form of bleeding diathesis. A petechia is a nonraised, pinpoint area of bleeding, whereas an ecchymosis is a larger, nonelevated area of hemorrhage. A hematoma is a localized collection of extravasated blood within a tissue space that produces clinical swelling (-oma is Greek for swelling). Submucosal hemorrhage is most often reddish-purple but also may appear blue or bluish-black. Because the blood is free within the soft tissues, it should not blanch when compressed. In some instances, hemorrhagic lesions may be a sign of an underlying bleeding diathesis, such as hemophilia, leukemia, thrombocytopenia, or anticoagulant therapy. Most areas of hemorrhage will organize with granulation tissue and resolve without treatment. Large hematomas may have to be surgically incised and drained.

### Figure 5.1
**LINEA ALBA**
Elevated white line along the occlusal plane.

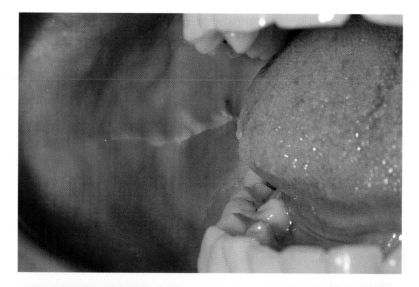

### Figure 5.2
**MORSICATIO BUCCARUM**
Macerated appearance of buccal mucosa in areas where the teeth can reach it.

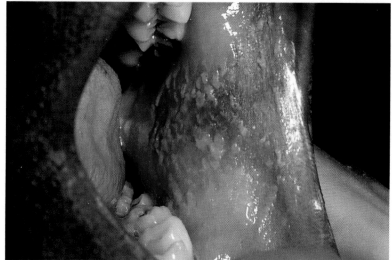

### Figure 5.3
**SUBMUCOSAL HEMORRHAGE**
Diffuse area of ecchymosis on the buccal mucosa after a tooth extraction. (Courtesy of Dr. Robert Gellin.)

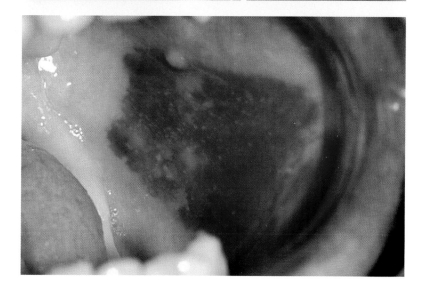

## Figs. 5.4, 5.5, and 5.6

Trauma-induced ulcerations of the oral cavity are frequently encountered by the clinician. The most common source of ulcers is probably self-induced trauma in which the patient inadvertently bites the buccal mucosa, lip, or tongue. Other causes include ill-fitting dentures, jagged teeth, toothbrush trauma, accidents, and iatrogenic injuries such as those that may occur during a dental or surgical procedure. Usually, traumatic ulcers can be readily diagnosed by their clinical features and history. They will usually heal within several weeks if the source of the irritation is removed. An ulcer that fails to heal will usually require biopsy to rule out the possibility of malignancy.

The clinician should always bear in mind the possibility of a self-inflicted injury as a symptom of underlying emotional disturbance. In such cases, patients may purposefully and secretly injure themselves to seek out medical or dental care (Munchausen syndrome). Such behavior may result from a desire for attention and sympathy or to obtain drugs. Psychiatric counseling is usually necessary in these cases.

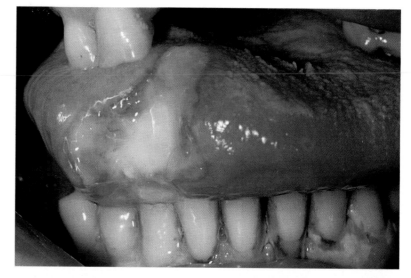

▶ **Figure 5.4**
**TRAUMATIC ULCER**
Ulcer of the tongue secondary to intubation for surgery.

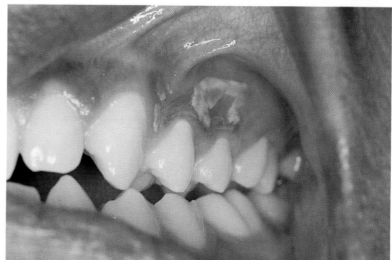

▶ **Figure 5.5**
**COTTON ROLL ULCER**
Gingival lesion caused by removal of dry cotton roll adherent to the mucosa.

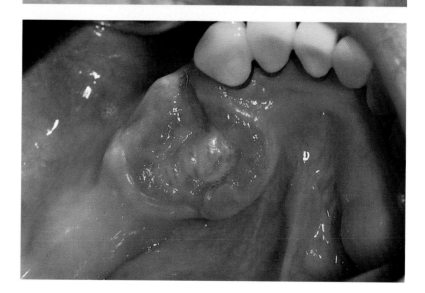

▶ **Figure 5.6**
**FACTITIAL ULCER**
Chronic ulceration of the mandibular alveolar ridge secondary to self-induced trauma.

PHYSICAL AND CHEMICAL INJURIES

# TRAUMATIC GRANULOMA (TRAUMATIC ULCERATIVE GRANULOMA WITH STROMAL EOSINOPHILIA, EOSINOPHILIC ULCER OF THE ORAL MUCOSA, RIGA-FEDE DISEASE)

**Fig. 5.7**

Some traumatic ulcerations of the oral mucosa are associated with a more florid and pseudoinvasive inflammatory reaction that extends deeper into the fibrous connective tissue and underlying skeletal muscle. This inflammatory infiltrate characteristically includes numerous eosinophils and histiocytes. These lesions are known by a variety of names, including traumatic granuloma, traumatic ulcerative granuloma with stromal eosinophilia, and eosinophilic ulcer. Riga-Fede disease (see Fig. 2.22) represents a distinctive form of traumatic granuloma in infants that occurs on the anterior ventral tip of the tongue secondary to trauma from the primary mandibular incisor teeth during feeding. Traumatic granulomas tend to be slow to resolve and, therefore, may be difficult to distinguish from carcinoma. For this reason, biopsy is often indicated to establish the diagnosis and promote healing. In infants with Riga-Fede disease, extraction of the anterior primary teeth is not recommended. Discontinuation of nursing or use of a protective shield will usually allow the lesion to resolve.

## ANESTHETIC NECROSIS

**Fig. 5.8**

On rare occasions, focal tissue necrosis may be produced at the site of injection of local anesthetics. The most common location for such lesions is the hard palate, where the mucosal tissues are tightly bound to the underlying bone. Usually such lesions present as well-circumscribed, punched-out ulcers that appear within a few days of the injection. The ulcer is created by ischemic necrosis that is probably induced by the direct trauma of the anesthetic solution being injected into the tissues, vasoconstriction from epinephrine in the anesthetic, or both. The ulcer often takes several weeks to heal and sometimes becomes chronic. Local stimulus, such as a cytologic smear, may be sufficient to induce healing in these cases.

## SOFT-TISSUE EMPHYSEMA

**Fig. 5.9**

Soft-tissue emphysema is a rare phenomenon in which air or gas is introduced into the soft tissues. In the orofacial region, soft-tissue emphysema most often is associated with the use of an air syringe or air-driven turbine handpiece with which air is forcefully blown into a surgical site, laceration, or salivary gland duct. Other possible causes include trauma, violent coughing, Valsalva maneuvers, and playing wind instruments. The introduced air may dissect along tissue planes, producing a sudden swelling. The presence of crepitation, or a crackling sound on palpation, is a helpful clinical sign. Emphysema in the neck can spread downward and produce a pneumomediastinum. Patients with soft-tissue emphysema should be treated with antibiotics to prevent secondary infection. Most cases resolve in 1 to 2 weeks.

**Figure 5.7**
**TRAUMATIC GRANULOMA**
Large, irregular area of ulceration on the tongue.

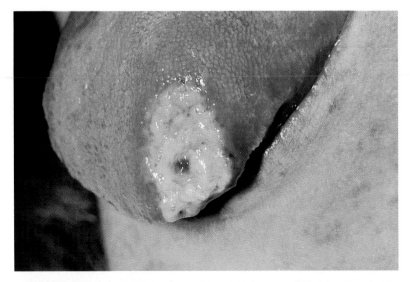

**Figure 5.8**
**ANESTHETIC NECROSIS**
Site of a palatal injection.

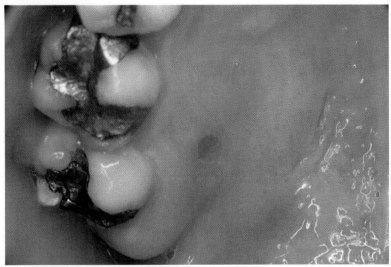

**Figure 5.9**
**SOFT-TISSUE EMPHYSEMA**
Facial and periorbital swelling caused by air-driven handpiece used during third molar removal.

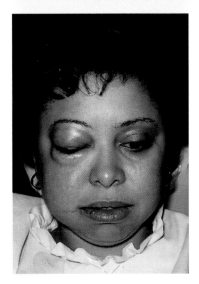

PHYSICAL AND CHEMICAL INJURIES

## Figs. 5.10, 5.11, and 5.12

Burns of the oral mucous membranes may be caused by injudicious use of a variety of drugs and chemical agents. The most common of these is the aspirin burn produced when a patient unwisely uses an aspirin tablet or aspirin powders topically for relief of a toothache. Usually the patient will place the aspirin in the buccal or labial sulcus so it can be held directly against the painful tooth. As it dissolves, a painful white area of epithelial necrosis is produced, which may slough off and leave a raw, red, bleeding ulceration. We have seen similar burns produced by the use of over-the-counter medications for toothaches and by other innovative topical home remedies such as rubbing alcohol, hydrogen peroxide, ice, and gasoline. Iatrogenic burns also can be produced by a variety of agents used in dentistry and medicine, such as silver nitrate, phenol, and eugenol. Treatment for oral chemical burns consists of elimination of the causative agent to allow normal healing to occur.

▶ **Figure 5.10**
**ASPIRIN BURN**
White lesion of buccal mucosa.

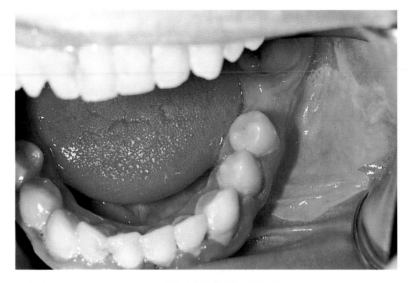

▶ **Figure 5.11**
**RUBBING ALCOHOL BURN**
White lesion of buccal mucosa.

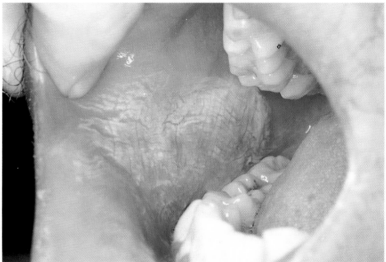

▶ **Figure 5.12**
**CHEMICAL BURN**
This patient repeatedly applied Anbesol to treat a toothache.

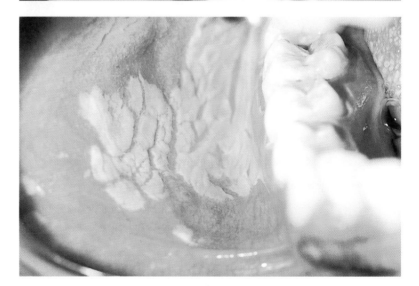

**Figs. 5.13 and 5.14**

The amalgam tattoo is a common pigmented lesion of the oral mucosa caused by the inadvertent introduction of dental amalgam particles into the soft tissues. Such lesions may be produced in several different ways: (1) during placement of a silver amalgam restoration, particles may be condensed into abraded gingiva or deposited in an accidental laceration of the mucosa; (2) during removal of old amalgam restorations, particles may be deposited in accidental lacerations or forcefully propelled through intact mucosa by high-speed drills; (3) during root canal therapy with a retrograde amalgam, particles may be incorporated into the surgical wound; or (4) during tooth extraction, fragments of amalgam restoration may fall into the tooth socket.

Clinically, amalgam tattoos present as macular areas of pigmentation that are usually described as gray, blue, or black. Most are less than 1 cm in size, but occasionally they can be quite large. The most common sites are the gingiva, alveolar mucosa, and buccal mucosa. Small radiopaque flecks may be visible on radiographs in some cases, but often the radiographic results will be negative because of the small size of the amalgam particles. Diagnosis usually can be made on a clinical basis, but biopsy may be necessary for unusual cases. Amalgam tattoos of the anterior gingiva may be aesthetically displeasing and may require surgical removal with gingival grafting. One recent report also documents the successful use of a Q-switched ruby laser for the treatment of an amalgam tattoo of the anterior maxillary gingiva.

## SMOKER'S MELANOSIS

**Fig. 5.15**

Individuals who smoke may develop benign areas of hyperpigmentation of the oral mucosa. Depending on the number of cigarettes smoked daily, as many as 31% of smokers may develop clinically visible areas of melanin pigmentation. Smoker's melanosis is seen more often in females and most frequently affects the anterior mandibular and maxillary gingiva. However, virtually any oral site may be affected. The pigmentation varies from light to dark brown and may appear diffuse or be more localized in nature. The diagnosis often can be made by correlating the smoking history with the clinical presentation of the lesions. However, biopsy should be considered for pigmented lesions in unusual locations, such as the hard palate, or for pigmented lesions with an unusual clinical appearance. Smoker's melanosis usually will disappear gradually during a 3-year period after cessation of smoking.

**Figure 5.13**
**AMALGAM TATTOO**
Bluish-gray pigmentation in the alveolar mucosa.

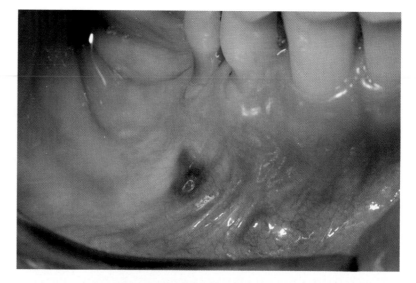

**Figure 5.14**
**AMALGAM TATTOO**
Grayish-black pigmentation in the floor of the mouth. (Courtesy of Dr. Brian Blocher.)

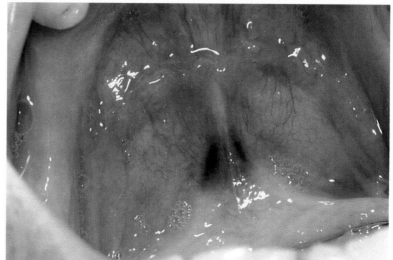

**Figure 5.15**
**SMOKER'S MELANOSIS**
Diffuse pigmentation of the maxillary facial gingiva.

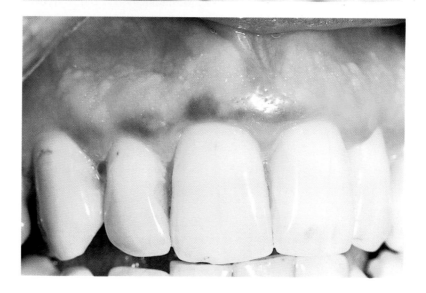

## ANTIMALARIAL PIGMENTATION

### Fig. 5.16

In addition to their use in the treatment of malaria, antimalarial drugs such as quinacrine, chloroquine, hydroxychloroquine, and amodiaquine have found widespread use in the treatment of rheumatoid arthritis, lupus erythematosus, and other skin disorders. One of the occasional side effects of these drugs is the development of hyperpigmented lesions of the oral mucosa, usually on the hard palate. This pigment usually is described as gray or bluish-black, often with a sharp line of demarcation at the junction of the unaffected soft palate. The nail beds and conjunctiva also may be affected, and a yellow pigmentation may occur on the skin. Similar pigmentation also has been reported in association with quinidine, a chemically similar drug used to treat patients with cardiac arrhythmia.

## TRAUMATIC LESIONS FROM OROGENITAL SEX

### Figs. 5.17 and 5.18

The practice of orogenital sex is common today, both in the form of fellatio (oral stimulation of the penis) and cunnilingus (oral stimulation of the female genitals). During the course of these sexual practices, traumatic lesions may occur to the oral mucosa. Fellatio may result in erythematous, petechial, or ecchymotic lesions near the junction of the hard and soft palate. It is theorized that such lesions are the result of direct trauma, negative pressure, or both, resulting in hemorrhage in the tissues. Differential diagnosis includes prodromal mononucleosis, upper respiratory infections, hemorrhagic disorders, and other types of suction trauma. The area usually resolves in 7 to 10 days.

During cunnilingus, traumatic ulceration may occur on the midportion of the lingual frenum as the tongue is protruded forward and rubbed over the lower incisor teeth. These lingual ulcers usually heal within 1 week, although chronic trauma may lead to fibrous hyperplasia. Similar ulcers can occur in patients after otolaryngologic examination, when the tongue is pulled out as far as possible to allow examination of the pharynx and larynx.

*COLOR ATLAS OF CLINICAL ORAL PATHOLOGY*

## Figure 5.16
### ANTIMALARIAL PIGMENTATION
Palatal hyperpigmentation secondary to chloroquine therapy. (Courtesy of Giansanti JS, Tillery DE, Olansky S. Oral mucosal pigmentation resulting from antimalarial therapy. Oral Surg Oral Med Oral Pathol 1971;31:66.)

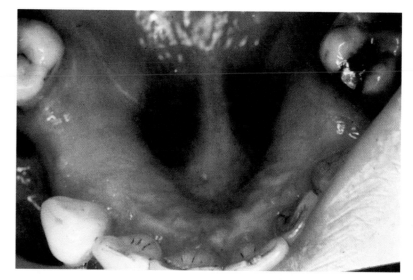

## Figure 5.17
### PALATAL ECCHYMOSIS SECONDARY TO FELLATIO
(Courtesy of Damm DD, White DK, Brinker CM. Variations of palatal erythema secondary to fellatio. Oral Surg Oral Med Oral Pathol 1981;52:417.)

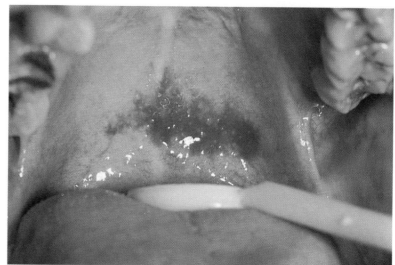

## Figure 5.18
### TRAUMA FROM CUNNILINGUS
Repeated irritation led to hyperkeratinized fibrous hyperplasia of the lingual frenum.

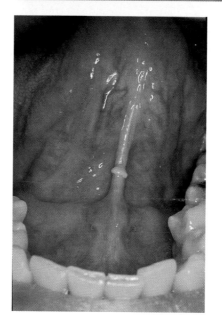

## PSEUDOCYST OF THE MAXILLARY SINUS (SINUS MUCOCELE)

**Fig. 5.19**

The pseudocyst of the maxillary sinus appears as a dome-shaped, homogeneous radiopacity arising from the floor of the sinus. Such lesions are common, having been found radiographically in 1.5 to 10.0% of the population. The terms "sinus mucocele" and "retention cyst" have been used for this entity; however, these terms are inaccurate because the lesion is not related to mucin accumulation but is most likely inflammatory in origin. (True sinus mucoceles and retention cysts can occur in the maxillary sinus but are much less common.) The pseudocyst represents an accumulation of fluid below the periosteum of the floor of the sinus that results in separation and elevation of the sinus mucosal lining from the bony wall. The fluid appears to be an inflammatory exudate that may on occasion represent extension of adjacent dental infection, for which the patient should be evaluated. Generally, the patient will have no symptoms. The lesion often regresses on its own, and no treatment is necessary in most cases.

## EFFECTS OF RADIATION THERAPY

**Figs. 5.20 and 5.21**

Radiation therapy is used widely for the treatment of oral and paraoral malignancies and often is associated with transient or permanent side effects. One of the first manifestations is the development of oral erythema and edema, which may occur within the first 2 weeks of therapy. As treatment continues, the mucosa becomes ulcerated and covered by a fibrinoid exudate. The mouth is quite painful, making eating difficult and contributing to nutritional impairment. Radiation mucositis will persist throughout therapy, but it typically resolves several weeks after treatment is completed.

Patients who receive radiation therapy also develop xerostomia secondary to the direct effect on salivary glands in the fields of irradiation. The degree of xerostomia is related to the dose and ports of radiation, and it may be permanent. This alteration of salivary flow may later contribute to the development of xerostomia-related caries or "radiation caries," a rampant form of tooth decay occurring at the cervical margins of the teeth. Other side effects associated with oral radiotherapy include loss of taste, trismus, candidiasis, possible development of osteoradionecrosis (see Figures 4.17 and 4.18), and arrested development of teeth (see Figure 2.7).

Caring for the patient who receives radiation therapy can be complex and requires a multidisciplinary approach involving a radiation oncologist, a general dentist, an oral and maxillofacial surgeon, and a dental hygienist. All patients who are to receive radiation therapy to the head and neck should have a dental consultation as soon as possible before the onset of therapy. At this time, nonsalvageable teeth can be removed, oral foci of infection treated, dental prophylaxis performed, and oral hygiene instructions emphasized. During and after the radiation therapy, oral management often includes oral rinses and antibiotics to treat mucositis; saliva substitutes and sialogogues to treat xerostomia; frequent prophylaxis and topical fluoride applications to prevent caries and periodontal disease; and exercises to prevent trismus.

COLOR ATLAS OF CLINICAL ORAL PATHOLOGY

### ▶ Figure 5.19
### PSEUDOCYST OF THE MAXILLARY SINUS
Dome-shaped, radiopaque lesion of the floor of the sinus.

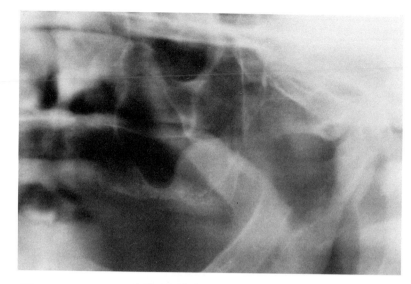

### ▶ Figure 5.20
### RADIATION MUCOSITIS
Painful ulceration of the tongue. (Courtesy of Dr. Rich Daniel.)

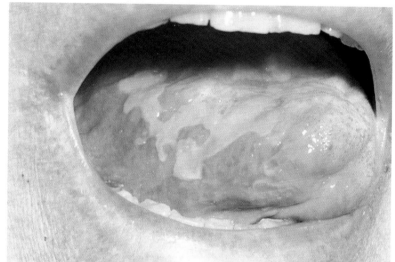

### ▶ Figure 5.21
### XEROSTOMIA-RELATED CARIES
Extensive cervical decay in a patient with previous radiation therapy of the head and neck.

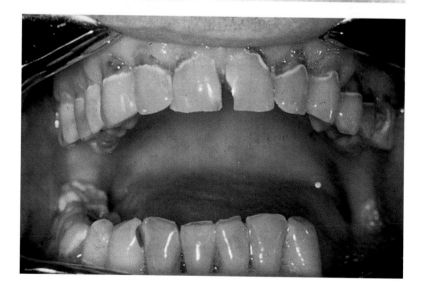

# SUGGESTED READINGS

## Linea Alba

Kashani HG, Mackenzie IC, Kerber PE. Cytology of linea alba using a filter imprint technique. Clin Prevent Dent 1980;2:21.

Neville BW, Damm DD, Allen CM, Bouquot JE. Oral & maxillofacial pathology. Philadelphia: WB Saunders, 1995:211.

## Morsicatio Buccarum

Hjørting-Hansen E, Holst E. Morsicatio mucosae oris and suctio mucosae oris: an analysis of oral mucosal changes due to biting and sucking habits. Scand J Dent Res 1970;78:492.

Van Wyk CW, Staz J, Farman AG. The chewing lesion of the cheeks and lips: its features and prevalence among a selected group of adolescents. J Dent 1977;5:193.

Walker RS, Rogers WA. Modified maxillary occlusal splint for prevention of cheek biting: a clinical report. J Prosthet Dent 1992;67:581.

## Submucosal Hemorrhage

Neville BW, Damm DD, Allen CM, Bouquot JE. Oral & maxillofacial pathology. Philadelphia: WB Saunders, 1995:223.

Wood NK, Goaz PW. Differential diagnosis of oral and maxillofacial lesions. 5th ed. St. Louis: CV Mosby, 1997:187.

## Traumatic Ulcers

Blanton PL, Hurt WC, Largent MD. Oral factitious injuries. J Periodontol 1977;48:33.

Fusco MA, Freedman PD, Black SM, et al. Munchausen's syndrome: report of case. J Am Dent Assoc 1986;112:210.

Heasman PA, MacLeod I, Smith DG. Factitious gingival ulceration: a presenting sign of Munchausen's syndrome? J Periodontol. 1994;65:442.

## Traumatic Granuloma

El-Mofty SK, Swanson PE, Wick MR, et al. Eosinophilic ulcer of the oral mucosa: report of 38 new cases with immunohistochemical observations. Oral Surg Oral Med Oral Pathol 1993;75:716.

Elzay RP. Traumatic ulcerative granuloma with stromal eosinophilia (Riga-Fede's disease and traumatic eosinophilic granuloma). Oral Surg Oral Med Oral Pathol 1983;55:497.

Mezei MM, Tron VA, Stewart WD, et al. Eosinophilic ulcer of the oral mucosa. J Am Acad Dermatol 1995;33:734.

## Anesthetic Necrosis

Carroll MJ. Tissue necrosis following a buccal infiltration. Br Dent J 1980;149:209.

Giunta J, Tsamsouris A, Cataldo E, et al. Postanesthetic necrotic defect. Oral Surg Oral Med Oral Pathol 1975;40:590.

## Soft-Tissue Emphysema

Horowitz I, Hirshberg A, Freedman A. Pneumomediastinum and subcutaneous emphysema following surgical extraction of mandibular third molars: three case reports. Oral Surg Oral Med Oral Pathol 1987;63:25.

Oliver AJ, Diaz EM, Helfrick JF. Air emphysema secondary to mandibular fracture: case report. J Oral Maxillofac Surg 1993;51:1143.

Sansevere JJ, Badwal RS, Najjar TA. Cervical and mediastinal emphysema secondary to mandible fracture: case report and review of the literature. Int J Oral Maxillofac Surg 1993;22:278.

Spaulding CR. Soft tissue emphysema. J Am Dent Assoc 1979;98:587.

Takenoshita Y, Kawano Y, Oka M. Pneumoparotis, an unusual occurrence of parotid gland swelling during dental treatment: report of a case with a review of the literature. J Craniomaxillofac Surg 1991;19:362.

## Chemical Burns

Baruchin AM, Lustig JP, Nahlieli O, et al. Burns of the oral mucosa: report of 6 cases. J Craniomaxillofac Surg 1991;19:94.

Kawashima Z, Flagg RH, Cox DE. Aspirin-induced oral lesion: report of case. J Am Dent Assoc 1975;91:130.

Maron FS. Mucosal burn resulting from chewable aspirin: report of case. J Am Dent Assoc 1989;119:279.

## Amalgam Tattoo

Ashinoff R, Tanenbaum D. Treatment of an amalgam tattoo with the Q-switched ruby laser. Cutis 1994;54:269.

Buchner A, Hansen LS. Amalgam pigmentation (amalgam tattoo) of the oral mucosa: a clinicopathologic study of 268 cases. Oral Surg Oral Med Oral Pathol. 1980;49:139.

Owens BM, Johnson WW, Schuman NJ. Oral amalgam pigmentations (tattoos): a retrospective study. Quintessence Int 1992;23:805.

Weathers DR, Fine RM. Amalgam tattoo of oral mucosa. Arch Dermatol 1974;110:727.

## Smoker's Melanosis

Axéll T, Hedin CA. Epidemiologic study of excessive oral melanin pigmentation with special reference to the influence of tobacco habits. Scand J Dent Res 1982;90:434.

Brown FH, Houston GD. Smoker's melanosis: a case report. J Periodontol 1991;62:524.

Hedin CA. Smoker's melanosis: occurrence and localization in the attached gingiva. Arch Dermatol 1977;113:1533.

Hedin CA, Axéll T. Oral melanin pigmentation in 467 Thai and Malaysian people with special emphasis on smoker's melanosis. J Oral Pathol Med 1991;20:8.

Hedin CA, Pindborg JJ, Axéll T. Disappearance of smoker's melanosis after reducing smoking. J Oral Pathol Med 1993;22:228.

## Antimalarial Pigmentation

Birek C, Main JHP. Two cases of oral pigmentation associated with quinidine therapy. Oral Surg Oral Med Oral Pathol 1988;66:59.

Giansanti JS, Tillery DE, Olansky S. Oral mucosal pigmentation resulting from antimalarial therapy. Oral Surg Oral Med Oral Pathol 1971;31:66.

## Traumatic Lesions From Orogenital Sex

Damm DD, White DK, Brinker CM. Variations of palatal erythema secondary to fellatio. Oral Surg Oral Med Oral Pathol 1981;52:417.

Giansanti JS, Cramer JR, Weathers DR. Palatal erythema: another etiologic factor. Oral Surg Oral Med Oral Pathol 1975;40:379.

Mader CL. Lingual frenum ulcer resulting from orogenital sex. J Am Dent Assoc 1981;103:888.

## Pseudocyst of the Maxillary Sinus

Allard RHB, van der Kwast WAM, van der Waal I. Mucosal antral cysts: review of the literature and report of a radiographic survey. Oral Surg Oral Med Oral Pathol. 1981;51:2.

Casamassimo PS, Lilly GE. Mucosal cysts of the maxillary sinus: a clinical and radiographic study. Oral Surg Oral Med Oral Pathol 1980;50:282.

Gardner DG. Pseudocysts and retention cysts of the maxillary sinus. Oral Surg Oral Med Oral Pathol 1984;58:561.

Halstead CL. Mucosal cysts of the maxillary sinus: report of 75 cases. J Am Dent Assoc 1973;87:1435.

MacDonald A, Newton CW. Pseudocyst of the maxillary sinus. J Endod 1993;19:618.

## Effects of Radiation Therapy

Al-Joburi, W, Clark DC, Fisher R. A comparison of the effectiveness of two systems for the prevention of radiation caries. Clin Prevent Dent 1991;13:15.

Al-Tikriti U, Martin MV, Bramley PA. A pilot study of the clinical effects of irradiation on the oral tissues. Br J Oral Maxillofac Surg 1984;22:77.

Fleming TJ. Oral tissue changes of radiation-oncology and their management. Dent Clin North Am 1990;34:223.

Jansma J, Vissink A, Spijkervet FKL, et al. Protocol for the prevention and treatment of oral sequelae resulting from head and neck radiation therapy. Cancer 1992;70:2171.

Rubin RL, Doku HC. Therapeutic radiology—the modalities and their effects on oral tissues. J Am Dent Assoc 1976;92:731.

Schuller DE, Stevens, P, Clausen KP, et al. Treatment of radiation side effects with oral pilocarpine. J Surg Oncol 1989;42:272.

# chapter 6

# ALLERGIES AND IMMUNOLOGIC DISEASES

**Figs. 6.1 and 6.2**

Aphthous ulcerations are recurring lesions of the oral cavity and oropharynx and can be classified into three types: minor, major, and herpetiform. Minor aphthous ulcerations are the most common form of the disease and account for 80% of all cases. Minor aphthae arise almost exclusively on nonkeratinized movable mucosa and exhibit yellow fibrinopurulent membranes surrounded by erythematous halos. The ulcerations are typically less than 1 cm in diameter, are usually extremely painful, and tend to heal without scarring. Most patients have from one to five ulcerations during each episode. The lesions arise quickly, heal within 10 to 14 days, and exhibit a highly variable recurrence interval.

The cause of aphthous ulcerations is unknown, but the damage seems to be mediated by both the humoral and the cell-mediated immune systems. What elicits the immune response is unknown and may vary from person to person. Heredity, stress, local trauma, vitamin deficiencies, and food allergens may be responsible in some cases. Bacteria, especially the L-form streptococci, have been implicated by some investigators, and one recent investigation suggests that recurrences may be associated with reactivation of varicella-zoster virus or cytomegalovirus. Increased keratinization of the oral mucosa associated with tobacco use has been known to reduce the prevalence of aphthae.

A variety of therapies have been used in patients with aphthous ulcers. Topical steroid elixirs and gels seem to be the most consistently effective treatments. Levamisole, colchicine, tetracycline rinses, and chlorhexidine gluconate rinses have all been used with variable success. Cautery of the ulcerations with concentrated silver nitrate should be discouraged because of potential significant adverse effects, such as severe localized necrosis.

# RECURRENT MAJOR APHTHOUS ULCERATIONS

**Fig. 6.3**

Major aphthae are recurrent mucosal ulcerations that appear similar to minor aphthae but that tend to be larger, to recur more often, and to take longer to heal. They account for about 10% of all aphthous ulcerations. Major aphthae arise predominantly on movable mucosa and are larger than 1 cm, with many reaching several centimeters, in diameter. Typically, 1 to 10 lesions are present at one time. Because of their larger size, the ulcers may require up to 6 weeks to heal. Many patients are rarely free of ulcerations because of the short recurrence interval and the long healing time. Usual topical corticosteroid treatment is often not as beneficial for patients with major aphthae as for those with minor aphthae. Treatment with higher potency steroid elixirs, intralesional steroids, and systemic steroids has been successful in producing remissions. Despite its potential teratogenic effects, thalidomide has been shown to be effective in treating patients with extremely severe cases of aphthous stomatitis.

### Figure 6.1
**RECURRENT MINOR APHTHOUS ULCERATIONS**

Area of ulceration with surrounding erythema present on movable mucosa of the left maxillary mucobuccal fold.

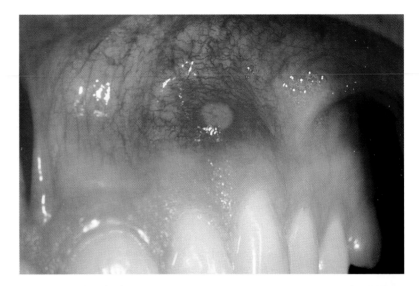

### Figure 6.2
**RECURRENT MINOR APHTHOUS ULCERATIONS**

Two areas of ulceration and erythema located on the mucosa of the anterior maxillary mucolabial fold.

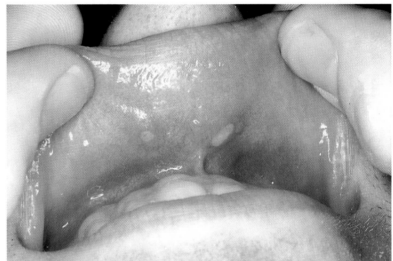

### Figure 6.3
**RECURRENT MAJOR APHTHOUS ULCERATIONS**

Large, deep ulceration of the right lateral soft palate and anterior tonsillar pillar.

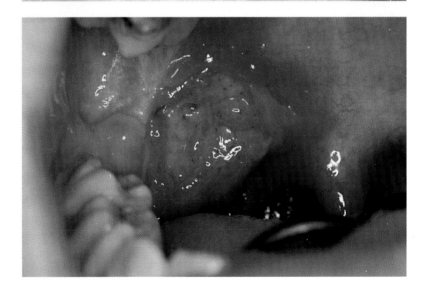

### Figs. 6.4 and 6.5

Herpetiform aphthous ulcerations occur in about 10% of patients with aphthous stomatitis. These ulcers are clinically similar to minor aphthous ulcerations but are typically smaller and occur in greater numbers. The lesions are generally 2 mm or less in size, and outbreaks usually consist of 10 to 100 individual ulcers. These extremely painful, pinhead-sized ulcers tend to cluster and coalesce with time. Any oral mucosal surface may be involved. The clinical presentation is similar to that of primary herpes simplex infection, but the intense gingival erythema is absent and the lesions are recurrent. The cause of these ulcerations is unknown. No virus has been cultured from these ulcers, and biopsy examination fails to reveal the typical cytopathologic effects seen in herpes virus infections. As with all aphthous ulcerations, other conditions that may mimic aphthae should be ruled out. The possibility of Crohn's disease, Behçet's disease, blood dyscrasia, and nutritional deficiency should be investigated. A 2% tetracycline rinse has been used successfully, but it is not effective in all patients and may become ineffective in some patients after a period of use. Topical steroid elixirs and gels are the treatment of choice for temporary remission; as with all aphthae, there is no permanent cure.

## BEHÇET'S DISEASE

### Fig. 6.6

Behçet's disease is included on many authors' lists of aphthous ulcerations because the oral lesions are morphologically indistinguishable from those of typical aphthae. The lesions occur at any oral mucosal site and vary in size from a few millimeters to more than 1 cm. Although oral lesions may occur initially, Behçet's disease historically demonstrates a triple symptom complex of recurrent oral ulcerations, recurrent genital ulcerations, and ocular inflammation. In addition, vasculitis, meningoencephalitis, joint pain, gastrointestinal pain, diarrhea, and skin lesions may be present. The cause of Behçet's disease is unknown, but it seems to have an immunogenetic background because of its strong association with certain HLA types. The disease is most common in Japan and in eastern Mediterranean countries, with a lower prevalence in the United States and northern Europe. Potent topical corticosteroids are often helpful in the management of oral ulcerations. In addition, systemic therapy is often necessary, including the use of colchicine, dapsone, prednisone, methotrexate, azathioprine, or thalidomide.

**▶ Figure 6.4**
**RECURRENT HERPETIFORM APHTHOUS ULCERATIONS**
Multiple pinhead ulcerations with surrounding erythema on the soft palate.

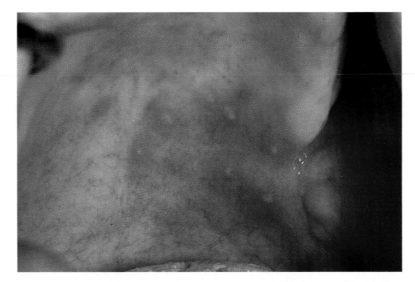

**▶ Figure 6.5**
**RECURRENT HERPETIFORM APHTHOUS ULCERATIONS**
Multiple pinhead ulcerations of the lower labial mucosa.

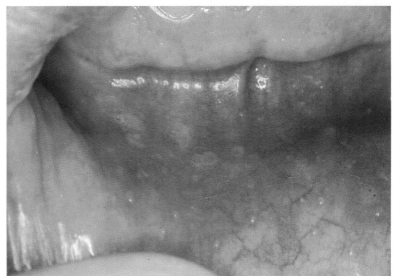

**▶ Figure 6.6**
**BEHÇET'S DISEASE**
Multiple large ulcerations of the right anterior buccal mucosa. The patient has similar genital lesions.

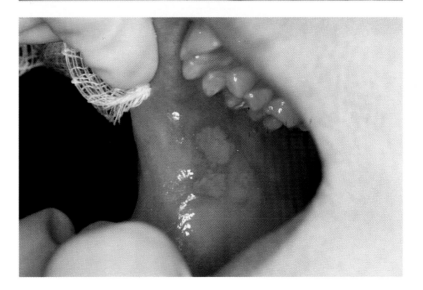

## Figs. 6.7 and 6.8

Wegener's granulomatosis is a multisystem inflammatory disease characterized by necrotizing and granulomatous vasculitis. The classic form of the disease shows a triad of upper respiratory, lower respiratory, and renal lesions, although limited forms of the disease also may be seen. The disease usually has an insidious onset, with clinical symptoms of weight loss, fatigue, and low-grade fever. Upper respiratory involvement is often similar to that of "midline lethal granuloma," being characterized by sinusitis, rhinitis, nasal obstruction, and necrotic, destructive lesions of the nasal and oral cavities. Palatal destruction with resultant oral-nasal communication may occur, but less frequently than in midline lethal granuloma (see Fig. 11.18). The most common oral lesion is a reddish-purple hyperplastic gingivitis, often exhibiting a friable, granular surface with many petechiae (strawberry gingivitis). Alveolar bone loss and tooth mobility may also occur. Granulomatous lesions of the salivary glands may result in parotid gland enlargement. Lung involvement may produce cough and dyspnea, with hemoptysis occurring in rare cases. Skin involvement is seen in about half of the patients, most commonly in the form of ulcerative or papular lesions.

A helpful laboratory marker for the diagnosis of Wegener's granulomatosis is the presence of antineutrophil cytoplasm antibodies. These antibodies are found in more than 90% of patients with acute generalized disease, but they are not always found in those with more limited forms of the disease. Renal failure was formerly a common cause of death, but most patients now have a good prognosis with cyclophosphamide and corticosteroid therapy.

# SARCOIDOSIS

## Fig. 6.9

Sarcoidosis is a disease of unknown cause that presents with multifocal areas of noncaseating granulomatous inflammation. Numerous causes, including mycobacteria, viruses, and a host of different foreign materials, have been suggested. The disease is more common among women and blacks, and the diagnosis is usually made in patients between the ages of 20 and 35 years. The most frequent sites of involvement are the lymph nodes and the lungs. Bilateral hilar lymphadenopathy often is seen on chest radiographs. Violaceous plaques may occur on the skin, and salivary involvement can result in glandular enlargement and xerostomia. Intraoral lesions are rarely seen; when noted, they present as nodular, papular, or granular lesions that may be brownish-red, violaceous, or normal in color. Intrabony granulomatous lesions within the jaws may also occur. Salivary gland biopsy is sometimes performed as a diagnostic aid in suspected cases of sarcoidosis. Elevated levels of angiotensin-converting enzyme (ACE) strongly support the diagnosis.

### Figure 6.7
**WEGENER'S GRANULOMATOSIS**

Palatal ulceration. (Courtesy of Allen CM, Camisa C, Salewski C, et al. Wegener's granulomatosis: report of three cases with oral lesions. J Oral Maxillofac Surg 1991;49:294.)

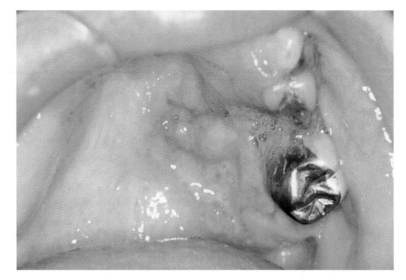

### Figure 6.8
**WEGENER'S GRANULOMATOSIS**

Same patient as in Figure 6.7 exhibiting red, granular gingivitis with petechial hemorrhage. (Courtesy of Allen CM, Camisa C, Salewski C, et al. Wegener's granulomatosis: report of three cases with oral lesions. J Oral Maxillofac Surg 1991;49:294.)

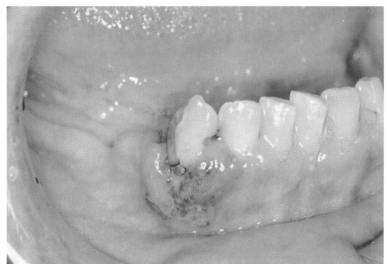

### Figure 6.9
**SARCOIDOSIS**

Multiple papules and plaques on the facial skin around the eyes and nose. (Courtesy of Dr. Marty Burtner.)

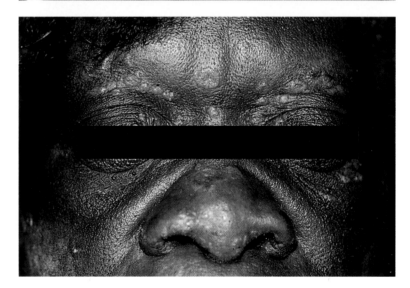

## Figs. 6.10, 6.11, and 6.12

Orofacial granulomatosis is a term used to describe unexplained granulomatous inflammatory lesions of the oral and facial regions. The diagnosis requires exclusion of systemic granulomatous processes that may have oral or facial involvement, including tuberculosis, sarcoidosis, and Crohn's disease. Although the cause is unknown in most instances, some reported cases have been etiologically related to adjacent odontogenic infections or to exposure to certain foods or food additives.

Orofacial granulomatosis is predominantly characterized by recurring episodes of swelling of the mouth and face that may result in permanent enlargement. One of the best known clinical presentations is a diffuse enlargement of one or both lips known as "cheilitis granulomatosa." This enlargement may appear clinically similar to that of angioneurotic edema; however, the swelling is produced not only by edema but also by infiltration of the connective tissue and minor salivary glands by noncaseating granulomatous inflammation. The lip enlargement may be associated with scaling and fissuring of the vermilion border. Some patients may develop swelling, erythema, or erosion of other sites, including the buccal mucosa, palate, or floor of the mouth. Other patterns include granulomatous gingivitis and linear hyperplastic tissue in the mucobuccal fold. If fissured tongue and facial nerve paralysis occur in association with cheilitis granulomatosa, the condition is referred to as "Melkersson-Rosenthal syndrome."

The course of the lesions in orofacial granulomatosis is variable. Exacerbations of the swellings may last from hours to months at a time. Over time, the rate of recurrence and extent of the swellings may gradually diminish, but some degree of permanent enlargement may persist. In any patient with orofacial granulomatosis, systemic granulomatous disease processes, such as Crohn's disease, chronic granulomatous disease, sarcoidosis, and granulomatous infectious diseases, should be ruled out before any treatment.

Treatment of orofacial granulomatosis is often disappointing. The most common treatment consists of intralesional injections of corticosteroids. Systemic steroids have also sometimes been used. Cosmetic surgical reduction of the enlarged tissues has sometimes been performed, but such resections should probably be reserved for those patients whose disease is in a quiescent stage. In cases related to adjacent odontogenic infections or exposure to certain foods, elimination of these causative factors may lead to resolution of the swellings.

**OROFACIAL GRANULOMATOSIS (CHEILITIS GRANULOMATOSA)**

Young adult female exhibiting diffuse, firm enlargement of the upper lip.

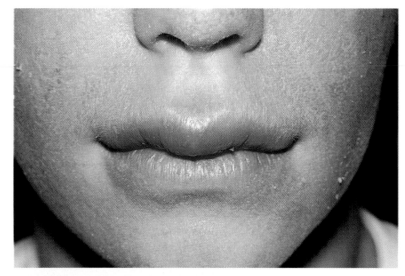

▶ **Figure 6.11**

**MELKERSSON-ROSENTHAL SYNDROME**

Adult male with diffuse enlargement of both lips and right facial paralysis. Note the lack of eyebrow raise and forehead wrinkle on the right side.

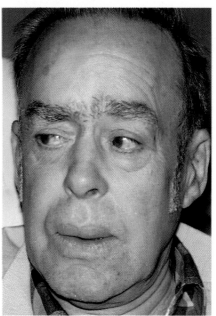

▶ **Figure 6.12**

**MELKERSSON-ROSENTHAL SYNDROME**

Dorsal tongue of the same patient depicted in Figure 6.11. Note the numerous fissures radiating out from the midline.

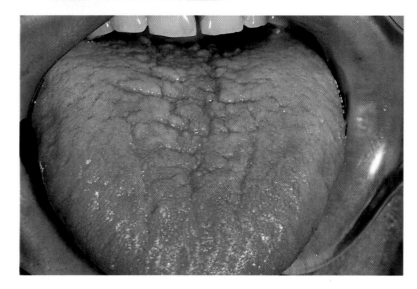

## ALLERGIC DRUG REACTIONS (STOMATITIS MEDICAMENTOSA)

### Fig. 6.13

Allergic mucosal reactions to the administration of systemic drugs are referred to as "stomatitis medicamentosa." A long list of medications is capable of producing such reactions; antibiotics such as penicillin and sulfa drugs are among the more common culprits. Allergic drug reactions can affect any oral site and may appear as areas of erythema and edema, vesiculobullous lesions, or frank ulcerations. Erythema multiforme (see Figures 13.55, 13.56, and 13.57) is one specific pattern that may occur. Anaphylactic reactions can be associated with skin urticaria and life-threatening respiratory difficulties. Allergic mucosal reactions may also clinically and microscopically mimic lichen planus, lupus erythematosus, or pemphigus. The diagnosis of stomatitis medicamentosa requires a careful medical history relating the clinical lesions to the drugs the patient is taking. After consultation with the patient's physician, if the medication can be discontinued, the lesions should resolve. Topical corticosteroids may be helpful in the treatment of localized reactions. Systemic anaphylactic reactions may require administration of epinephrine, corticosteroids, or antihistamines.

## ANGIOEDEMA (ANGIONEUROTIC EDEMA)

### Figs. 6.14 and 6.15

Angioedema is an acute condition characterized by sudden, rapid tissue swelling. Two major categories of angioedema are recognized: hereditary and acquired. Both result in soft-tissue edema, which can arise within a matter of minutes or hours. The lack of pain, heat, and erythema help to rule out an infectious process.

Two rare autosomal-dominant hereditary forms of angioedema are recognized. Type I is caused by a lack of C1 esterase inhibitor of the complement system. Without this important inhibitor, patients are susceptible to massive inflammatory responses because of the unimpeded action of C1, C2, and C4 of the complement system. Type II is characterized by normal levels of C1 esterase inhibitor, but this protein is dysfunctional. Attacks of hereditary angioedema may be frequent and are often precipitated by trauma or stress.

The most common type of acquired angioedema is an IgE-mediated hypersensitivity reaction characterized by mast cell degranulation and associated histamine release. Episodes can be precipitated by a variety of factors, including exposure to various drugs, foods, plants, dust, heat, cold, or emotional stress. Patients using angiotensin-converting enzyme inhibitors can develop a nonallergic form of acquired angioedema because these medications may result in increased levels of bradykinin. Acquired angioedema can also occur in patients with certain lymphoproliferative disorders or in patients who develop autoantibodies to C1 esterase inhibitor. Attacks of acquired angioedema have been reported that were precipitated by dental procedures.

Milder cases of allergic angioedema usually respond well to treatment with oral antihistamines. When tongue, pharyngeal, or laryngeal involvement threatens the airway, parenteral epinephrine therapy is indicated. When the airway is involved, the condition may be life-threatening: the patient may asphyxiate if prompt therapy is not initiated, including intubation or tracheostomy in some instances. Intravenous corticosteroids also may be needed.

Patients with angioedema related to angiotensin-converting enzyme inhibitors or C1 esterase inhibitor deficiency may not respond to treatment with antihistamines, epinephrine, or corticosteroids. Tracheostomy or intubation may be required for patients with laryngeal involvement. C1 esterase inhibitor concentrate and esterase-inhibiting drugs are also used for cases related to C1 esterase inhibitor deficiency. Preventive treatment consists of synthetic androgens to raise C1 esterase inhibitor levels. Before dental surgery, fresh frozen plasma or purified C1 esterase inhibitor can be administered prophylactically.

### Figure 6.13
**ALLERGIC DRUG REACTION**
Diffuse ulceration of the lateral tongue secondary to oxaprozin treatment.

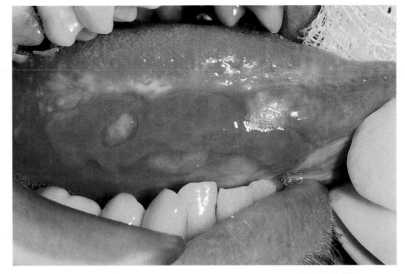

### Figure 6.14
**ANGIOEDEMA**
Diffuse swelling of the lower lip.

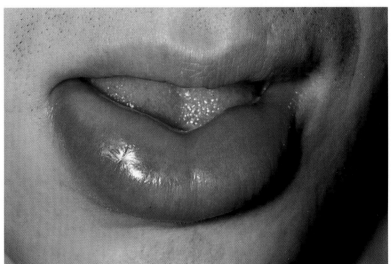

### Figure 6.15
**ANGIOEDEMA**
Same patient as in Figure 6.14 after antihistamine therapy.

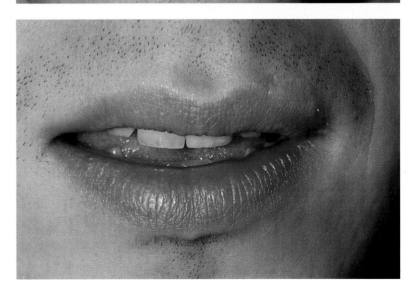

## ALLERGIC CONTACT REACTIONS (STOMATITIS/DERMATITIS VENENATA)

### Figs. 6.16 and 6.17

Contact stomatitis (stomatitis venenata) is an allergic reaction of the oral mucous membranes that arises at the site of exposure to the causative agent. The analogous reaction on the skin is termed "contact dermatitis." The affected area usually appears red and inflamed, sometimes with the formation of vesicles and erosions. Although contact stomatitis is uncommon, a variety of substances may produce such reactions, including toothpastes, mouthrinses, topical drugs, foods, and dental materials. True allergy to dental acrylic is exceedingly uncommon, and some cases of "denture sore mouth" (see Figures 4.25, 4.26, and 4.27) are associated with candidal colonization. Even in examples in which *Candida* cannot be implicated, the reaction may actually be caused by the leaching out of unpolymerized monomer or by denture cleansers and other substances absorbed by the denture base. Treatment for allergic contact reactions consists of elimination of the causative agent and possibly administration of topical corticosteroids.

## EXFOLIATIVE CHEILITIS

### Fig. 6.18

Exfoliative cheilitis is characterized by chronic dryness, scaling, and fissuring of the lip vermilion. In severe cases, the vermilion may be covered by a thickened, yellowish hyperkeratotic crust that can become cracked and hemorrhagic. Both lips or only the lower lip may be involved. Most cases are factitial in origin, being caused by lip licking, biting, picking, or sucking. Many affected patients have an underlying psychological problem or abnormal thyroid function. On occasion, the condition may result from photosensitivity or from a contact allergy to various substances. Secondary candidiasis (cheilocandidiasis) may develop in some cases. In factitial cases, treatment may require psychotherapy with mild tranquilization and reduction of stress. In cases related to contact allergy, identification and elimination of the causative allergen should allow resolution of the lesions. Application of protective moisturizing ointments also may be helpful in some cases.

### Figure 6.16
**CONTACT STOMATITIS TO ACRYLIC**
Mucosal ulceration adjacent to temporary acrylic bridge. The patient developed similar reactions to other temporary acrylic crowns.

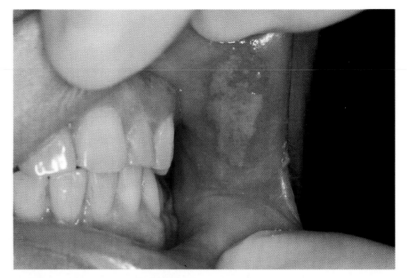

### Figure 6.17
**ALLERGIC CONTACT DERMATITIS**
Marked inflammation of the perioral skin secondary to the use of antibiotic ointment on the lips. (Courtesy of Dr. John LeMaster.)

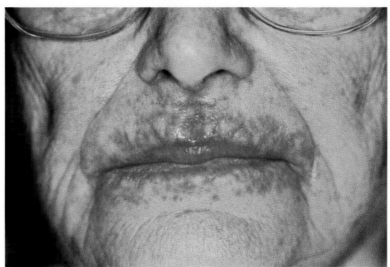

### Figure 6.18
**EXFOLIATIVE CHEILITIS**
Dry, scaly lesions on the lip vermilion.

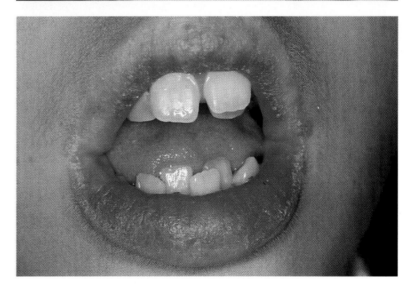

## PERIORAL DERMATITIS

### Fig. 6.19

Perioral dermatitis is a persistent erythematous eruption that is characterized by the development of multiple papules, vesicles, or pustules on the skin around the mouth. Lesions may additionally affect the periorbital areas, the nasolabial folds, the cheeks, the forehead, and the neck. The condition occurs primarily in young women and may be related to acne rosacea.

Perioral dermatitis is most commonly related to the overuse of potent topical corticosteroids. Sometimes such medications are initially prescribed for treatment of a mild skin eruption, or patients may misuse steroid preparations prescribed for another area of the body or for another patient. If the patient tries to stop using the medication, there is often a rebound flare and worsening of the disease. Some cases of perioral dermatitis may be related to the use of topical antibiotics (see Fig. 6.17) or various cosmetics. The use of tartar control toothpastes has also been reported to cause circumoral dermatitis and cheilitis.

The treatment of perioral dermatitis can prove frustrating. Topical steroid use should be discontinued; this often leads to a temporary flaring of the disease, but the lesions should then slowly resolve over several months. Management of the poststeroid flare can be best accomplished using oral tetracycline. Topical metronidazole treatment also may be effective. Dermatitis and cheilitis related to use of topical antibiotics or tartar control toothpaste usually resolve after discontinuation of the offending drug or dentifrice.

## CONTACT STOMATITIS TO CINNAMON FLAVORING

### Figs. 6.20 and 6.21

Cinnamon is a common flavoring agent that frequently results in contact stomatitis. Such reactions are most often associated with chewing cinnamon-flavored gum, but they also may arise in patients who habitually eat candy or use toothpaste or dental floss containing this flavor. Reactions to cinnamon-flavored gum or candy characteristically occur along the bite line of the buccal mucosa and the lateral border of the tongue. The lesions present as irregular white plaques that may occur on an erythematous base. The surface often seems ragged and macerated, being easily confused with morsicatio. Sometimes buccal mucosal lesions exhibit a somewhat lacy, striated appearance that can mimic lichen planus. Lingual lesions may suggest the possibility of hairy leukoplakia or squamous cell carcinoma. The patient often complains of tenderness or burning of the areas but may not associate the symptoms with cinnamon exposure. Cinnamon-flavored toothpastes may result in generalized gingival inflammation that can resemble "plasma cell gingivitis" (see Figure 3.23). Contact reactions to cinnamon are easily managed by discontinuation of the cinnamon-containing product, which typically results in rapid resolution of the lesions.

### Figure 6.19
### PERIORAL DERMATITIS
Erythematous rash of the perioral skin.

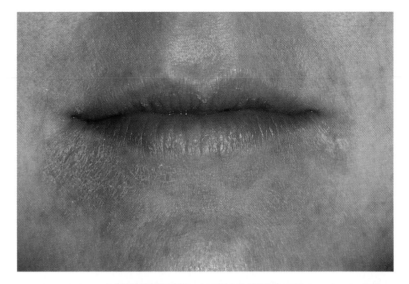

### Figure 6.20
### CONTACT STOMATITIS TO CINNAMON FLAVORING
Mixed white and red lesion of the buccal mucosa along the bite line.

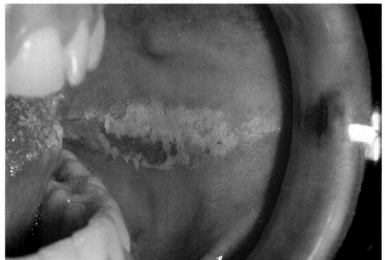

### Figure 6.21
### CONTACT STOMATITIS TO CINNAMON FLAVORING
White lesion of the lateral border of the tongue. Such a lesion could easily be mistaken for leukoplakia or hairy leukoplakia.

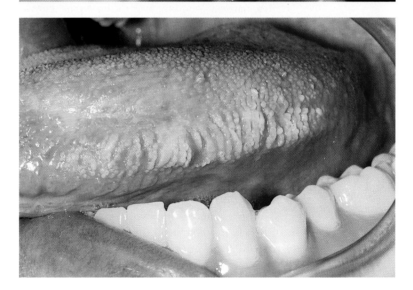

## CONTACT STOMATITIS TO DENTAL AMALGAM

**Fig. 6.22**

Dental amalgam has long been used as a restorative material and rarely produces any significant adverse health effects. However, some patients may develop chronic allergic contact reactions of the oral mucosa to amalgam restorations. Although such reactions were once speculated to be caused by electrogalvanic currents developed between different restorative metals, it is now believed that such lesions are the result of hypersensitivity to one of the metals in the amalgam. Although any of the metals may be responsible, the most frequently suspected is mercury, and some affected patients demonstrate positive results on skin patch tests to mercury. Clinically, these lesions are most common on the posterior buccal mucosa and lateral/ventral surface of the tongue in areas that come into direct contact with large buccal or lingual amalgams. However, sometimes the lesions may involve broader areas of the mucosa that are not in direct contact with the restorations. They present as white, red, or mixed white and red patches that may be asymptomatic or may be associated with erosion and tenderness. Some lesions demonstrate white striations that mimic lichen planus. The microscopic appearance is also lichenoid, and it is probable that many contact amalgam reactions are mistakenly diagnosed as lichen planus. Removal of the offending amalgam(s) should result in resolution or improvement of the lesion.

## GRAFT-VERSUS-HOST DISEASE

**Figs. 6.23 and 6.24**

Graft-versus-host disease (GVHD) is a common complication of allogeneic bone marrow transplantation, a procedure performed to treat such life-threatening diseases as leukemia, aplastic anemia, and metastatic carcinoma. In this procedure, cytotoxic medications and radiation therapy are used to destroy the malignant cells in the body; in doing so, the patient's normal hematopoietic cells are also destroyed. To replace this tissue, the patient must receive a bone marrow transplant from an HLA-matched donor. However, the HLA match is often not exact, and despite the use of immunosuppressive drugs, the transplanted immune cells may recognize that they are in a "foreign" environment and may attack the patient's other tissues, producing GVHD.

Acute GVHD occurs within the first 100 days of transplantation and is characterized by diarrhea, nausea, vomiting, liver dysfunction, skin rash, or sloughing of the skin that resembles toxic epidermal necrolysis. Chronic GVHD may represent a continuation of acute GVHD or may develop later than 100 days after transplantation. The symptoms often mimic one of the autoimmune diseases, such as lupus erythematosus, Sjögren syndrome, or primary biliary cirrhosis. Skin lesions are common and may resemble lichen planus or systemic sclerosis. Oral involvement occurs in 80% of individuals with chronic GVHD. The lesions are most commonly characterized by white plaques and striations of the buccal mucosa, labial mucosa, and tongue that may resemble lichen planus. Tender, eroded areas are not uncommon. Patients also sometimes complain of a generalized burning sensation of the oral mucosa, which must be differentiated from a secondary candidiasis. Xerostomia may occur as a result of salivary gland involvement.

Patients with GVHD are usually already taking potent systemic immunosuppressive medications such as cyclosporine and prednisone. Therefore, any specific treatment of oral lesions of chronic GVHD should be coordinated with the patient's hematologist/oncologist. Use of topical anesthetics can provide temporary relief to facilitate eating, and topical corticosteroid treatment may help promote healing of the oral lesions. Topical cyclosporine A has also been used to treat oral lesions. If xerostomia is present, topical fluoride applications may be indicated to help prevent xerostomia-related caries.

**Figure 6.22**
**CONTACT STOMATITIS TO DENTAL AMALGAM**
White plaque of the posterior buccal mucosa adjacent to a tooth that has a large amalgam extending onto the buccal surface.

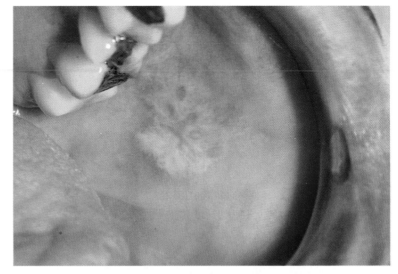

**Figure 6.23**
**CHRONIC GRAFT-VERSUS-HOST DISEASE**
Scaly lesions of the lip vermilion.

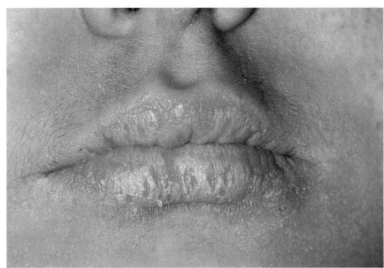

**Figure 6.24**
**CHRONIC GRAFT-VERSUS-HOST DISEASE**
Ulcerated lesion with lichenoid striations on the buccal mucosa.

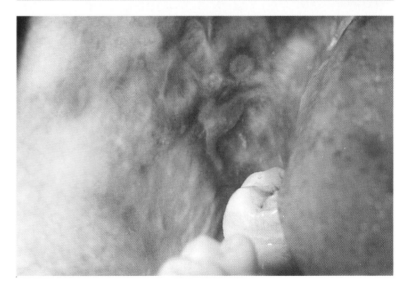

## Aphthous Ulcerations

Brooke RI, Sapp, JP. Herpetiform ulceration. Oral Surg Oral Med Oral Pathol 1976;42:182.

Frost DE, Barkmeier WW, Abrams H. Aphthous ulcer—a treatment complication: report of a case. Oral Surg Oral Med Oral Pathol 1978;45:863.

Pedersen A. Recurrent aphthous ulceration: virological and immunological aspects. APMIS 1993;101(Suppl 37):1.

Pedersen A, Hornsleth A. Recurrent aphthous ulceration: a possible clinical manifestation of reactivation of varicella zoster or cytomegalovirus infection. J Oral Pathol Med 1993;22:64.

Porter SR, Scully C. Aphthous stomatitis: an overview of aetiopathogenesis and management. Clin Exp Dermatol 1991;16:235.

Ship JA. Recurrent aphthous stomatitis: an update. Oral Surg Oral Med Oral Pathol Oral Radiol Endod 1996;81:141.

Vincent SD, Lilly GE. Clinical, historic, and therapeutic features of aphthous stomatitis. Oral Surg Oral Med Oral Pathol 1992;74:79.

## Behçet's Disease

Helm TN, Camisa C, Allen C, et al. Clinical features of Behçet's disease: report of four cases. Oral Surg Oral Med Oral Pathol 1991;72:30.

Jorizzo JL, Abernethy JL, White WL, et al. Mucocutaneous criteria for the diagnosis of Behçet's disease: an analysis of clinicopathologic data from multiple international centers. J Am Acad Dermatol 1995;32:968.

Main DMG, Chamberlain MA. Clinical differentiation of oral ulceration in Behçet's disease. Br J Rheumatol 1992;31:767.

Mangelsdorf HC, White WL, Jorizzo JL. Behçet's disease: report of twenty-five patients from the United States with prominent mucocutaneous involvement. J Am Acad Dermatol 1996;34:745.

Schiffman L, Giansiracusa D, Calabro JJ, et al. Behçet's syndrome. Compr Ther 1986;12:62.

## Wegener's Granulomatosis

Allen CM, Camisa C, Salewski C, et al. Wegener's granulomatosis: report of three cases with oral lesions. J Oral Maxillofac Surg 1991;49:294.

Burlacoff SG, Wong FSH. Wegener's granulomatosis—the great masquerade: a clinical presentation and literature review. J. Otolaryngol 1993;22:94.

Cohen RE, Cardoza TT, Drinnan AJ, et al. Gingival manifestations of Wegener's granulomatosis. J Periodontol 1990;61:705.

Handlers JP, Waterman J, Abrams AM, et al. Oral features of Wegener's granulomatosis. Arch Otolaryngol 1985;111:267.

Hansen LS, Silverman S, Pons VG, et al. Limited Wegener's granulomatosis: report of a case with oral, renal, and skin involvement. Oral Surg Oral Med Oral Pathol 1985;60:524.

Lustmann J, Segal N, Markitziu A. Salivary gland involvement in Wegener's granulomatosis: a case report and review of the literature. Oral Surg Oral Med Oral Pathol 1994;77:254.

Patten SF, Tomecki KJ. Wegener's granulomatosis: cutaneous and oral mucosal disease. J Am Acad Dermatol 1993;28:710.

## Sarcoidosis

Blinder D, Yahatom R, Taicher S. Oral manifestations of sarcoidosis. Oral Surg Oral Med Oral Pathol Oral Radiol Endod 1997;83:458.

Hildebrand J, Plezia RA, Rao SB. Sarcoidosis: report of two cases with oral involvement. Oral Surg Oral Med Oral Pathol 1990;69:217.

Mandel L, Kaynar A. Sialadenopathy—a clinical herald of sarcoidosis: report of two cases. J Oral Maxillofac Surg 1994;52:1208.

Marx RE, Hartman KS, Rethman KV. A prospective study comparing incisional labial to incisional parotid biopsies in the detection and confirmation of sarcoidosis, Sjögren's disease, sialosis and lymphoma. J Rheumatol 1988;15:621.

Nessan VJ, Jacoway JR. Biopsy of minor salivary glands in the diagnosis of sarcoidosis. N Engl J Med 1979;301:922.

Steinberg MJ, Mueller DP. Treating oral sarcoidosis. J Am Dent Assoc 1994;125:76.

## Orofacial Granulomatosis

Oliver AJ, Rich AM, Reade PC, et al. Monosodium glutamate-related orofacial granulomatosis. Oral Surg Oral Med Oral Pathol 1991;71:560.

Sakuntabhai A, MacLeod RI, Lawrence CM. Intralesional steroid injection after nerve block anesthesia in the treatment of orofacial granulomatosis. Arch Dermatol 1993;129:477.

Wiesenfeld D, Ferguson MM, Mitchell DN, et al. Oro-facial granulomatosis: a clinical and pathological analysis. Q J Med 1985;54:101.

Worsaae N, Christensen KC, Schiødt M, et al. Melkersson-Rosenthal syndrome and cheilitis granulomatosa: a clinicopathologic study of thirty-three patients with special reference to their oral lesions. Oral Surg Oral Med Oral Pathol 1982;54:404.

Zimmer WM, Rogers RS III, Reeve CM, et al. Orofacial manifestations of Melkersson-Rosenthal syndrome. Oral Surg Oral Med Oral Pathol 1992;74:610.

## Allergic Drug Reactions

Felder RS, Millar SB, Henry RH. Oral manifestations of drug therapy. Spec Care Dent 1988;8:119.

Matthews TG. Medication side effects of dental interest. J Prosthet Dent 1990;64:219.

Robertson WD, Wray D. Ingestion of medication among patients with oral keratosis including lichen planus. Oral Surg Oral Med Oral Pathol 1992;74:183.

Wright JM. Oral manifestations of drug reactions. Dent Clin North Am 1984;28:529.

## Angioedema

Atkinson JC, Frank MM. Oral manifestations and dental management of patients with hereditary angio-edema. J Oral Pathol Med 1991;20:139.

Greaves M, Lawlor F. Angioedema: manifestations and management. J Am Acad Dermatol 1991;25:155.

Ogbureke KUE, Cruz C, Johnson JV, et al. Perioperative angioedema in a patient on long-term angiotensin-converting enzyme (ACE)-inhibitor therapy. J Oral Maxillofac Surg 1996;54:917.

Rees SR, Gibson J. Angioedema and swellings of the orofacial region. Oral Dis 1997;3:39.

Sturdy KA, Beastall RH, Grisius RJ, et al. Hereditary angioedema controlled with danazol. Oral Surg Oral Med Oral Pathol 1979;48:418.

## Allergic Contact Reactions

Alanko K, Kanerva L, Jolanki R, et al. Oral mucosal diseases investigated by patch testing in a dental screening series. Contact Derm 1996;34:263.

Eversole LR. Allergic stomatitides. J Oral Med 1979;34:93.

Koch P, Baum H-P. Contact stomatitis due to palladium and platinum in dental alloys. Contact Derm 1996;34:253.

Reese JA, ed. Effects and side-effects of dental restorative materials: an NIH technology assessment conference. Adv Dent Res 1992;6(theme issue) pp. 1-144.

Turrell AJW. Allergy to denture-base materials—fallacy or reality. Br Dent J 1966;120:415.

## Exfoliative Cheilitis

Brooke RI. Exfoliative cheilitis. Oral Surg Oral Med Oral Pathol 1978;45:52.

Reade PC, Sim R. Exfoliative cheilitis—a factitious disorder? Int J Oral Maxillofac Surg 1986;15:313.

Thomas JR, Greene SL, Dicken CH. Factitious cheilitis. J Am Acad Dermatol 1983;8:368.

## Perioral Dermatitis

Beacham BE, Kurgansky D, Gould WM. Circumoral dermatitis and cheilitis caused by tartar control dentifrices. J Am Acad Dermatol 1990;22:1029.

Manders SM, Lucky AW. Perioral dermatitis in childhood. J Am Acad Dermatol 1992;27:688.

Veien NK, Munkvad JM, Nielsen AO, et al. Topical metronidazole in the treatment of perioral dermatitis. J Am Acad Dermatol 1991;24:258.

Wells K, Brodell RT. Topical corticosteroid "addiction": a cause of perioral dermatitis. Postgrad Med 1993;93:226.

## Contact Stomatitis to Cinnamon Flavoring

Allen CM, Blozis GG. Oral mucosal reactions to cinnamon-flavored chewing gum. J Am Dent Assoc 1988;116:664.

Miller RL, Gould AR, Bernstein ML. Cinnamon-induced stomatitis venenata: clinical and characteristic histopathologic features. Oral Surg Oral Med Oral Pathol 1992;73:708.

## Contact Stomatitis to Dental Amalgam

Henriksson E, Mattsson U, Håkansson J. Healing of lichenoid reactions following removal of amalgam: a clinical follow-up. J Clin Periodontol 1995;22:287.

Larsson Å, Warfvinge G. The histopathology of oral mucosal lesions associated with amalgam or porcelain-fused-to-metal restorations. Oral Dis 1995;1:152.

Östman P-O, Anneroth G, Skoglund A. Oral lichen planus lesions in contact with amalgam fillings: a clinical, histologic, and immunohistochemical study. Scand J Dent Res 1994;102:172.

Östman P-O, Anneroth G, Skoglund A. Amalgam-associated oral lichenoid reactions: clinical and histologic changes after removal of amalgam fillings. Oral Surg Oral Med Oral Pathol Oral Radiol Endod 1996;81:459.

## Graft-Versus-Host Disease

Curtis JW, Caughman GB. An apparent unusual relationship between rampant caries and the oral mucosal manifestations of chronic graft-versus-host disease. Oral Surg Oral Med Oral Pathol 1994;78:267.

Epstein JB, Reece DE. Topical cyclosporin A for treatment of oral chronic graft-versus-host disease. Bone Marrow Transplant 1994;13:81.

Hiroki A, Nakamura S, Shinohara M, et al. Significance of oral examination in chronic graft-versus-host disease. J Oral Pathol Med 1994;23:209.

Rodu B, Gockerman JP. Oral manifestations of the chronic graft-v-host reaction. JAMA 1983;249:504.

Schubert MM, Williams BE, Lloid ME, et al. Clinical assessment scale for the rating of oral mucosal changes associated with bone marrow transplantation: development of an oral mucositis index. Cancer 1992;69:2469.

# chapter 7

# BENIGN AND MALIGNANT LESIONS OF
# EPITHELIAL ORIGIN

## PAPILLOMA (SQUAMOUS PAPILLOMA)

### Figs. 7.1, 7.2, and 7.3

The papilloma (squamous papilloma) is a benign, exophytic proliferation of stratified squamous epithelium arranged in fingerlike projections. Clinically, this configuration may appear cauliflowerlike. The base may be either pedunculated or sessile. The color ranges from that of normal mucosa to white or red. Papillomas are generally less than 1 cm in diameter, but they have grown as large as 2 to 3 cm. Human papillomavirus subtypes 6 and 11 have been identified in this epithelial proliferation in more than 50% of lesions probed for viral DNA.

The papilloma develops in all age groups but is most often seen in the third to fifth decades of life. It is most commonly seen on the hard and soft palate–uvula complex but is often seen on the ventral and dorsal tongue, the gingiva, and the buccal mucosa. In most situations, the lesion is solitary; however, an occasional patient will have multiple papillomas. In addition, multiple papillomalike epithelial proliferations may develop in immunocompromised persons. Treatment is conservative surgical excision, including a small amount of normal epithelium at the base. Recurrence is rare.

### Figure 7.1
**PAPILLOMA**

Pink, pedunculated, and papillary lesion attached to the lingual frenum.

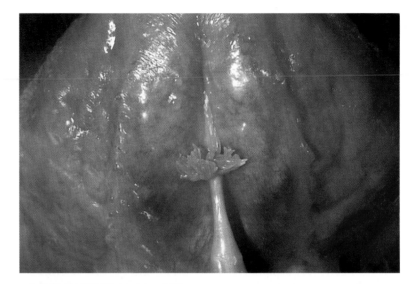

### Figure 7.2
**PAPILLOMA**

Pink, papillary growth attached to the soft palate by a stalk.

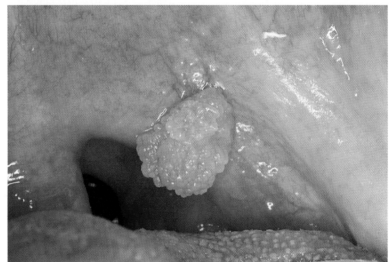

### Figure 7.3
**PAPILLOMA**

White, exophytic growth with papillary projections exhibiting a cauliflower appearance.

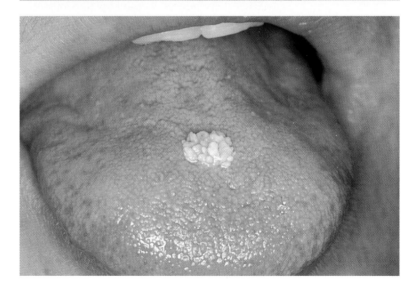

## VERRUCA VULGARIS

**Fig. 7.4**

The verruca vulgaris is a benign hyperplasia of squamous epithelium that is induced by subtypes 2, 4, and 40 of the human papillomavirus. It is a common problem on skin and is referred to as the common skin wart. The lesion appears as a papillary or rough-surfaced papule or nodule. The color ranges from tan to white and it often is seen on the skin of the hands and not infrequently on the face and perioral skin. The verruca vulgaris may occur as a single lesion or as multiple lesions. It most often is seen in children, but it also occurs in adults. It is contagious and can be spread to other skin and mucosal sites by autoinoculation.

Oral mucosal involvement is much less common than skin lesions and usually is seen on the labial mucosa, the tongue, and the palate. Oral verrucae present as white, papillary nodules that are clinically indistinguishable from the much more common squamous papilloma. Oral lesions occur with greater frequency in immunocompromised or immunosuppressed persons. Treatment for oral verrucae is conservative surgical removal, cryotherapy, or electrosurgery. Skin lesions are treated by a variety of means, including surgery, liquid nitrogen, cryotherapy, or topical application of keratinolytic agents. Recurrence may be seen and spontaneous regression can occur.

## CONDYLOMA ACUMINATUM (VENEREAL WART)

**Fig. 7.5**

Condyloma acuminatum is the name given to a benign proliferation of urogenital squamous epithelium caused by several subtypes of the human papillomavirus. It is sexually transmitted and can be spread by autoinoculation. Occasionally condyloma acuminatum develops on oral mucosa where contact with infected genital tissue has occurred.

Condyloma acuminatum typically is seen in teenagers and young adults, and the oral lesion appears as a sessile, exophytic growth with blunt projections. The lesion may be single or multiple, and coalescence of nearby lesions may occur. Its color ranges from pink to white, and it may appear similar to the squamous papilloma; however, its attachment to mucosa is generally broader than that of the papilloma.

Common oral sites are the lips, the floor of the mouth, the tongue, and the palate. Condylomalike lesions induced by the human papillomavirus are rather common in human immunodeficiency virus–positive patients.

Treatment of oral lesions is by conservative surgical excision. Large lesions may require laser therapy. Recurrence is common.

## FOCAL EPITHELIAL HYPERPLASIA (HECK'S DISEASE)

**Fig. 7.6**

Focal epithelial hyperplasia is a proliferation of oral squamous epithelium caused by the human papillomavirus subtypes 13 and 32. It was first observed in Navajo Indians, but it has been seen in many ethnic groups throughout the world. It almost always is seen in children and is characterized by the presence of multiple, slightly raised papules on the lower lip, the buccal mucosa, and the tongue. Other oral sites are infrequently affected. The lesions also can be papillary, and the individual lesion usually is less than 1.0 cm. in diameter. Their distribution often is somewhat symmetrical, and the color ranges from pink to white. The lesions often undergo spontaneous regression but may persist for several years. Multifocal papular lesions closely resembling this disease may occur in human immunodeficiency virus–infected patients.

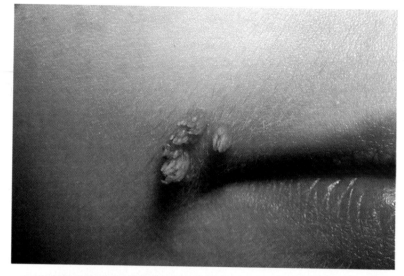

### Figure 7.4
### VERRUCA VULGARIS
Multiple white, exophytic verrucae with fingerlike projections on the lip.

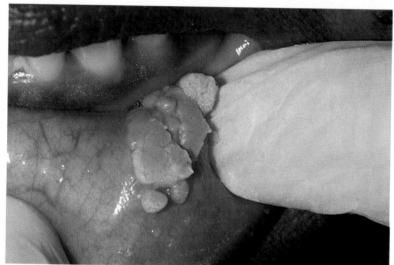

### Figure 7.5
### CONDYLOMA ACUMINATUM
Multiple broad-based lesions of mucosa with a delicate papillary surface.

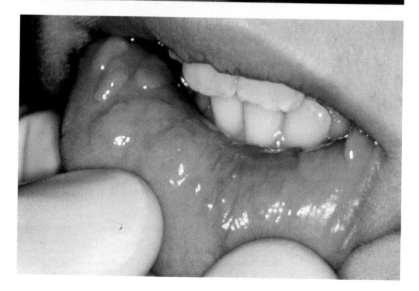

### Figure 7.6
### FOCAL EPITHELIAL HYPERPLASIA
### (HECK'S DISEASE)
Multiple smooth nodules of the lower lip. (Courtesy of Dr. Brad Rodu.)

## MOLLUSCUM CONTAGIOSUM

**Fig. 7.7**

Molluscum contagiosum is a benign proliferation of stratified squamous epithelium caused by the poxvirus. It is generally seen in children and young adults, mostly males. It is usually seen on the skin of the trunk, neck, face, and anogenital area. The mouth is rarely involved, but it has occurred on the lips, buccal mucosa, and palate. Molluscum contagiosum may develop as a single papule or nodule, but it is often multiple. The surface appearance varies from smooth to lobulated, and the center may be depressed (umbilicated) or may contain a keratinlike plug. Molluscum contagiosum is contracted by direct contact, including sexual contact, and may be spread by autoinoculation. Usually, the lesion heals spontaneously within several months of development, although it may persist for some time. It is a common lesion in human immunodeficiency virus–infected persons.

## VERRUCIFORM XANTHOMA

**Fig. 7.8**

The verruciform xanthoma is a benign hyperplasia of squamous epithelium accompanied by an infiltrate of histiocytes in the subadjacent connective tissue. It primarily is a disease of oral mucosa but has occurred on the skin. Its cause is unknown, but it may be related to damage to squamous epithelial cells resulting in the release of lipid and subsequent accumulation of foamy histiocytes (xanthoma cells). Its clinical appearance is variable. Its color ranges from white to cream to red and the surface texture ranges from flat to rough or pebbly like a papilloma. The verruciform xanthoma typically occurs in adults and usually develops on gingiva and alveolar mucosa. There is a female predilection. It usually develops as an isolated lesion but has occurred in association with other mucosal diseases, such as lichen planus, pemphigus vulgaris, and carcinoma-in-situ. Treatment is surgical excision and recurrence is rare.

## ACTINIC CHEILOSIS (ACTINIC KERATOSIS OF THE LIP)

**Fig. 7.9**

Actinic cheilosis is an alteration of lip mucosa that microscopically ranges from hyperkeratosis with degeneration of superficial connective tissue to significant levels of epithelial dysplasia. It develops most often in light-complexioned persons who have long-term exposure to the ultraviolet radiation of sunlight. It is analogous to actinic keratosis of the skin, and its importance is the potential progression to squamous cell carcinoma. This process evolves slowly and is seen in adults. The early changes consist of pallor and a loss of the well-defined border that exists between the mucosa and skin portions of the lip. As the process progresses, the mucosa becomes blotchy, and, eventually, discrete white and red areas are seen. Thickened areas may become scaly. Ulceration may develop at the site of trauma or spontaneously and may be a harbinger to the development of squamous cell carcinoma. Treatment depends on the extent of both clinical and microscopic alterations. Early changes are often watched, and a sunscreen is used to slow or halt the process. However, existing cellular damage is probably permanent. The concept of when to perform a biopsy is not well-defined, but biopsy should be performed when discrete changes are present. Even subtle clinical changes may contain a squamous cell carcinoma. Treatment includes surgical excision, cryosurgery, carbon dioxide laser surgery, and the use of topical cancer chemotherapeutic agents such as 5-fluorouracil. The existence of a squamous cell carcinoma modifies the therapy.

### Figure 7.7
### MOLLUSCUM CONTAGIOSUM

Several grayish-white nodules on skin and lip mucosa, the largest exhibiting a lobulated surface. (Courtesy of Dr. Yoshifumi Tajima.)

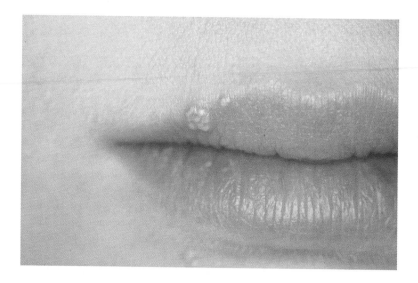

### Figure 7.8
### VERRUCIFORM XANTHOMA

A circumscribed red and yellow pebbly lesion of the palatal mucosa. (Courtesy of Neville BW. The verruciform xanthoma: a review and report of 8 new cases. Am J Dermatopathol 1986;8:247.)

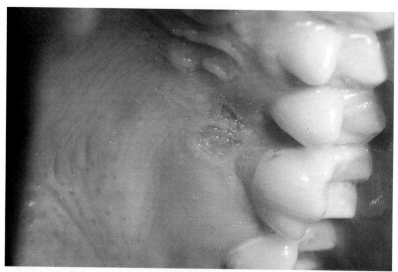

### Figure 7.9
### ACTINIC CHEILOSIS (ACTINIC KERATOSIS OF THE LIP)

Severe actinic change of the lower lip with an indistinct vermilion border and discrete areas of keratosis overlying an erythematous base.

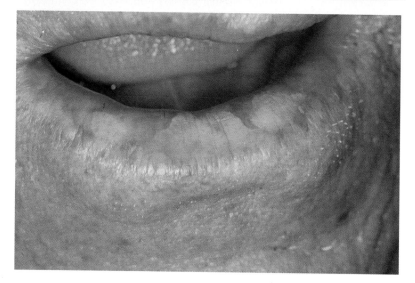

## FRICTIONAL (MECHANICAL) KERATOSIS

### Fig. 7.10

Chronic mechanical irritation of oral mucosa often results in thickening of surface epithelium that manifests clinically as a white change. Microscopically, there is thickening of the surface keratin with or without a thickening of the spinous cell layer (acanthosis). This is a protective mechanism and is analogous to callus formation on skin. In most situations, the cause is evident on clinical examination or is uncovered by reviewing the patient's history. Common causes include chronic mucosal biting, such as in the development of morsicatio buccarum (see Figure 5.2); vigorous tooth brushing of gingival tissue; using an edentulous ridge as an occlusal table; and movement of a denture over alveolar mucosa.

Frequently involved sites are the lips, the buccal mucosa, the tongue, the gingiva, the edentulous alveolar ridge, and the retromolar pad. With the redefining of the term "leukoplakia," frictional keratosis is not included in this definition; it should not be considered a premalignant or potentially malignant lesion.

In most cases, treatment consists of removing the cause and observing the patient for healing. The tissue change often regresses when the source of the trauma is eliminated. Biopsy of the lesion should be considered if the area persists or continues to progress after correcting the cause or if the patient has a high-risk factor for the development of oral squamous cell carcinoma, e.g., the use of tobacco or the abuse of alcohol. Occurrence on the lower lip, the floor of the mouth, the ventral and lateral tongue, and the soft palate–tonsillar pillar complex should also be viewed with suspicion.

## NICOTINE STOMATITIS

### Figs. 7.11 and 7.12

Nicotine stomatitis is a benign thickening of oral mucosa typically associated with tobacco smoking. It usually is seen in pipe smokers but also may develop in cigarette and cigar smokers. It also can be seen in persons who drink very hot beverages and do not smoke tobacco of any kind. The alterations typically develop on the hard and soft palates but infrequently can be seen on the retromolar pad and the posterior buccal mucosa. The typical presentation is that of multiple white, circular papules exhibiting red centers that may be slightly depressed. The erythematous portion represents dilated salivary gland duct orifices that are inflamed and exhibit squamous metaplasia. The surrounding white surface represents hyperkeratosis. The nodules are initially separated by normal mucosa, but the individual nodules coalesce, resulting in a diffuse white area interspersed with erythematous dots. The changes can extend to the gingiva, where the tissue appears white and thickened. The keratosis may be smooth or fissured.

In the western world, nicotine stomatitis is not considered a precancerous condition, but patients should be carefully observed for changes in the involved area and for alterations at other mucosal sites that could represent precancerous or cancerous alterations. This process may resolve on smoking cessation. Similar but more severe palatal changes may be seen in reverse smokers, who hold the burning end of the cigarette inside the mouth. This habit, which is not rare in India and some other Southeast Asian and South American countries, has been associated with the development of dysplasia and squamous cell carcinoma.

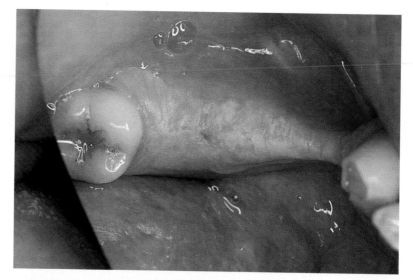

### ▶ Figure 7.10
### FRICTIONAL (MECHANICAL) KERATOSIS
White, rough-surfaced, edentulous alveolar ridge used as an occlusal table.

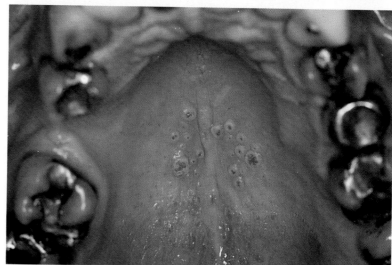

### ▶ Figure 7.11
### NICOTINE STOMATITIS
Multiple nodules of the palate, each with a white periphery and a red, depressed center.

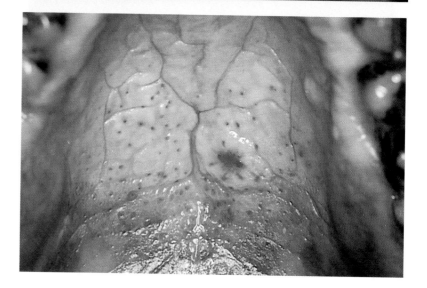

### ▶ Figure 7.12
### NICOTINE STOMATITIS
Advanced case with diffuse keratosis of the palate and multiple red dots.

### Figs. 7.13, 7.14, and 7.15

The placement of smokeless tobacco, either snuff or chewing tobacco, in the mouth can result in direct alterations of the oral mucosa. It occurs in all age groups, including childhood and adolescence. Typically, the lesion is found in the vestibule where the tobacco is placed, and it may extend onto the gingiva and buccal mucosa. The changes range from a wrinkling of tissue that disappears on stretching, to a granular surface with mild keratosis, to a greatly thickened tissue with well-developed fissures and keratosis. The extent of the changes depends on host susceptibility, the form and quantity of tobacco used, and the number of years of use. The gingiva may be inflamed and exhibit recession.

Persons who use smokeless tobacco are at higher risk for oral carcinoma than non-tobacco users. Well-documented cases exist of squamous cell carcinoma or verrucous carcinoma developing within tobacco pouches (see Fig. 7.37). These carcinomas usually present as large, exophytic lesions that develop at the site of tobacco placement. However, some patients develop cancer at other oral mucosal sites. Although such tumors usually are quite obvious, more subtle clinical changes also can show atypical or dysplastic alterations. Most carcinomas that develop in smokeless tobacco users occur in older individuals who have practiced the habit for many years, typically 30 years or more.

Many tobacco pouches are readily reversible once the habit is discontinued. Histopathologic examination of the involved tissue is recommended if the patient will not stop using tobacco or if tissue changes persist after the patient has stopped the habit. Biopsy also is indicated if the clinical lesion is markedly papillary or demonstrates areas of redness or ulceration.

**Figure 7.13**
**TOBACCO POUCH**
Young adult male with a faintly white and granular pouch. The patient has gingivitis and gingival recession. Placement of snuff in this area was reported.

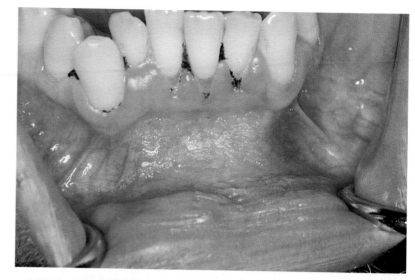

**Figure 7.14**
**TOBACCO POUCH**
Adult user of snuff with diffuse thickened and white mucosal change exhibiting significant ridges.

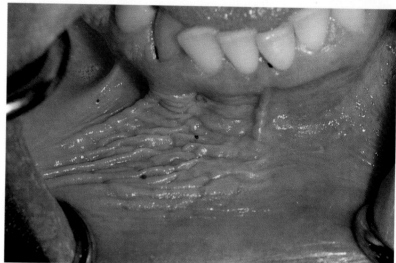

**Figure 7.15**
**TOBACCO POUCH**
Sixteen-year-old male with an extensive white pouch that is deeply fissured.

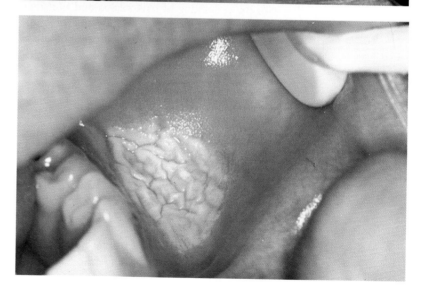

Leukoplakia is a term used to describe certain white changes of oral mucosa. The concept of leukoplakia has undergone extensive study and review in recent years, and the definition used in this section represents a modification of the World Health Organization's, which was proposed at a recent symposium of international leaders in the field. The definition used in this book reads as "a predominantly white lesion of the oral mucosa that cannot be characterized as any other definable lesion."

This definition excludes those white changes in which a specific clinical diagnosis or non-tobacco related cause can be established, e.g., frictional keratosis, mucosal biting, chemical injury, lichen planus, or candidiasis. The term does not imply a distinct histologic picture, and histopathologic diagnosis of a specific disease entity would exclude the use of leukoplakia as a clinical diagnosis. The cause of leukoplakia has been subdivided into idiopathic and tobacco associated. However, nicotine stomatitis has been excluded because of its unique clinical presentation and prognosis. Some investigators also have removed smokeless tobacco pouches from this definition because such lesions have an identifiable, direct cause and a distinct clinical picture.

Leukoplakia is subclassified into two clinical presentations: homogeneous and nonhomogeneous. The homogeneous variety exhibits a fairly uniform, consistent texture and the nonhomogeneous type exhibits irregularities in surface architecture that may include smooth, flat, rough-surfaced, papillary (verrucous), fissured, and nodular areas. Nonhomogeneous leukoplakia also may have areas of erythema (erythroplakia) interspersed, and this presentation has been referred to as erythroleukoplakia. Leukoplakia may be small and localized, diffuse, or multifocal. Nonhomogeneous leukoplakias with erythroplakic, nodular, or papillary areas have a greater risk of exhibiting dysplasia, carcinoma-in-situ, or squamous cell carcinoma. However, homogeneous leukoplakias may also have these histopathological changes.

Leukoplakia is more common in males and is most often seen in the fifth to seventh decades of life. All areas of the mouth can be involved, but leukoplakia most often occurs on the buccal mucosa, the floor of the mouth, the labial commissures, the lateral borders of the tongue, and the alveolar ridges. Microscopically, leukoplakia ranges from benign keratosis, epithelial dysplasia, carcinoma-in-situ, and squamous cell carcinoma. Studies have indicated that approximately 20% of oral leukoplakias exhibit dysplastic and cancerous changes. However, with the redefining of leukoplakia and the removal of frictional keratosis from the definition, the actual percentage is no doubt much higher. Areas of leukoplakia at considerable risk for being dysplasia or squamous cell carcinoma are the floor of the mouth, the tongue, and the soft palate–tonsillar complex.

Management of leukoplakia is dependent on the clinical characteristics, cause, and microscopic diagnosis. Patients with a microscopic diagnosis of keratosis are still at risk for progression to dysplasia and/or squamous cell carcinoma, especially those who have no recognizable cause. Tobacco smokers should be encouraged to quit and patients should be closely followed, with repeat biopsies performed if there is clinical change. Total removal of such lesions may also be considered, especially if they occur in high-risk locations such as the lateral tongue and the floor of the mouth.

Those patients with the microscopic diagnosis of moderate dysplasia or worse should be managed by removal of the lesion if possible. This may be accomplished by excisional surgery, laser ablation, electrocautery, or cryosurgery. Systemic retinoids recently have been used in the management of oral leukoplakia. Although some studies have shown promise, further investigation is necessary to confirm the effectiveness of this mode of therapy.

Malignant transformation of leukoplakia is an acknowledged problem, but there is considerable variation in the reported prevalence. Older studies indicated that it happened in 4 to 6% of the cases. However, recent studies have suggested a range of 9 to 17%. This increase in the transformation rate is expected with the use of the new, more narrow definition of leukoplakia. Future studies should help to substantiate this significant consequence. Lesions that show a red component or that exhibit microscopic evidence of dysplasia show a much greater risk of progressing to squamous cell carcinoma.

Proliferative verrucous leukoplakia is a term given to a progressive, spreading leukoplakia that predominantly occurs in elderly females who usually are not tobacco users. The buccal mucosa is the most common site in women and the tongue is the most common site in men. It starts out as a single area of white change that slowly but persistently spreads and often becomes multifocal. The lesions tend to become thickened and papillary or verrucous in nature. Microscopically, proliferative verrucous leukoplakia exhibits a spectrum from benign keratosis to verrucous or squamous cell carcinoma. Despite surgical excision, the lesions show a high rate of recurrence and frequent development of invasive carcinoma.

### Figure 7.16
### LEUKOPLAKIA

Irregular white alterations of the left buccal mucosa in a heavy smoker. Biopsy results revealed carcinoma-in-situ with areas of early invasive squamous cell carcinoma.

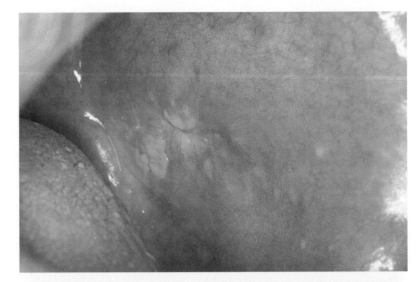

### Figure 7.17
### LEUKOPLAKIA

Adult patient with multifocal areas of flat and thick leukoplakia of the posterior lateral border of the tongue and of the floor of the mouth. Areas represent mild epithelial dysplasia.

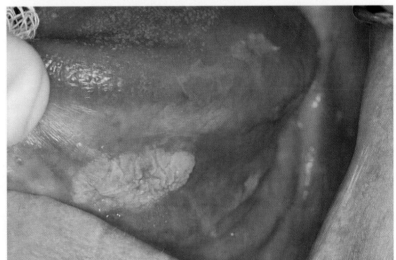

### Figure 7.18
### LEUKOPLAKIA

Diffuse leukoplakia of the floor of the mouth and ventral tongue in an adult. Area represents mild epithelial dysplasia.

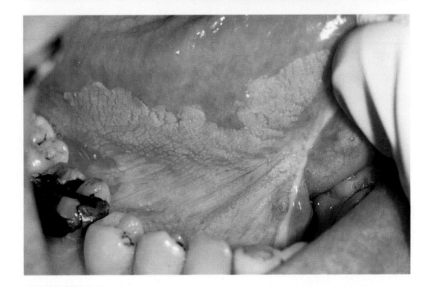

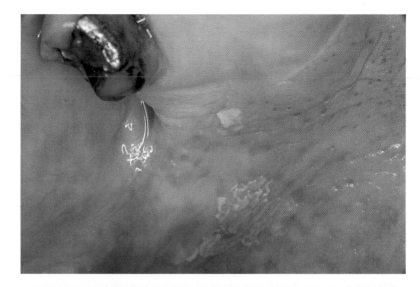

**Figure 7.19**
**LEUKOPLAKIA**
Localized white area of the right soft palate in a heavy smoker. Biopsy results revealed mild dysplasia.

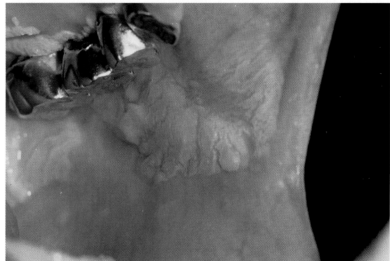

**Figure 7.20**
**PROLIFERATIVE VERRUCOUS LEUKOPLAKIA**
Diffuse areas of leukoplakia of palatal gingiva and buccal mucosa in an older adult female with no known etiologic factors. The lesion has recurred after initial excision and is progressive.

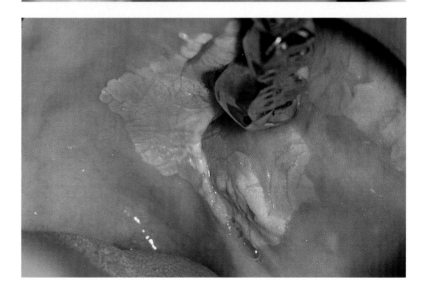

**Figure 7.21**
**PROLIFERATIVE VERRUCOUS LEUKOPLAKIA**
The same patient shown in Figure 7.20 with diffuse involvement of the posterior buccal mucosa and the soft palate.

### Figs. 7.22, 7.23, and 7.24

Erythroplakia is a term used to designate a red patch of oral mucosa that cannot be diagnosed as any specific disease. It is usually seen in the sixth and seventh decades of life, and most affected patients use tobacco and chronically consume alcoholic beverages. Any area of oral mucosa can be affected, but erythroplakia is most commonly seen on the floor of the mouth, the retromolar pad–tonsillar pillar complex, and the soft palate. The lesions may be single or multiple, smooth or pebbly. The color ranges from subtle to bright red. In addition, some lesions may contain areas of focal leukoplakia and have been designated as speckled erythroplakias. The difference between this clinical term and erythroleukoplakia is based on the degree of each color change, but both indicate a potentially serious lesion.

The significance of erythroplakia is that histopathologically it usually represents various degrees of dysplasia, carcinoma-in-situ, or squamous cell carcinoma. Published articles indicate that up to 90% of patients with erythroplakia will exhibit severe epithelial dysplasia, carcinoma-in-situ, or squamous cell carcinoma. Therefore, any red area of mucosa that cannot be associated with injury or a specific cause should undergo microscopic examination to establish a definitive diagnosis. Treatment of erythroplakia depends on the extent of cellular changes and it is managed in a similar fashion as leukoplakia.

Subtle, ill-defined red area of the floor of the mouth histopathologically representing carcinoma-in-situ.

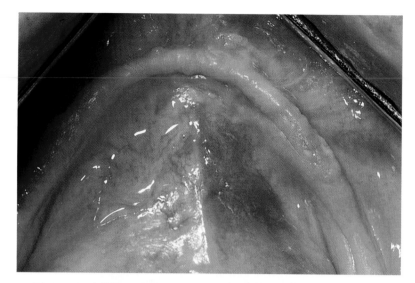

► **Figure 7.23**
**SPECKLED ERYTHROPLAKIA**
Discrete red lesion with numerous centrally placed white specks. Biopsy results revealed invasive squamous cell carcinoma.

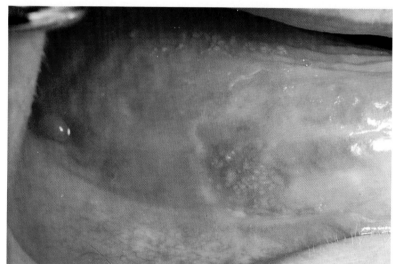

► **Figure 7.24**
**ERYTHROPLAKIA**
Red, granular lesion of the posterior lateral border of the tongue with central white areas. Biopsy specimen showed invasive squamous cell carcinoma at the site of ulceration and cavitation.

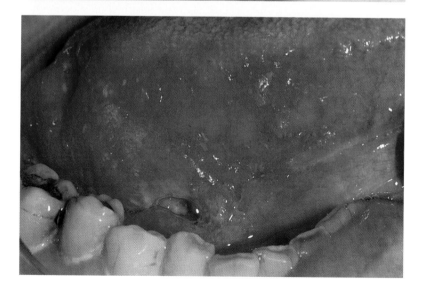

# SQUAMOUS CELL CARCINOMA (EPIDERMOID CARCINOMA)

## Figs. 7.25 to 7.36

Squamous cell carcinoma is the cancer of stratified squamous epithelium. It accounts for approximately 90% of all oral cancers and is characterized by the invasion of supporting connective tissue and adjacent structures by malignant squamous epithelial cells. It has the capacity to invade vascular and lymphatic channels and metastasize to lymph nodes and distant organs.

A number of causative factors have been implicated in the development of oral squamous cell carcinoma. The most compelling statistical and clinical evidence supports tobacco and alcohol as primary factors. Eighty percent of oral squamous cell carcinomas develop in smokers, and the development of carcinoma in tobacco pouches is well documented. The use of tobacco is further supported by the high prevalence of squamous cell carcinoma in persons in India and Southeast Asia who have specialized tobacco habits such as reverse smoking or chewing betel quid. In these parts of the world, oral carcinoma is one of the most common of all cancers. Those persons who combine the use of tobacco and the chronic use of alcohol seem to have a synergistic risk rather than an additive one. Ultraviolet radiation from sunlight has been implicated as the principal factor in the development of squamous cell carcinoma of the lip.

Other factors also may play a promoting or supporting role in the development of oral carcinoma. At one time, carcinoma of the tongue was associated with syphilis; however, its development may have been associated with arsenic and other heavy metals that were used to treat syphilis before the advent of modern antibiotics. However, recent studies indicate that there is indeed an increased prevalence of tongue carcinoma in patients who have positive test results for *Treponema* antibodies and who have not been treated with heavy metal therapy.

Human papillomavirus genotypes have been identified in human epithelial dysplasias and oral squamous cell carcinomas, but its significance in the development of this cancer has not been determined. A link between oral squamous cell carcinoma and herpes simplex virus has been suggested, but little clinical and statistical evidence is available to support this contention. Laboratory studies indicate that *Candida albicans* has the ability to be a promoting factor in the proliferation of squamous cells, but little clinical evidence is available to support its being a true cofactor. Persons with Plummer-Vinson syndrome (see Figure 10.7)—a severe form of iron deficiency anemia in women of Scandinavian descent—have an increased risk for squamous cell carcinoma of the esophagus and oropharynx. Chronically immunosuppressed persons also are at risk for development of oral carcinoma because of their inability to generate an immune response against aberrant host cell development.

Most patients with oral squamous cell carcinoma are 45 years of age or older; but the disease also occurs in earlier decades of life, including the first. The tumor is very aggressive in the younger age groups and is often misdiagnosed because of a lack of suspicion by health care professionals.

Early squamous cell carcinoma of the lip vermilion may begin as thickened white plaques or areas of erythema as seen in actinic cheilosis. More advanced lesions usually consist of an ulcer or a fixed, crusted area surrounded by a raised, rolled border. The ulcer may scab over and appear to be healing, but the tissue invariably breaks down again. There is a significant male predilection, and almost all cases arise on the lower lip.

Intraoral squamous cell carcinoma is more common in males, but there has been a significant decrease in the male-to-female ratio in recent years. Nearly every area of the oral cavity may be involved, but the sites most frequently affected are the ventral and lateral portions of the tongue, the floor of the mouth, and the soft palate–tonsillar pillar complex. The alveolar ridge–vestibule–buccal mucosa complex is often involved in smokeless tobacco users. Patients may have multiple concurrent primary tumors. The gingiva is a less common location, but it often mimics inflammation and is treated as gingivitis or periodontitis. Gingival carcinomas often spread in a lateral fashion but also may invade the alveolar bone, causing loose teeth. There is a female predilection, and the patient is frequently a nonsmoker.

Considerable variation in the clinical presentation of oral squamous cell carcinoma exists. The early lesion is usually flat and smooth or granular and appears red, white, or a mixture of both. Almost all have a red (erythroplakic) component. As the lesion progresses and infiltrates deeper and lateral tissues, there is no distinct separation between it and normal tissue, thus the feeling of fixation to normal tissue. The area feels firm and thickened. As the tumor continues to grow, it may become elevated above the normal surface, and a mass may be present. Ulceration also may be present over the mass, or the process may present as a cavitated and ulcerated area. Some carcinomas initially grow in an exophytic fashion and exhibit a papillary or deeply furrowed surface. Pain may or may not be present.

The treatment of primary squamous cell carcinoma consists of surgery, radiation therapy, or combinations of both, depending on the site of occurrence, the size of the primary tumor, and the presence of lymph node metastasis. Chemotherapy is usually used only in advanced disease and is only palliative. Approximately 20% of patients have regional lymph node metastasis at the time of diagnosis, and only a very small percent have distant metastasis that usually involves the lungs, bone, and liver.

Similar to therapy, the prognosis also depends on the location, the size, and the spread of the tumor. The 5-year survival rate varies from more than 90% for patients with localized, lower lip lesions to approximately 10% for those who have oral disease and distant metastasis. The 5-year survival rate for patients with localized intraoral disease is approximately 75%, but those with cervical lymph node involvement only have a 40% rate. Detection of early lesions dramatically influences the course of this disease. Patients with intraoral carcinoma also have a significant risk for development of a subsequent second intraoral or upper aerodigestive tract carcinoma. This risk seems to be higher than in any other primary cancer.

▶ **Figure 7.25**
**SQUAMOUS CELL CARCINOMA**
Area of ulceration of the lower lip proven
to be superficial squamous cell carcinoma.
Adjacent areas of flat red and white
changes exhibited epithelial dysplasia.
(Courtesy of Dr. Carl Allen.)

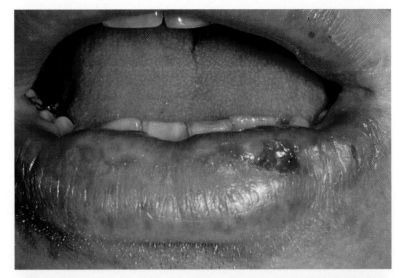

▶ **Figure 7.26**
**SQUAMOUS CELL CARCINOMA**
Firm, dished-out lesion of the lower lip that
was fixed to adjacent tissue and exhibited
surface ulceration. (Courtesy of Dr. Dan
Sarasin.)

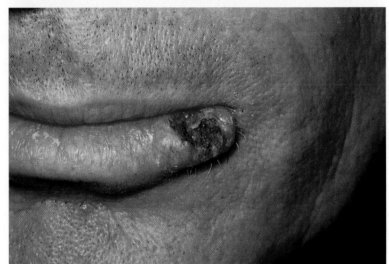

▶ **Figure 7.27**
**SQUAMOUS CELL CARCINOMA**
Advanced, ulcerated carcinoma involving
most of the lower lip. Prognosis is significantly lower than that for the patient
shown in Figure 7.25.

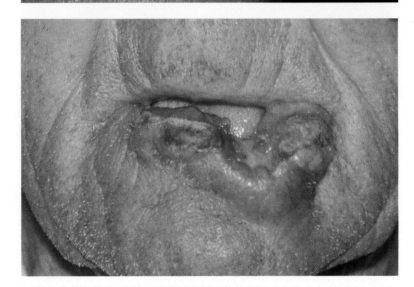

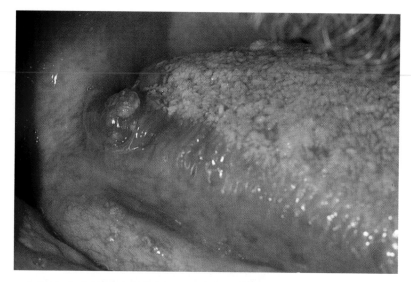

► **Figure 7.28**
**SQUAMOUS CELL CARCINOMA**
Small, exophytic tumor of the posterior lateral border of the tongue. This lesion could easily be mistaken for lymphoid hyperplasia.

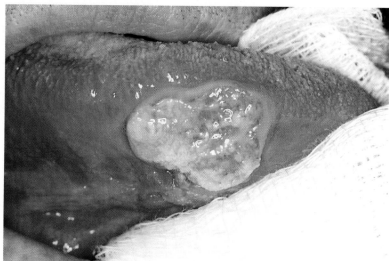

► **Figure 7.29**
**SQUAMOUS CELL CARCINOMA**
Chronic, asymptomatic, and well-defined area of ulceration of the right lateral border and ventral surface of the tongue

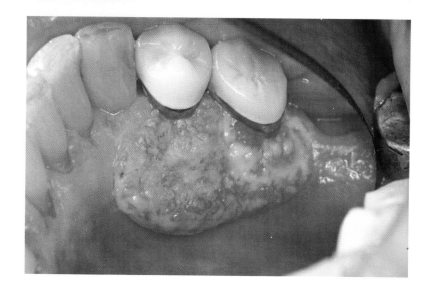

► **Figure 7.30**
**SQUAMOUS CELL CARCINOMA**
Exophytic, red, white, and granular mass of the lingual mandibular gingiva.

**Figure 7.31**
**SQUAMOUS CELL CARCINOMA**
Large ulcerative and proliferative lesion of the vental surface of the tongue.

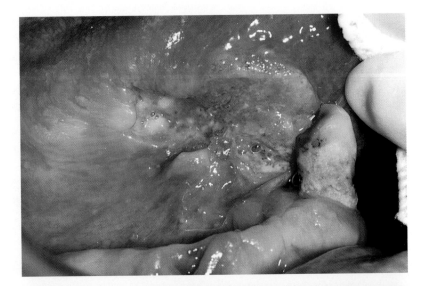

**Figure 7.32**
**SQUAMOUS CELL CARCINOMA**
Raised, granular-appearing white lesion of the soft palate and tonsillar pillar with surface ulceration.

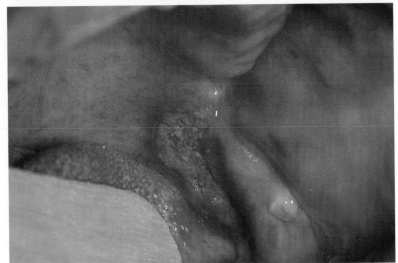

**Figure 7.33**
**SQUAMOUS CELL CARCINOMA**
Large, exophytic, white, red, and granular mass of the hard palate.

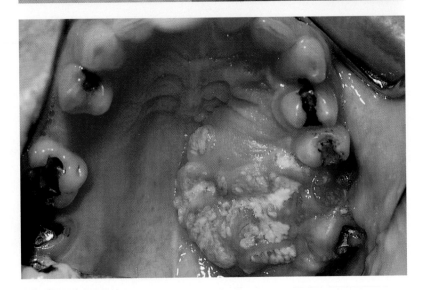

COLOR ATLAS OF CLINICAL ORAL PATHOLOGY

### Figure 7.34
### SQUAMOUS CELL CARCINOMA
Large, white, erythematous, ulcerated, and exophytic mass of the left posterior buccal mucosa. The patient did not smoke or consume alcohol but was a long-term user of smokeless tobacco.

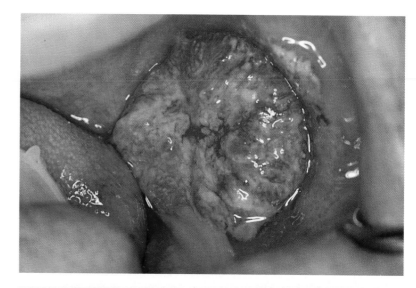

### Figure 7.35
### SQUAMOUS CELL CARCINOMA
Diffuse ulcerated and granular enlargement that involved the entire surface of the tongue. The tongue was deeply indurated and firmly bound to the adjacent structures.

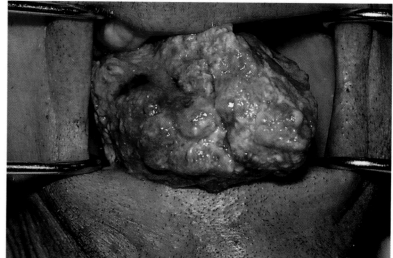

### Figure 7.36
### SQUAMOUS CELL CARCINOMA
Erythema and ulceration of the right neck as the result of direct extension from a primary squamous cell carcinoma of the right floor of the mouth. (Courtesy of Dr. D. E. Kenady.)

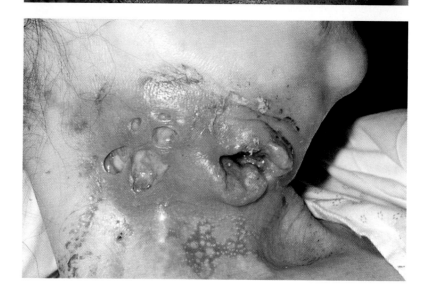

## VERRUCOUS CARCINOMA

### Figs. 7.37 and 7.38

Verrucous carcinoma is a special form of well-differentiated squamous cell carcinoma that exhibits a characteristic histopathologic picture and clinical behavior pattern. Histopathologically, the tumor is composed of well-differentiated squamous cells that lack the usual cytologic changes associated with malignancy. The tumor, though, penetrates into the underlying connective tissue with a blunt, well-defined border. The lesion is slow-growing, spreads primarily by lateral extension, and is destructive locally. Some authorities believe it lacks the ability to metastasize. Early lesions may appear as white, roughened plaques; advanced lesions are bulky, papillary growths. Some squamous cell carcinomas also exhibit a papillary pattern. Verrucous carcinoma occurs in older persons, with most patients in their sixth to eighth decades of life. It represents only a small percentage of intraoral carcinomas.

Most affected patients use tobacco, whether in the form of snuff, chewing tobacco, or cigarettes, but not all give a history of tobacco use. Human papillomavirus DNA has been identified in cells of verrucous carcinoma, but its significance is undetermined. This lesion is more common in men, except in the southeastern United States. Most lesions develop in the buccal mucosa–vestibule–alveolar ridge complex, where smokeless tobacco has been placed. Multiple lesions may be present. The recommended treatment is surgical removal or laser therapy. Radiation therapy can be effective and should be considered for lesions not amenable to surgery. Although earlier reports suggested that radiation therapy could be associated with dedifferentiation of the lesion into anaplastic carcinoma, recent analysis suggests that this threat may have been overstated. Prognosis is generally considered to be good. However, recurrence can be a problem, and some lesions are relentless in growth and can reach a considerable size.

## NASOPHARYNGEAL CARCINOMA

### Fig. 7.39

Nasopharyngeal carcinoma is the name given to the cancer that develops from the epithelial lining of the nasopharynx. It is an aggressive cancer that exhibits varying forms of differentiation. It usually occurs in the fifth, sixth, and seventh decades of life but may occur in the second and third decades. The cause is unknown, but the Epstein-Barr virus has been implicated as a factor. It also is believed that environmental factors are influential. There is a significant predilection for males, and it is rare outside of southern China, where it is endemic. Its most common initial presentation is a neck mass that represents metastasis to regional lymph nodes. Other signs and symptoms include nasal congestion and obstruction, epistaxis, headache, otitis media, and hearing loss. Even with these obvious problems, the primary tumor, usually in the lateral or posterior pharyngeal walls, may be small and difficult to find. Treatment primarily consists of radiation therapy.

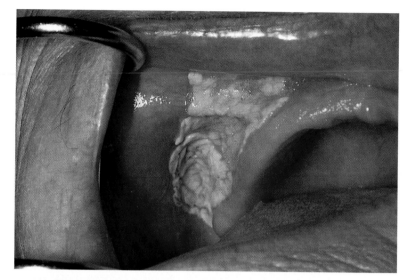

▶ **Figure 7.37**
**VERRUCOUS CARCINOMA**
Extensive, thick, white plaque of vestibule associated with the placement of chewing tobacco.

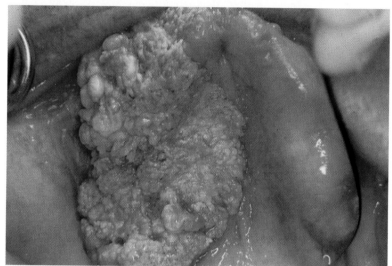

▶ **Figure 7.38**
**VERRUCOUS CARCINOMA**
Diffuse, exophytic, and papillary mass of the hard palate.

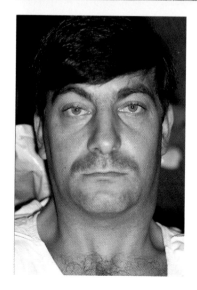

▶ **Figure 7.39**
**NASOPHARYNGEAL CARCINOMA**
Metastatic nasopharyngeal carcinoma in a left cervical lymph node.

# MAXILLARY SINUS CARCINOMA

## Figs. 7.40 and 7.41

Maxillary sinus carcinoma is an aggressive cancer that arises from the lining epithelium of the sinus or mucous glands in the subjacent connective tissue. Most are squamous cell carcinomas that vary from well-differentiated or keratinizing lesions to nonkeratinizing or poorly differentiated lesions. There is a male predilection, and the tumor tends to occur in older adults, usually in the sixth to eighth decades of life. Most patients will present with advanced disease because the initial signs and symptoms of dull, unilateral facial pain and nasal discharge are misinterpreted as an inflammatory process or sinusitis, and the tumor grows unchecked. As the tumor fills the sinus and invades the bony walls, the more obvious signs of advanced disease occur. These include paresthesia, nasal obstruction and hemorrhage, facial expansion, displacement and bulging of the eye, and oral cavity involvement.

A variety of changes can occur with extension into the oral cavity. Pain simulating a toothache may be felt in the posterior maxilla, and posterior teeth may become loose because of maxillary alveolar bone destruction. A mass of the alveolar ridge or hard palate may develop, which may ulcerate. Radiographs generally will show a clouding or opacification of the sinus cavity and destruction of the bony walls.

Treatment consists of hemimaxillectomy and/or radiation therapy. The prognosis is poor.

# ORAL SUBMUCOUS FIBROSIS

## Fig. 7.42

Oral submucous fibrosis is a chronic, progressive inflammatory and scarring disorder that is associated with the chronic contact of oral mucosa with hot peppers (chilies) and the chewing of betel quid, a combination of areca nut and slaked lime that also may contain native herbs and tobacco. The latter mixture seems to be the chief etiologic agent. Genetic predisposition also may play a role. It is primarily seen in persons from India and Southeast Asia, where the use of these materials is popular.

There is a female predilection, and the use of betal quid may begin as early as childhood. Common locations of involvement are the buccal mucosa, the lips, and the soft palate. Occasionally, the tongue and pharynx may be involved. The mucosa becomes inflamed, and ulcerations and vesicles may develop. With continued contact, the tissue appears blotchy, and areas of keratinization occur. Patients may complain of a burning sensation, pain, and xerostomia. With chronic use, the connective tissue at the exposed sites becomes fibrotic and scarlike, and there is limitation of movement of these tissues that limits the ability to open the mouth. The teeth may exhibit extensive staining from the betel quid (see Figure 2.17).

The damage to the tissue seems to be permanent even if use of the agent is discontinued. Treatment has included surgery to remove the binding, scarlike areas, the use of intralesional and systemic corticosteroids to impede the inflammatory process and scar formation, and the use of intralesional proteolytic enzymes to treat the fibrosis. Persons with this condition have a higher prevalence of oral squamous cell carcinoma.

COLOR ATLAS OF CLINICAL ORAL PATHOLOGY

### Figure 7.40
**SINUS CARCINOMA**

Extension of cancer beyond the maxillary sinus causing expansion of the cheek and displacement of the eye.

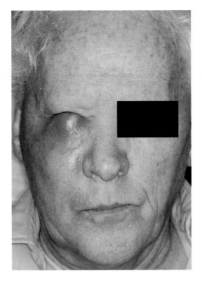

### Figure 7.41
**SINUS CARCINOMA**

Extension into the palate and alveolar ridge with an erythematous and ulcerated mass.

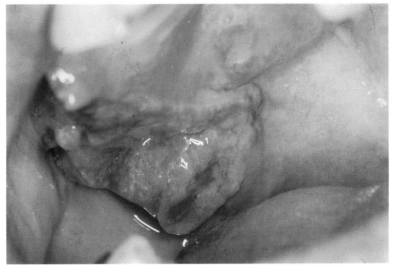

### Figure 7.42
**ORAL SUBMUCOUS FIBROSIS**

Patient with a white-appearing and atrophic soft palate that was limited in movement. The uvula has retained its normal color.

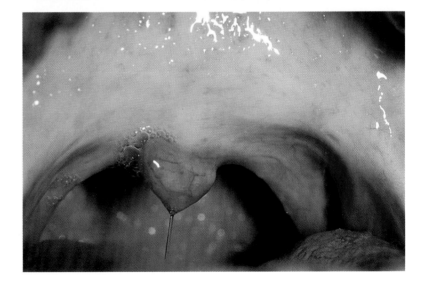

### Figs. 7.43, 7.44, and 7.45

Basal cell carcinoma is the most common type of skin cancer. Most lesions occur in adult males on the skin of the head and neck; the middle one-third of the face, forehead, and ears are particularly vulnerable. This tumor is most common in light-complexioned persons, and most are associated with chronic sun exposure. Dark-skinned persons are rarely affected. Basal cell carcinoma develops from surface and hair follicle epithelium and is an invasive and locally destructive neoplasm. It may cause death by involvement of adjacent vital structures but rarely metastasizes. It does not develop from oral mucosa, but lip mucosa may become involved by peripheral extension of an adjacent tumor.

The clinical picture is variable. Most lesions develop as nodules that have increased vascularity over the surface (telangiectasia). The color may be pearl-like. The tumor may ulcerate or develop a keratin-filled crater. The lesion grows slowly, with deep and lateral extension, giving rise to a rounded or rolled border. Ulcerated lesions may exhibit attempts at healing, but they eventually break down again. In other instances, basal cell carcinoma develops as a scaly, erythematous plaque or a scarlike area. It is not unusual for a person to develop multiple lesions. Basal cell carcinoma has become a problem in immunocompromised patients because of their diminished host-defense mechanisms against tumorigenesis.

A variety of methods are used to treat basal cell carcinoma, including surgical excision, irradiation therapy, electrodesiccation, and cryotherapy. Surgical techniques that use concomitant frozen section determinations to evaluate margins (Mohs micrographic surgery) have allowed for the removal of basal cell carcinomas with minimal morbidity and with a reduced chance of recurrence.

### Figure 7.43
### BASAL CELL CARCINOMA
Raised, nodular, and fixed lesion of the skin of the temple that exhibits a grayish hue.

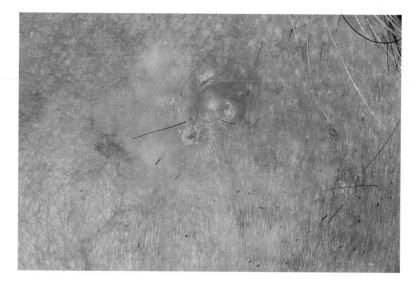

### Figure 7.44
### BASAL CELL CARCINOMA
Firm nodule of the face with a central crater and rolled borders.

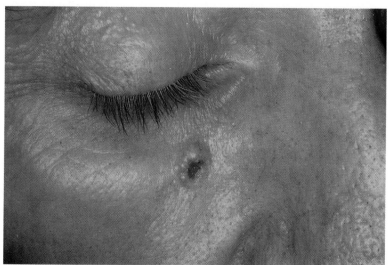

### Figure 7.45
### BASAL CELL CARCINOMA
Large lesion of the right inner canthus of the eye, which demonstrated indurated and rolled borders with central ulceration and scab formation. (Courtesy of Dr. D. E. Kenady.)

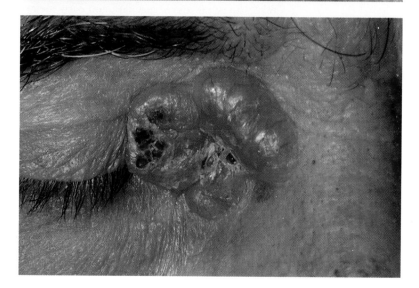

## KERATOACANTHOMA

**Fig. 7.46**

The keratoacanthoma is a proliferation of squamous epithelium that clinically and microscopically resembles squamous cell carcinoma. In fact, some authorities believe that it actually represents a well-differentiated carcinoma. The cause remains unknown. Several clinical forms exist, and the most common is a solitary nodule that develops on sun-exposed skin. Several other rare types involve the occurrence of multiple lesions that have widespread skin distribution and oral cavity involvement. The solitary form is common and often occurs on the face. There is a male predilection, and it usually arises in older adults. It typically develops as a rapidly growing nodule with a well-circumscribed, rolled border and a keratin-filled crater in the center. Frequently, spontaneous regression occurs within 4 to 6 months, but a scar may be left. Solitary keratoacanthomas are often removed because of their close resemblance to skin cancer and for cosmetic purposes. Keratoacanthoma occasionally develops on the lip vermilion and appears similar to squamous cell carcinoma. Diagnosis is determined by biopsy. Keratoacanthomas have been reported to occur on oral mucosa in rare instances, but squamous cell carcinoma and other specific keratoses should be completely ruled out before this diagnosis is accepted.

## ACQUIRED MELANOCYTIC NEVUS

**Fig. 7.47**

The acquired melanocytic nevus is a benign proliferation of cells of neural crest origin generally accepted to be melanocytes. Acquired melanocytic nevi usually develop on the skin after 6 months of life. The head and neck are common sites. There are three common types: junctional, intradermal (intramucosal), and compound. The names are derived from the distribution of the nevus cells within the involved tissue. Their color ranges from tan to brown to black, and they may be flat to nodular depending on the placement of cells within the epithelium and connective tissue. Some nevi do not produce pigmentation. They may lose their color with age and can undergo regression.

Melanocytic nevi are not common within the oral cavity. When they occur on the oral mucosa, they usually develop on the palate and gingiva. They can be confused clinically with amalgam tattoos, melanotic macules, and early melanoma (Fig. 7.49). Because of the latter possibility, unexplained intraoral pigmentation should undergo biopsy to rule out this condition.

## BLUE NEVUS

**Fig. 7.48**

The blue nevus is a benign proliferation of dermal melanocytes that is normally present at birth or that appears in childhood. It is more common on skin, but it is the second most common intraoral melanocytic nevus, following the intramucosal nevus. The most common intraoral location is the hard palate, but it has occurred on the buccal mucosa, lips, and soft palate. Clinically, it appears as a single, well-circumscribed, slightly raised nodule that varies in color from brown to blue to black. It also may have a grayish hue. Most lesions are less then 1.0 cm in diameter. Malignant transformation has been reported in extraoral blue nevi. Since the intraoral blue nevus can mimic an early developing melanoma, pigmented lesions of the palatal mucosa should be removed to rule out the latter condition.

### Figure 7.46
### KERATOACANTHOMA

Elevated and crusted dome-shaped nodule of the right aspect of the nose.

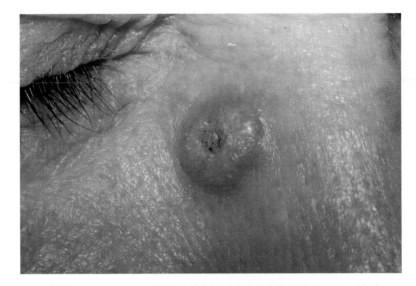

### Figure 7.47
### ACQUIRED MELANOCYTIC NEVUS

Well-delineated, homogeneously brown nevus in a 3-year-old female.
Biopsy results revealed junctional melanocytic nevus.

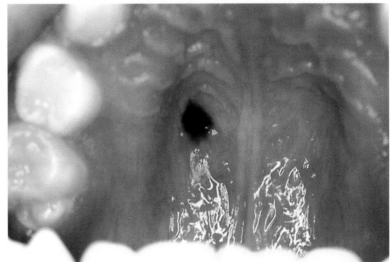

### Figure 7.48
### BLUE NEVUS

Raised, discrete area of blue-gray color of the vermilion border of the lower lip.

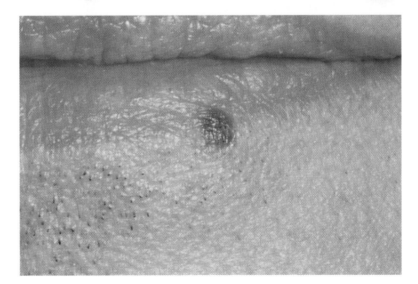

## Figs. 7.49, 7.50, and 7.51

Malignant melanoma is the cancer of melanocytes that primarily occurs on skin but occasionally develops from oral mucosa. The cause of intraoral melanoma is unknown, but there is strong evidence that the development of cutaneous melanomas is related to sun exposure, particularly in areas where sunburns have occurred. Genetic predisposition also is a factor. Intraoral melanomas are rare compared with cutaneous melanomas. They are usually diagnosed in adults between the ages of 40 and 60 years, and there is a male predilection. The most common locations are the palate and maxillary gingiva. The color ranges from tan to brown to blue-black and may be homogeneous or a mixture of colors. The lesion may be flat, nodular, or ulcerated. The outline may be somewhat well-delineated or irregular with adjacent areas of pigmentation (satellite lesions). The tumor may present as a single lesion or as multiple areas of increased melanin pigmentation interspersed with normal-appearing mucosa. Early intraoral melanoma may mimic areas of innocuous-appearing, benign melanosis or amalgam tattoos.

Treatment for primary melanoma is surgical excision. Radiation therapy, chemotherapy, and immunotherapy are used as adjuvant modalities, depending on the extent of the disease. The prognosis of oral melanoma is considered worse than its cutaneous counterpart because it often presents with metastasis to regional lymph nodes and distant organs. This is possibly due to anatomic considerations and the lack of recognition of the initial changes of melanoma when atypical melanocytes are still confined within the epithelium and no invasion has taken place.

### Figure 7.49
**MALIGNANT MELANOMA**

Small, flat area of dark brown pigmentation of hard palate similar to a melanotic macule (Fig. 13.17) or a melanocytic nevus (Fig. 7.47).

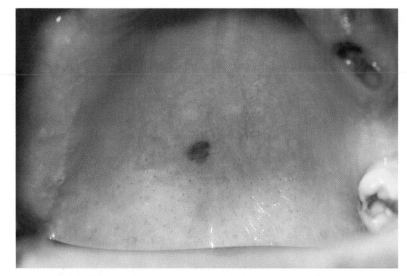

### Figure 7.50
**MALIGNANT MELANOMA**

Large, black, exophytic mass originating from the facial maxillary gingiva. (Courtesy of Dr. L. Costa.)

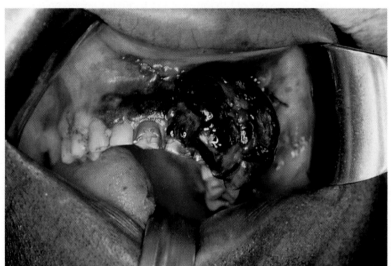

### Figure 7.51
**MALIGNANT MELANOMA**

Large, darkly pigmented ulceration of the hard palate.

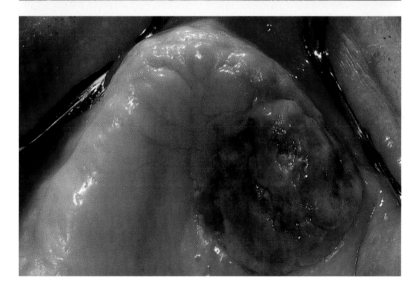

## Figs. 7.52, 7.53, and 7.54

Metastatic cancer to the oral cavity results from the hematogenous spread of cancers from distant primary sites. It is believed that this occurs through a paravertebral grouping of veins called Batson's plexus, which allows the cancer cells to bypass the lungs and continue into the arterial system. Most persons with intraoral metastasis are older adults, but metastasis can occur from cancers in children and young adults. Nearly every type of cancer, including sarcomas, can give rise to oral metastasis, but it is the more common types of carcinoma—lung, breast, colon, and prostate cancer—that are usually seen.

Oral metastases are expressed in a variety of ways. The most common presentation is a poorly delineated, destructive lesion of the posterior mandible. Pathologic fracture may be present. Teeth may be loose if alveolar bone is involved, and metastatic disease may mimic inflammatory periodontal bone loss. Occasionally, the process causes extrusion of teeth. Some types of cancer, such as breast, prostate, thyroid, and lung, may induce new bone formation, giving the lesion a mixed radiolucent/radiopaque appearance. The patient may also complain of pain and paresthesia of the lower lip; in some instances, pain may be the initial symptom, with no demonstrable changes seen on dental radiographs.

Swelling may or may not be present. The maxilla is much less frequently involved, but the signs and symptoms are the same. Extraction of teeth in an unsuspected involved area can result in proliferation of tumor out of the socket.

Soft-tissue involvement can also occur. The gingiva and alveolar mucosa are the most common soft-tissue locations, followed by the tongue. These often appear much like a reactive lesion such as the pyogenic granuloma. Metastasis to the mouth may be the first demonstrable sign of the cancer, with the patient being unaware of the primary tumor. Prognosis is poor because the metastasis is indicative of disseminated disease.

### Figure 7.52
**METASTATIC CARCINOMA**
Erythematous swelling of the gingiva representing metastatic colon cancer. (Courtesy of Dr. R. J. Lee.)

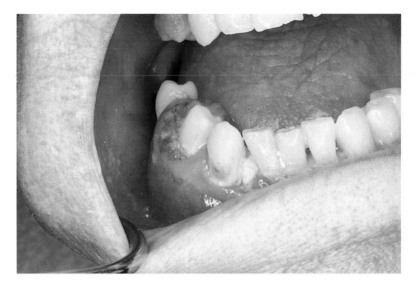

### Figure 7.53
**METASTATIC CARCINOMA**
Enlarged brown and necrotic mass of the tonsil from malignant melanoma of the skin of the shoulder.

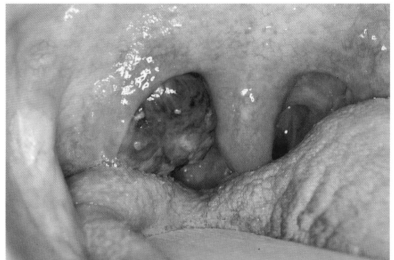

### Figure 7.54
**METASTATIC CARCINOMA**
Destructive radiolucency of the mandible with a recent history of loose teeth caused by metastatic adenocarcinoma.

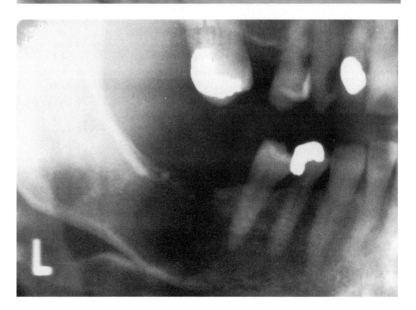

### Papilloma, Verruca Vulgaris, and Condyloma Acuminatum

Abbey LM, Page DG, Sawyer DR. The clinical and histopathologic features of a series of 464 oral squamous cell papillomas. Oral Surg Oral Med Oral Pathol 1980;49:419.

Barasch A, Eisenberg E, D'Ambrosio N, et al. Oral verruca vulgaris in a bone marrow transplant patient: a case report and review of literature. Eur J Cancer Oral Oncol 1996;32B:137.

Barone R, Ficarra G, Gaglioti D, et al. Prevalence of oral lesions among HIV-infected intravenous drug abusers and other risk groups. Oral Surg Oral Med Oral Pathol 1990;69:169.

Eversole LR, Laipis PJ, Green TL. Human papillomavirus type 2 DNA in oral and labial verruca vulgaris. J Cutan Pathol 1987;14:319.

Eversole LR, Laipis PJ, Merrill P, et al. Demonstration of human papillomavirus DNA in oral condyloma acuminatum. J Oral Pathol 1987;16:266.

Gonzalez-Moles MA, Ruiz-Avila I, Gonzalez-Moles S, et al. Detection of HPV DNA by in situ hybridization in benign, premalignant and malignant lesions of the oral mucosa. Bull Group Int Rech Sci Stomatol Odontol 1994;37:79.

Green TL, Eversole LR, Leider AS. Oral and labial verruca vulgaris: clinical, histologic and immunohistochemical evaluation. Oral Surg Oral Med Oral Pathol 1986;62:410.

Itin PH, Lautenschlager S. Viral lesions of the mouth in HIV-infected patients. Dermatology 1997;194:1.

Miller CS, White DK, Royse DD. In situ hybridization analysis of human papillomavirus in orofacial lesions using a consensus biotinylated probe. Am J Dermatopathol 1993;15:256.

Premoli-de-Percoco G, Galindo I, Ramirez JL, et al. Detection of human papillomavirus-related oral verruca vulgaris among Venezuelans. J Oral Pathol Med 1993;22:113.

Swan RH, McDaniel RK, Rome WC. Condyloma acuminatum involving the oral mucosa. Oral Surg Oral Med Oral Pathol 1981;51:503.

Ward KA, Napier SS, Winter PC, et al. Detection of human papilloma virus DNA sequences in oral squamous cell papillomas by the polymerase chain reaction. Oral Surg Oral Med Oral Pathol Oral Radiol Endod 1995;80:63.

Wysocki GP, Hardie J. Ultrastructural studies of intraoral verruca vulgaris. Oral Surg Oral Med Oral Pathol 1979;47:58.

Young SK, Min KW. In situ DNA hybridization analysis of oral papillomas, leukoplakias, and carcinomas for human papillomavirus. Oral Surg Oral Med Oral Pathol 1991;71:726.

Zeuss MS, Miller CS, White DK. In situ hybridization analysis of human papillomavirus DNA in oral mucosal lesions. Oral Surg Oral Med Oral Pathol 1991;71:714.

Zunt SL, Tomich CE. Oral condyloma acuminatum. J Dermatol Surg Oncol 1989;15:591.

### Focal Epithelial Hyperplasia (Heck's Disease)

Archard HO, Heck JW, Stanley HR. Focal epithelial hyperplasia: an unusual oral mucosal lesion found in Indian children. Oral Surg Oral Med Oral Pathol 1965;20:201.

Carlos R, Sedano HO. Multifocal papilloma virus epithelial hyperplasia. Oral Surg Oral Med Oral Pathol 1994;77:631.

Harris AM, van Wyk CW. Heck's disease (focal epithelial hyperplasia): a longitudinal study. Community Dent Oral Epidemiol 1993;21:82.

Padayachee A, van Wyk CW. Human papillomavirus (HPV) DNA in focal epithelial hyperplasia by in situ hybridization. J Oral Pathol Med 1991;20:210.

Vilmer C, Cavelier-Balloy B, Pinquier L, et al. Focal epithelial hyperplasia and multifocal human papillomavirus infection in an HIV-seropositive man. J Am Acad Dermatol 1994;30:497.

Viraben R, Aquilina C, Brousset P, et al. Focal epithelial hyperplasia (Heck disease) associated with AIDS. Dermatology 1996;193:261.

### Molluscum Contagiosum

Laskaris G, Sklavounov A. Molluscum contagiosum of the oral mucosa. Oral Surg Oral Med Oral Pathol 1984;58:688.

Lowy DR. Milker's nodules, molluscum contagiosum. In: Fitzpatrick TB, et al., eds. Dermatology in general medicine. 4th ed. New York: McGraw-Hill, 1993:2608–2610.

Schwartz JJ, Myskowski PL. Molluscum contagiosum in patients with human immunodeficiency virus infection: a review of twenty-seven patients. J Am Acad Dermatol 1992;27:583.

Whitaker SB, Wiegand SE, Budnick SD. Intraoral molluscum contagiosum. Oral Surg Oral Med Oral Pathol 1991;72:334.

## Verruciform Xanthoma

Drummond JF, White DK, Damm DD, et al. Verruciform xanthoma present within carcinoma-in-situ. J Oral Maxillofac Surg 1989;47:398.

Gehrig RD, Baughman RA, Collins JF. Verruciform xanthoma in a young male patient with a past history of pemphigus vulgaris. Oral Surg Oral Med Oral Pathol 1983;55:58.

Iamaroon A, Vickers RA. Characterization of verruciform xanthoma by in situ hybridization and immunohistochemistry. J Oral Pathol Med 1996;25:395.

Miyamoto Y, Nagayama M, Hayashi Y. Verruciform xanthoma occurring within oral lichen planus. J Oral Pathol Med 1996;25:188.

Mostafa KA, Takata T, Ogawa I, et al. Verruciform xanthoma of the oral mucosa: a clinicopathological study with immunohistochemical findings related to pathogenesis. Virchows Arch A Pathol Anat Histopathol 1993;423:243.

Neville BW. The verruciform xanthoma: a review and report of 8 new cases. Am J Dermatopathol 1986;8:247.

Nowparast B, Howell FV, Rick GM. Verruciform xanthoma: a clinicopathologic review and report of fifty-four cases. Oral Surg Oral Med Oral Pathol 1981;51:619.

## Actinic Cheilosis (Actinic Keratosis of the Lip)

Cataldo E, Doku HC. Solar cheilitis. J Dermatol Surg Oncol 1981;7:989.

Dufresne RG Jr, Curlin MU. Actinic cheilitis: a treatment review. Dermatol Surg 1997;23:15.

Main JH, Pavone M. Actinic cheilitis and carcinoma of the lip. J Can Dent Assoc 1994;60:113.

Picascia DD, Robinson JK. Actinic cheilitis: a review of the etiology, differential diagnosis, and treatment. J Am Acad Dermatol 1987;17:255.

Schmitt CK, Folsom TC. Histologic evaluation of degenerative changes of the lower lip. J Oral Surg 1968;26:51.

Warnock GR, Fuller RP Jr, Pelleu GB. Evaluation of 5-fluorouracil in the treatment of actinic keratosis of the lip. Oral Surg Oral Med Oral Pathol 1981;52:501.

Zelickson BD, Roenigk RK. Actinic cheilitis: treatment with the carbon dioxide laser. Cancer 1990;65:1307.

## Frictional (Mechanical) Keratosis

Corbet EF, Holmgren CJ, Phillipsen HP. Oral mucosal lesions in 65-74-year-old Hong Kong Chinese. Community Dent Oral Epidemiol 1994;22:392.

Daley TD. Common acanthotic and keratotic lesions of the oral mucosa: a review. J Can Dent Assoc 1990;56:407.

Macigo FG, Mwaniki DL, Gunthua SW. Prevalence of oral mucosal lesions in a Kenyan population with special reference to oral leukoplakia. East Afr Med J 1995;72:778.

Neville BW, Damm DD, Allen CM, Bouquot JE. Oral and maxillofacial pathology. 1st ed. Philadelphia: WB Saunders, 1995:282.

Regezi JA, Sciubba J. Oral pathology: Clinical-pathologic correlations. 2nd ed. Philadelphia: WB Saunders, 1993:98–99.

## Nicotine Stomatitis

Pindborg JJ, Mehta FS, Gupta PC, et al. Reverse smoking in Andhra Pradesh, India: a study of palatal lesions among 10,169 villagers. Br J Cancer 1971;25:10.

Reddy CR, Kameswari VR, Ramulu PG. Histopathological study of stomatitis nicotina. Br J Cancer 1971;25:403.

Rossie KM, Guggenheimer J. Thermally induced nicotine stomatitis: a case report. Oral Surg Oral Med Oral Pathol 1990;70:597.

Thoma KH. Stomatitis nicotina and its effect on the palate. Am J Orthod Oral Surg 1941;27:38.

## Tobacco Pouch

Connolly GN, Winn DM, Hecht SS, et al. The reemergence of smokeless tobacco. N Engl J Med 1986;314:1020.

Creath CJ, Shelton WO, Wright JT, et al. The prevalence of smokeless tobacco use among adolescent male athletes. J Am Dent Assoc 1988;116:43.

Creath CJ, Cutter G, Bradley DH, et al. Oral leukoplakia and adolescent smokeless tobacco use. Oral Surg Oral Med Oral Pathol 1991;72:35.

Daniels TE, Hansen LS, Greenspan JS, et al. Histopathology of smokeless tobacco lesions in professional baseball players. Oral Surg Oral Med Oral Pathol 1992;73:720.

Frithiof L, Anneroth G, Lasson U, et al. The snuff-induced lesion: a clinical and morphological study of a Swedish material. Acta Odontol Scand 1983;41:53.

Ghosh S, Shukla HS, Mohapatra SC, et al. Keeping chewing tobacco in the cheek pouch overnight (night quid) increases risk of cheek carcinoma. Eur J Surg Oncol 1996;22:359.

Grady D, Greene J, Daniel TE, et al. Oral mucosal lesions found in smokeless tobacco users. J Am Dent Assoc 1990;121:117.

Greer RO, Poulson TC, Boone ME, et al. Smokeless tobacco-associated oral changes in juvenile, adult and geriatric patients: clinical and histomorphologic features. Gerodontics 1986;2:87.

Kaugars GE, Mehailescu WL, Gunsolley JC. Smokeless tobacco use and oral epithelial dysplasia. Cancer 1989;64:1527.

Kaugars GE, Riley WT, Brandt RB, et al. The prevalence of oral lesions in smokeless tobacco users and evaluation of risk factors. Cancer 1992;70:2579.

McGuirt WF. Snuff dipper's carcinoma. Arch Otolaryngol 1983;109:757.

Sundström B, Mörnstad H, Axéll T. Oral carcinomas associated with snuff dipping: some clinical and histological characteristics of 23 tumors in Swedish males. J Oral Pathol 1982;11:245.

Winn DM, Blot WJ, Shy CM, et al. Snuff dipping and oral cancer among women in the southern United States. N Engl J Med 1981;304:745.

## Leukoplakia/Erythroplakia

Axéll T, Holmstrup P, Kramer IRH, et al. International seminar on oral leukoplakia and associated lesions related to tobacco habits. Community Dent Oral Epidemiol 1984;12:145.

Axéll T, Pindborg JJ, Smith CJ, et al. Oral white lesions with reference to precancerous and tobacco-related lesions: conclusions of an international symposium held in Uppsala, Sweden, May 18-21, 1994. J Oral Pathol Med 1996;25:49.

Bouquot JE, Whitaker SB. Oral leukoplakia: rationale for diagnosis and prognosis of its clinical subtypes or phases. Quint Int 1994;25:133.

Conley BA, Ord RA. Current status of retinoids in chemoprevention of oral squamous cell carcinoma: an overview. J Craniomaxillofac Surg 1996;24:339.

Garewal HS, Schantz S. Emerging role of beta-carotene and antioxidant nutrients in prevention of oral cancer. Arch Otolaryngol Head Neck Surg 1995;121:141.

Hansen LS, Olson JA, Silverman S. Proliferative verrucous leukoplakia. Oral Surg Oral Med Oral Pathol 1985;60:285.

Kaugars GE, Silverman S Jr, Lovas JG, et al. A review of the use of antioxidant supplements in the treatment of human oral leukoplakia. J Cell Biochem Suppl 1993;17F:292.

Lumerman H, Freedman P, Kerpel S. Oral epithelial dysplasia and the development of invasive squamous cell carcinoma. Oral Surg Oral Med Oral Pathol Oral Radiol Endod 1995;79:321.

Mashberg A. Erythroplasia: the earliest sign of asymptomatic oral cancer. J Am Dent Assoc 1978;96:615.

Palefsky JM, Silverman S Jr, Abdel-Salaam M, et al. Association between proliferative verrucous leukoplakia and infection with human papillomavirus type 16. J Oral Pathol Med 1995;24:193.

Pindborg JJ, Daftary DK, Mehta FS. A follow-up study of sixty-one oral dysplastic precancerous lesions in Indian villagers. Oral Surg Oral Med Oral Pathol 1977;43:383.

Shafer WG, Waldron CA. A clinical and histopathologic study of oral leukoplakia. Surg Gynecol Obstet 1961;112:411.

Shafer WG, Waldron CA. Erythroplakia of the oral cavity. Cancer 1975;36:1021.

Shear M. Erythroplakia of the mouth. Int Dent J 1972;22:460.

Silverman S Jr, Gorsky M. Proliferative verrucous leukoplakia: a follow-up study of 54 cases. Oral Surg Oral Med Oral Pathol Oral Radiol Endod 1997;84:154.

Silverman S Jr, Gorsky M, Lozada F. Oral leukoplakia and malignant transformation: a follow-up study of 257 patients. Cancer 1984;53:563.

Waldron CA, Shafer WG. Leukoplakia revisited: a clinicopathologic study of 3256 oral leukoplakias. Cancer 1975;36:1386.

WHO Collaborating Centre for Oral Precancerous Lesions. Definition of leukoplakia and related lesions: an aid to studies on oral precancer. Oral Surg Oral Med Oral Pathol 1978;46:518.

## Squamous Cell Carcinoma

Awde JD, Kogon SL, Morin RJ. Lip cancer: a review. J Can Dent Assoc 1996;62:634.

Blot WJ, McLauglin JK, Winn DM, et al. Smoking and drinking in relation to oral and pharyngeal cancer. Cancer Res 1988;48:3282.

Bouquot JE, Weiland LH, Kurland LT. Metastases to and from the upper aerodigestive tract in the population of Rochester, Minnesota, 1935-1984. Head Neck 1989;11:212.

Chen J, Eisenberg E, Krutchkoff DJ, et al. Changing trends in oral cancer in the United States, 1935 to 1985: a Connecticut Study. J Oral Maxillofac Surg 1991;49:1152.

Choi SY, Kahyo H. Effect of cigarette smoking and alcohol consumption in the aetiology of cancer of the oral cavity, pharynx and larynx. Int J Epidemiol 1991;20:878.

Day GL, Blot WJ. Second primary tumors in patients with oral cancer. Cancer 1992;70:14.

Flaitz CM, Nichols CM, Adler-Storthz K, et al. Intraoral squamous cell carcinoma in human immunodeficiency virus infection: a clinicopathologic study. Oral Surg Oral Med Oral Pathol Oral Radiol Endod 1995;80:55.

Hicks WL Jr, Loree TR, Garcia RI, et al. Squamous cell carcinoma of the floor of mouth: a 20 year review. Head Neck 1997;19:400.

Kassim KH, Daley TD. Herpes simplex virus Type 1 proteins in human oral squamous cell carcinoma. Oral Surg Oral Med Oral Pathol 1988;66:445.

Kessler S, Bartley MH. Spindle cell squamous carcinoma of the tongue in the first decade of life. Oral Surg Oral Med Oral Pathol 1988;66:470.

Krolls SO, Hoffman S. Squamous cell carcinoma of the oral soft tissues: a statistical analysis of 14,253 cases by age, sex and race of patients. J Am Dent Assoc 1976;92:571.

Mashberg A, Meyers H. Anatomical site and size of 222 early asymptomatic oral squamous cell carcinomas: a continuing prospective study of oral cancer: II. Cancer 1976;37:2149.

Mashberg A, Morrisey JB, Garfinkel L. A study of the appearance of early asymptomatic squamous cell carcinoma. Cancer 1973;32:1436.

Michalek AM, Mahoney MC, McLauglin CC, et al. Historical and contemporary correlates of syphilis and cancer. Int J Epidemiol 1994;23:381.

Miller CS, White DK. Human papillomavirus expression in oral mucosa, premalignant conditions, and squamous cell carcinoma: a retrospective review of the literature. Oral Surg Oral Med Oral Pathol Oral Radiol Endod 1996;82:57.

Nielsen H, Norrild B, Vedtofte P, et al. Human papillomavirus in oral premalignant lesions. Eur J Cancer Oral Oncol 1996;32B:264.

O'Grady JF, Reade PC. Candida albicans as a promoter of oral mucosal neoplasia. Carcinogenesis 1992;13:783.

Oliver AJ, Helfrick JF, Gard D. Primary oral squamous cell carcinoma: a review of 92 cases. J Oral Maxillofac Surg 1996;54:949.

Park N-H, Dokko H, Li S-L, et al. Synergism of herpes simplex virus and tobbaco-specific N'-nitrosamines in cell transformation. J Oral Maxillofac Surg 1991;49:276.

Paz IB, Cook N, Odom-Maryon T, et al. Human papillomavirus (HPV) in head and neck cancer: an association of HPV 16 with squamous cell carcinoma of Waldeyer's tonsillar ring. Cancer 1997;79:595.

Sankaranarayanan R. Oral cancer in India: an epidemiologic and clinical review. Oral Surg Oral Med Oral Pathol 1990;69:325.

Sarkaria JN, Harari PM. Oral tongue cancer in young adults less than 40 years of age: rationale for aggressive therapy. Head Neck 1994;16:107.

Silverman S Jr. Early diagnosis of oral cancer. Cancer 1988;62:1796.

Sundström B, Mörnstad H, Axéll T. Oral carcinomas associated with snuff dipping: some clinical and histological characteristics of 23 tumors in Swedish males. J Oral Pathol 1982;11:245.

Thomas DW, Seddon SV, Shepherd JP. Systemic immunosuppression and oral malignancy: a report of a case and review of the literature. Br J Oral Maxillofac Surg 1993;31:391.

Watts JM. The importance of the Plummer-Vinson syndrome in the aetiology of carcinoma of the upper gastro-intestinal tract. Postgrad Med J 1961;37:523.

Zitsch RP III, Park CW, Renner GJ, et al. Outcome analysis for lip carcinoma. Otolaryngol Head Neck Surg 1995;113:589.

### Verrucous Carcinoma

Batsakis JG, Hybels R, Crissman JD, et al. The pathology of head and neck tumors: verrucous carcinoma, part 15. Head Neck Surg 1982;5:29.

Jordan RC. Verrucous carcinoma of the mouth. J Can Dent Assoc 1995;61:797.

Jyothirmayi R, Sankaranarayanan R, Varghese C, et al. Radiotherapy in the treatment of verrucous carcinoma of the oral cavity. Oral Oncol 1997;33:124.

Kamath VV, Varma RR, Gadewar DR, et al. Oral verrucous carcinoma: an analysis of 37 cases. J Craniomaxillofac Surg 1989;17:309.

Lubbe J, Kormann A, Adams V, et al. HPV-11 and HPV-16-associated oral verrucous carcinoma. Dermatology 1996;192:217.

McDonald JS, Crissman JD, Gluckman JL. Verrucous carcinoma of the oral cavity. Head Neck Surg 1982;5:22.

Medina JE, Dichtel W, Luna MA. Verrucous-squamous carcinoma of the oral cavity: a clinicopathologic study of 104 cases. Arch Otolaryngol 1984;110:437.

Shroyer KR, Greer RO, Fankhouser CA, et al. Detection of human papillomavirus DNA in oral verrucous carcinoma by polymerase chain reaction. Mod Pathol 1993;6:669.

## Nasopharyngeal Carcinoma

Batsakis JG, Solomon AR, Rice CH. The pathology of head and neck tumors: carcinoma of the nasopharynx, part II. Head Neck Surg 1981;3:511.

Easton JM, Levine PH, Hyams VT. Nasopharyngeal carcinoma in the United States. Arch Otolaryngol 1980;106:88.

Epstein JB, Jones CK. Presenting signs and symptoms of nasopharyngeal carcinoma. Oral Surg Oral Med Oral Pathol 1993;75:32.

Hawkins EP, Krischer JP, Smith BE, et al. Nasopharyngeal carcinoma in children: a retrospective review and demonstration of Epstein-Barr viral genomes in tumor cell cytoplasm: a report of the Pediatric Oncology Group. Hum Pathol 1990;21:805.

Sham JS, Choy D. Prognostic factors of nasopharyngeal carcinoma: a review of 759 patients. Br J Radiol 1990;63:51.

Vasef MA, Ferlito A, Weiss LM. Nasopharngeal carcinoma, with emphasis on its relationship to Epstein-Barr virus. Ann Otol Rhinol Laryngol 1997;106:348.

Zheng X, Christensson B, Drettner B. Studies on etiological factors of nasopharyngeal carcinoma. Acta Otolaryngol (Stockh) 1993;113:455.

## Maxillary Sinus Carcinoma

Harbo G, Grau C, Bundgaard T, et al. Cancer of the nasal cavity and paranasal sinuses: a clinico-pathological study of 277 patients. Acta Oncol 1997;36:45.

Hone SW, O'Leary TG, Maguire A, et al. Malignant sinonasal tumors: the Dublin Eye and Ear Hospital experience. Ir J Med Sci 1995;164:139.

Jakobsen MH, Larsen SK, Kirkegaard J, et al. Cancer of the nasal cavity and paranasal sinuses: prognosis and outcome of treatment. Acta Oncol 1997;36:27.

Kenady DE. Cancer of the paranasal sinuses. Surg Clin North Am 1986;66:119.

Miyaguchi M, Sakai S, Mori N, et al. Symptoms in patients with maxillary sinus carcinoma. J Laryngol Otol 1990;104:557.

Sakata K, Aoki Y, Karasawa K, et al. Analysis of the results of combined therapy for maxillary carcinoma. Cancer 1993;71:2715.

St-Pierre S, Baker SR. Squamous cell carcinoma of the maxillary sinus: analysis of 66 cases. Head Neck Surg 1983;5:508.

Stern SJ, Goepfert H, Clayman G, et al. Squamous cell carcinoma of the maxillary sinus. Arch Otolaryngol Head Neck Surg 1993;119:964.

Weber AL, Stanton AC. Malignant tumors of the paranasal sinuses: radiologic, clinical and histopathologic evaluation of 200 cases. Head Neck Surg 1984;6:761.

## Oral Submucous Fibrosis

Canniff JP, Harvey W, Harris M. Oral submucous fibrosis: its pathogenesis and management. Br Dent J 1986;160:429.

Cox SC, Walker DM. Oral submucous fibrosis: a review. Aust Dent J 1996;41:294.

Gupta DG, Sharma SC. Oral submucous fibrosis: a new treatment regimen. J Oral Maxillofac Surg 1988;46:830.

Maher R, Lee AJ, Warnakulasuriya KAAS, et al. Role of areca nut in the causation of oral submucous fibrosis: a case-control study in Pakistan. J Oral Pathol Med 1994;23:65.

Morawetz G, Katsikeris N, Weinberg S, et al. Oral submucous fibrosis. Int J Oral Maxillofac Surg 1987;16:609.

Nair UJ, Obe G, Friesen M, et al. Role of lime in the generation of reactive oxygen species from betel-quid ingredient. Environ Health Perspect 1992;98:203.

Paissat DK. Oral submucous fibrosis. Int J Oral Surg 1981;10:307.

## Basal Cell Carcinoma

Blinder D, Taicher S. Metastatic basal cell carcinoma presenting in the oral cavity and auditory meatus: a case report and review of literature. Int J Oral Maxillofac Surg 1992;21:31.

Miller SJ. Biology of basal cell carcinoma, part 1. J Am Acad Dermatol 1991;24:1.

Miller SJ. Biology of basal cell carcinoma, part 2. J Am Acad Dermatol 1991;24:161.

Nguyen AV, Whitaker DC, Frodel J. Differentiation of basal cell carcinoma. Otolarynol Clin North Am 1993;26:37.

Preston DS, Stern RS. Nonmelanoma cancers of the skin. N Engl J Med 1992;327:1649.

Randle HW. Basal cell carcinoma. Identification and treatment of the high-risk patient. Dermatol Surg 1996;22:255.

Wang CY, Brodland DG, Su WP. Skin cancers associated with acquired immunodeficiency syndrome. Mayo Clin Proc 1995;70:766.

## Keratoacanthoma

Eversole LR, Leider AS, Alexander G. Intraoral and labial keratoacanthoma. Oral Surg Oral Med Oral Pathol 1982;54:663.

Goodwin RE, Fisher GH. Keratoacanthoma of the head and neck. Ann Otol Rhinol Laryngol 1980;89:72.

Habel G, O'Regan B, Eissing A, et al. Intra-oral keratoacanthoma: an eruptive variant and review of the literature. Br Dent J 1991;170:336.

Jaber PW, Cooper PH, Greer KE. Generalized eruptive keratoacanthoma of Grzybowski. J Am Acad Dermatol 1993;29:299.

Schwartz RA. Keratoacanthoma. J Am Acad Dermatol 1994;30:1.

Young SK, Larsen PE, Markowitz NR. Generalized eruptive keratoacanthoma. Oral Surg Oral Med Oral Pathol 1986;62:422.

## Acquired Melanocytic Nevus, Blue Nevus

Buchner A, Hansen LS. Pigmented nevi of the oral mucosa: a clinicopathologic study of 36 new cases and review of 155 cases from the literature: part I: a clinicopathologic study of 36 new cases. Oral Surg Oral Med Oral Pathol 1987;63:566.

Buchner A, Hansen LS. Pigmented nevi of the oral mucosa: a clinicopathologic study of 36 new cases and review of 155 cases from the literature: part II: analysis of 191 cases. Oral Surg Oral Med Oral Pathol 1987;63:676.

Buchner A, Leider AS, Merrell PW, et al. Melanocytic nevi of the oral mucosa: a clinicopathologic study of 130 cases from northern California. J Oral Pathol Med 1990;19:197.

Gonzalez-Campora R, Galera-Davidson H, Vazquez-Ramirez FJ, et al. Blue nevus: classical types and new related entities: a differential diagnostic review. Pathol Res Pract 1994;190:627.

Papanicolaou SJ, Pierrakou ED, Patsakas AJ. Intraoral blue nevus: review of the literature and a case report. J Oral Med 1985;40:32.

Rhodes AR. Neoplasms: benign neoplasia, hyperplasias and dysplasias of melanocytes. In: Fitzpatrick TB, et al, eds. Dermatology in general medicine. 4th ed. New York: McGraw-Hill, 1993:996–1048.

## Malignant Melanoma

Elwood JM. Melanoma and sun exposure. Semin Oncol 1996;23:650.

Manganaro AM, Hammond HL, Dalton MJ, et al. Oral melanoma: case reports and review of the literature. Oral Surg Oral Med Oral Pathol Oral Radiol Endod 1995;80:670.

Meyer LJ, Zone JH. Genetics of cutaneous melanoma. J Invest Dermatol 1994;103(Suppl 5):112S.

Rapini RP, Golitz LE, Greer RO, et al. Primary malignant melanoma of the oral cavity. Cancer 1985;55:1543.

Regezi JA, Hayward JR, Pickens TN. Superficial melanomas of oral mucous membranes. Oral Surg Oral Med Oral Pathol 1978;45:730.

Reintgen D, Balch CM, Kirkwood J, et al. Recent advances in the care of the patient with malignant melanoma. Ann Surg 1997;225:1.

Smyth AG, Ward-Booth RP, Avery EWH. Malignant melanoma of the oral cavity: an increasing clinical diagnosis. Br J Oral Maxillofac Surg 1993;31:230.

Tanaka N, Amagasa T, Iwaki H, et al. Oral malignant melanoma in Japan. Oral Surg Oral Med Oral Pathol 1994;78:81.

Umeda M, Shimada K. Primary malignant melanoma of the oral cavity: its histological classification and treatment. Br J Oral Maxillofac Surg 1994;32:39.

Van der Waal RI, Snow GB, Karim AB, et al. Primary malignant melanoma of the oral cavity: a review of eight cases. Br Dent J 1994;176:185.

## Metastatic Carcinoma

Allen CM, Neville B, Damm DD, et al. Leiomyosarcoma metastatic to the oral region: report of three cases. Oral Surg Oral Med Oral Pathol 1993;76:752.

Cohen DM, Green JG, Diekmann SL, et al. Maxillary metastasis of transitional cell carcinoma: report of a case. Oral Surg Oral Med Oral Pathol 1989;67:185.

Hashimoto N, Kurihara K, Yamasaki H, et al. Pathologic characteristics of metastatic carcinoma in the human mandible. J Oral Pathol 1987;16:362.

Hicks MJ, Smith JD Jr, Carter AB, et al. Recurrent intrapulmonary malignant small cell tumor of the thoracopulmonary region with metastasis to the oral cavity: review of literature and case report. Ultrastruc Pathol 1995;19:297.

Hirshberg A, Leibovich P, Buchner A. Metastases to the oral mucosa: analysis of 157 cases. J Oral Pathol Med 1993;22:385.

Hirshberg A, Leibovich P, Buchner A. Metastatic tumors to the jawbones: analysis of 390 cases. J Oral Pathol 1994;23:337.

Naylor GD, Auclair PL, Rathbun WA, et al. Metastatic adenocarcinoma of the colon presenting as periradicular periodontal disease: a case report. Oral Surg Oral Med Oral Pathol 1989;67:162.

Patton LL, Brahim JS, Baker AR. Metastatic malignant melanoma of the oral cavity: a retrospective study. Oral Surg Oral Med Oral Pathol 1994;78:51.

Zachariades N. Neoplasms metastatic to the mouth, jaws and surrounding tissues. J Craniomaxillofac Surg 1989;17:283.

# chapter 8

# SALIVARY GLAND PATHOLOGY

**Figs. 8.1 and 8.2**

The mucocele is an accumulation of mucus within the supporting connective tissue of minor salivary glands resulting from rupture of the ducts or glandular acini. The lesion affects all ages and occurs most commonly on the lower lip. Other common sites of involvement are the ventral tongue, the vestibule, and the buccal mucosa.

Small, blister-like mucoceles occur on the soft palate and tonsillar pillars, but well-developed ones seldom are encountered there. A mucocele of the upper lip or retromolar pad is rare, and a salivary gland neoplasm should be considered if a mucocele-like lesion is present in these locations. If the pooling of mucus is superficial, the lesion appears as a fluctuant mass that is blue-tinted and translucent. More deeply seated mucoceles may be firm and the color of normal mucosa. Treatment is surgical excision, including the adjacent salivary gland lobules.

# RANULA

**Fig. 8.3**

A ranula is a mucus extravasation phenomenon in the floor of the mouth, arising from the ducts of either the sublingual or submandibular glands. In most instances, it represents a mucocele arising from a break in one of the ducts of the sublingual gland. It appears as a significant, unilateral swelling of the floor of the mouth that is fluctuant and blue-tinted.

Mucoceles from minor glands of the floor of the mouth can occur and need to be differentiated from ones developing from the sublingual gland because of treatment differences. Also, vascular and salivary gland neoplasms may appear similar. Treatment includes marsupialization, surgical excision including the involved gland, and carbon dioxide laser excision. Rarely, this process may herniate through the muscles of the floor of the mouth and present as a cervical mass. This is referred to as a "plunging" or "cervical" ranula.

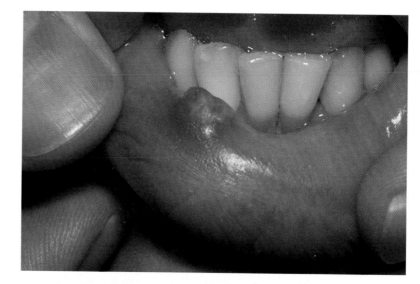

▶ **Figure 8.1**
**MUCOCELE**

Soft, fluid-filled mass of the lower lip.

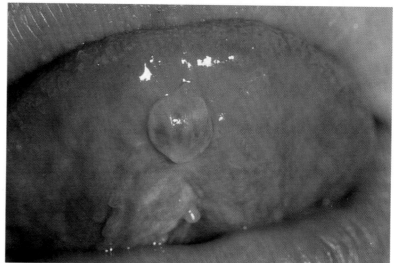

▶ **Figure 8.2**
**MUCOCELE**

Soft, exophytic mass of ventral tongue.

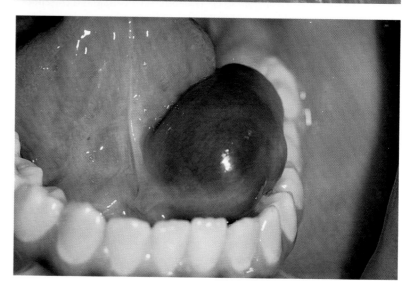

▶ **Figure 8.3**
**RANULA**

Soft, bluish swelling of the left side of the floor of the mouth. (Case courtesy of Dr. John Hann.)

## SALIVARY GLAND DUCT CYST (MUCUS RETENTION CYST, RETENTION MUCOCELE)

**Fig. 8.4**    The salivary gland duct cyst is an epithelium-lined cavity that arises from minor salivary gland duct epithelium within connective tissue of the oral cavity. It is much less common than the extravasation type of mucocele. The cyst most often is seen in adults and usually develops in the floor of the mouth, the upper lip, the buccal mucosa, or the vestibule. When superficially placed, it appears as a soft mass that is amber to yellow to light blue. Deeply seated cysts appear mucosal colored and often are detected only by palpation. In both situations, the cyst is indistinguishable from a true neoplasm, especially a salivary gland tumor. Treatment is surgical excision.

## SJÖGREN SYNDROME

**Figs. 8.5 and 8.6**    Sjögren syndrome is a chronic autoimmune disorder characterized principally by dry eyes (keratoconjunctivitis sicca) and dry mouth (xerostomia). These symptoms develop because of an intense lymphocytic infiltrate that destroys lacrimal and salivary gland parenchyma. In addition, other organs may be involved by the immunodestructive process and patients may exhibit dry skin, nephritis, lung fibrosis, nasal and vaginal dryness, Raynaud's phenomenon, vasculitis, and peripheral and central nervous system alterations. When associated with other autoimmune diseases, such as rheumatoid arthritis and systemic lupus erythematosus, it is termed "secondary Sjögren syndrome."

Sjögren syndrome primarily occurs in women between 30 and 65 years of age, but it may develop in children. The cause remains unknown, but the process tends to develop in certain HLA groups, and a viral cause has been hypothesized. However, definitive evidence is lacking. The autoimmune theory is supported by the presence of a number of circulating autoantibodies, particularly anti-SS-A and anti-SS-B, in affected patients.

About half of all patients exhibit parotid swelling, either unilateral or bilateral. The other major glands may exhibit swelling but less frequently than the parotid glands. The swelling may be persistent or intermittent. Minor salivary glands also may be affected by the immunologic infiltrate, but usually there is no noticeable swelling.

A number of changes may be seen in the oral cavity that are the result of the reduction of salivary flow. The mouth feels dry, and the mucosa may be erythematous. Candidiasis is a frequent complication. The tongue may be fissured and exhibit papillary atrophy. Patients may have altered taste sensation, and swallowing may be difficult. They also are susceptible to dental caries, especially cervical caries.

The diagnosis of Sjögren syndrome is based on a combination of clinical, microscopic, and serologic findings. The presence of dry eyes and dry mouth with ocular and oral mucosa alterations typically initiates the diagnostic process. Biopsy of the labial salivary glands or involved major salivary glands may be helpful in confirming the diagnosis, but minor salivary glands may not show the immunologic infiltrate even in patients with the disease. Correlation with signs and symptoms of other systemic diseases is helpful, and the presence of the SS-A and SS-B autoantibodies in conjunction with the appropriate clinical symptoms should fulfill the criteria for diagnosis. Sialograms of an involved parotid gland may show changes, but these are not diagnostic. It is important to note that bilateral parotid swelling alone is not diagnostic for Sjögren syndrome and that a variety of inflammatory, infectious, and neoplastic disorders can present in this fashion.

Treatment for Sjögren syndrome primarily is supportive in nature. Systemic corticosteroids may be used to contain the immunologic destruction, but they are not always effective. Artificial tears and saliva are helpful in managing dry mucosa, and pilocarpine may be helpful in stimulating salivary flow in patients who have salivary gland parenchyma remaining. The development of extensive dental caries is a common complication, and fluoride applications may help to contain the process. A significant consequence is the increased risk of developing malignant lymphoma, and patients should be followed up closely for the development of persistent lymphadenopathy, intraoral swelling, or an increase in the size of an involved major salivary gland.

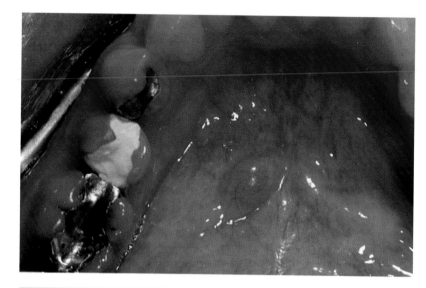

▶ **Figure 8.4**
**SALIVARY GLAND DUCT CYST**
Amber colored, translucent swelling of the
floor of the mouth.

▶ **Figure 8.5**
**SJÖGREN SYNDROME**
Adult female with bilateral parotid
swelling.

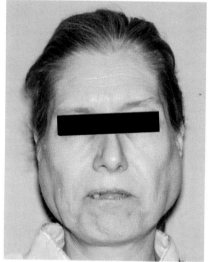

▶ **Figure 8.6**
**SJÖGREN SYNDROME**
Adult exhibiting loss of teeth from dental
caries and cervical decalcification of
remaining teeth.

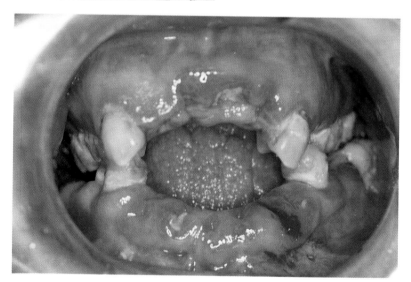

# Figs. 8.7, 8.8, 8.9, 8.10, 8.11, and 8.12

Sialolithiasis is the presence of a calcified structure (sialolith) within salivary gland ducts or, less frequently, within the glands. Calcium salts are deposited around a central nidus that provides the environment necessary for calcification to occur. In most cases, the sialolith, or stone, develops in the duct of the submandibular gland. The parotid and minor salivary gland ducts can also be affected. Most often, this process is seen in adults, but it can occur in children. Rarely, bilateral gland involvement is present. In most instances, sialolithiasis is not associated with systemic illnesses. However, results of a recent study indicate that these patients may be more prone to develop nephrolithiasis (kidney stones).

Symptoms of sialolithiasis are varied and may include soft-tissue swelling overlying the stone, swelling of the involved gland, and pain, particularly when food is ingested. The extent of symptoms depends on the amount of obstruction of the duct, the cessation of salivary flow, retention of saliva within the affected gland, and resultant inflammatory and degenerative changes. As with any chronic swelling of the oral cavity and head and neck, a neoplastic process should be included in a differential diagnosis. In most situations, the stone is visible on radiographs, but not all sialoliths are calcified sufficiently to be seen. Sialography may be helpful in identifying the blockage in these instances.

When the submandibular gland duct is involved, the stone may cause a firm swelling in the floor of the mouth. The gland may or may not be swollen. Deeply seated stones may not produce obvious intraoral swelling but can be found on radiographs, where the stone presents as a radiopaque mass in the floor of the mouth or superimposed on the mandible, simulating an intrabony alteration. A sialolith in the parotid duct may present as a hard mass in the buccal mucosa and as a radiopaque structure when a panoramic radiograph is taken. The parotid gland may or may not be enlarged. A minor salivary gland stone primarily presents as a firm dome-shaped or conical nodule of the upper lip or buccal mucosa and may appear yellowish. Typically, minor salivary gland stones are confused with salivary gland duct cysts, fibrous hyperplasia, or connective tissue tumors.

Some superficial stones may be expressed from the involved duct by simple manipulation, but most stones have to be removed by a more sophisticated method. Typically, surgical removal has been used, but now other modalities, such as a retrieval catheter with fluoroscopy, lasers, and extracorporeal electromagnetic shockwave lithotripsy, are being performed. Associated glands that have become symptomatic (swollen, inflamed, and fibrotic) generally require removal because of persistent pain and swelling.

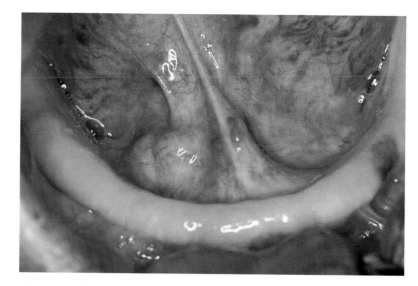

### Figure 8.7
### SIALOLITH
Firm unilateral swelling of the anterior floor of the mouth distal to submandibular gland duct orifice.

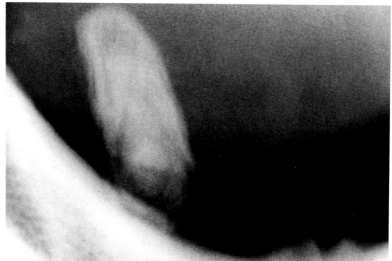

### Figure 8.8
### SIALOLITH
Occlusal radiograph of the patient depicted in Figure 8.7 that exhibits a large stone in the submandibular duct.

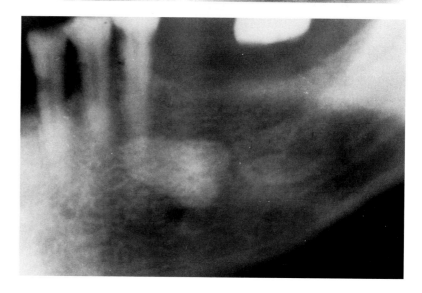

### Figure 8.9
### SIALOLITH
Stones of submandibular duct superimposed on the mandible on a panoramic radiograph. This was initially mistaken for an impacted tooth.

**Figure 8.10**

Gross appearance of sialoliths depicted in Figure 8.9. One of these stones exhibits a toothlike appearance.

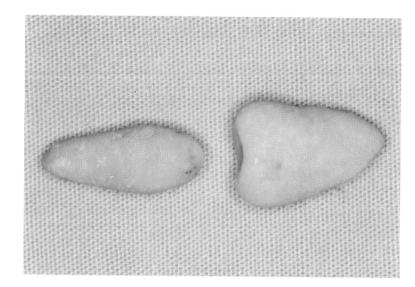

**Figure 8.11**
**SIALOLITH**

Firm, superficial nodule of the upper labial mucosa.

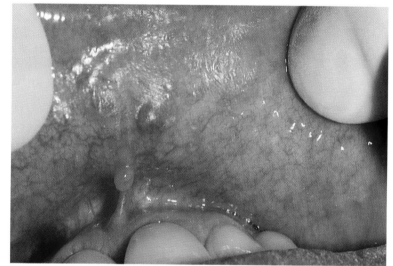

**Figure 8.12**
**SIALOLITH**

Radiograph of the upper lip in the patient shown in Figure 8.11 showing a small, calcified structure.

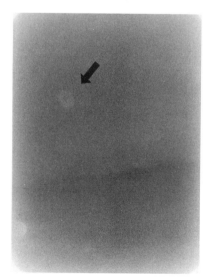

## Figs. 8.13, 8.14, 8.15, and 8.16

The pleomorphic adenoma is the most common salivary gland neoplasm. It derives its name from the varied histopathologic picture within the tumor. Histopathologically, it consists of an encapsulated proliferation of ductal and myoepithelial cells supported by a stroma that varies from dense hyalinized collagen to loosely arranged ground substance. Cartilage and bone may be present.

Pleomorphic adenomas may develop in patients of widely varying ages from the second decade onward, and there is a predilection among females. The parotid is the most common site, but the neoplasm may arise in any location where salivary gland tissue is present. The parotid pleomorphic adenoma usually develops in the superficial lobe and presents as a firm, slow-growing swelling anterior to the ear. A small number develop in the deep lobe and cause little facial asymmetry. However, they may exhibit swelling of the lateral pharyngeal wall that is noticeable on intraoral examination. Those that develop from the submandibular gland present as a firm, painless swelling of the upper neck overlying the involved gland.

The palate is the most common intraoral site, followed by the upper lip and the buccal mucosa. The intraoral tumor usually presents as a firm submucosal mass covered by intact epithelium. Ulceration may develop over large tumors. If a cystic component is present within the tumor, the lesion may have a bluish appearance and be indistinguishable clinically from a deeply seated mucocele or a mucoepidermoid carcinoma.

Treatment is complete surgical removal. In the major glands, lobectomy or total gland removal is the therapeutic choice to prevent recurrence. Intraoral lesions are treated best with surgical excision that includes a border of normal tissue. Malignant change is uncommon but has occurred in long-standing pleomorphic adenomas, and the tumor should not be considered a premalignant condition.

**Figure 8.13**
**PLEOMORPHIC ADENOMA**
Firm, unilateral swelling of the hard palate. A midline traumatic ulcer is present.

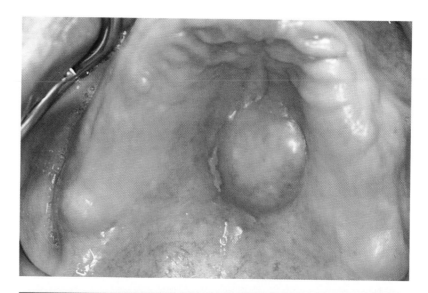

**Figure 8.14**
**PLEOMORPHIC ADENOMA**
Firm, submucosal mass of the upper labial mucosa. (Case courtesy of Dr. Karen Naples.)

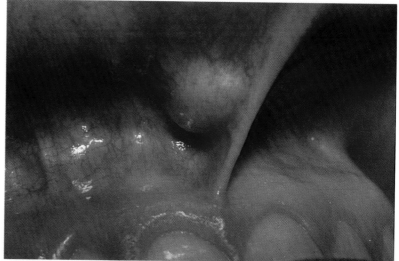

**Figure 8.15**
**PLEOMORPHIC ADENOMA**
Firm swelling of right parotid gland.

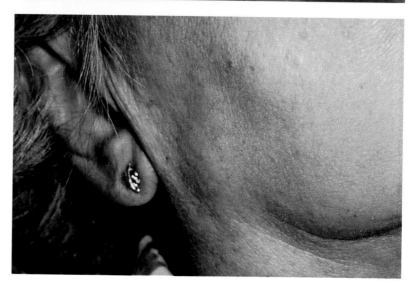

## CANALICULAR ADENOMA

**Fig. 8.17**

"Monomorphic adenoma" is a term applied to a group of benign neoplasms of salivary gland origin in which the histopathologic picture exhibits a uniform and distinctive appearance throughout the tumor. Several histopathologic variants occur, and there is movement toward using the more descriptive name rather than the generic term, monomorphic adenoma.

The canalicular variant typically arises from minor salivary glands of the upper lip. On rare occasions, it develops in the buccal mucosa and the hard palate. Multifocal tumors also have been described. The basal cell adenoma most often develops in the parotid gland but may arise from minor salivary glands.

The tumor is seen most often in patients in the sixth and seventh decades of life. When the lesion is deeply seated in oral mucosa or the parotid gland, it appears as a nonspecific mass, resembling any soft-tissue or glandular neoplasm. When arising in a superficial mucosal location, these tumors may appear fluctuant and blue-tinted, resembling a mucocele. The neoplasm is encapsulated and requires simple surgical removal, including the connective tissue capsule. The recurrence rate is low.

## WARTHIN'S TUMOR (PAPILLARY CYSTADENOMA LYMPHOMATOSUM)

**Fig. 8.18**

Warthin's tumor is a benign salivary gland neoplasm believed to arise from the proliferation of salivary gland tissue entrapped within lymphoid tissue. Alternately, it has been suggested that it may arise from the proliferation of antigenically changed ductal cells that elicit a chronic lymphoid immune reaction. It almost exclusively arises in the parotid gland, except for a few isolated cases reported in other major and minor salivary glands. Results of recent studies show a strong statistical association between cigarette smoking and the development of the tumor. Results of studies of atomic bomb victims in Japan show a slight increase in the prevalence of the tumor in survivors.

This tumor traditionally has been more common among men, but it now exhibits an increased prevalence among women. The tumor usually presents as a slow-growing, soft-tissue mass near the angle of the mandible, with peak incidence in patients in the sixth and seventh decades of life. A small percentage of patients develop bilateral parotid involvement, with the tumors occurring either simultaneously (synchronous) or at different times (metachronous). Multiple tumors within a single gland also have been described, and the tumor also has developed in association with other, different, salivary gland tumors.

Treatment is surgical excision. A recurrence rate of approximately 10% has been described, but this rate may be overstated because some of the recurrences actually may represent new tumor formation. Rare malignant transformation in the lymphoid or epithelial components has occurred.

▶ **Figure 8.16**
**PLEOMORPHIC ADENOMA**
Mass of the left parotid allowed to grow
for many years. (Courtesy of Dr. E. R.
Costich.)

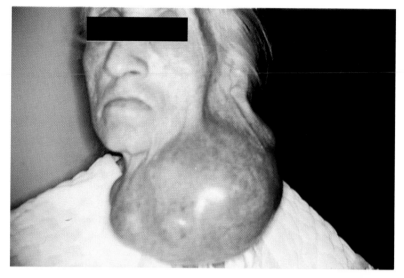

▶ **Figure 8.17**
**CANALICULAR ADENOMA**
Firm, submucosal mass of the upper lip.
(Courtesy of Dr. Jim C. Weir.)

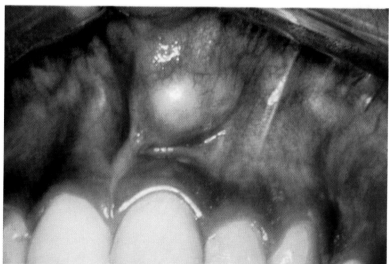

▶ **Figure 8.18**
**WARTHIN'S TUMOR**
Older male with firm swelling of left
parotid gland. The patient had a similar
tumor removed from the opposite side
7 years earlier.

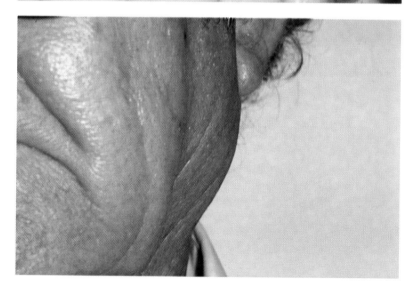

## Figs. 8.19 and 8.20

Mucoepidermoid carcinoma is a malignancy of the salivary glands composed of mucus-secreting and epidermoid cells in varying amounts and patterns. It is the most common salivary gland cancer, and it may be seen in patients at all ages, including children. There is a predilection among females. Ionizing radiation has been cited as a possible factor in the tumorigenesis of mucoepidermoid carcinoma from studies of atomic bomb survivors in Japan.

The palate and the retromolar pad are affected the most in the oral cavity; the parotid is the major gland affected most. Intraorally, mucoepidermoid carcinoma presents as a submucosal mass that may be mucosal colored or exhibit a bluish tint, not unlike a mucocele. Fast-growing lesions may cause surface ulceration. When it develops in the parotid or submandibular gland, the neoplasm usually presents as a soft-tissue mass.

The neoplasm has been divided histopathologically into low grade, intermediate grade, and high grade, depending on the cellular characteristics and the proportion of mucus-secreting to epidermoid cells. This grading system is used to help correlate the histologic picture with clinical behavior and prognosis. The low-grade variant usually is aggressive locally, and metastasis is uncommon but can occur. Treatment is complete excision, with a modest border of normal tissue. Prognosis is excellent. The high-grade variant is staged and treated like a squamous cell carcinoma of the same site. Surgery often combined with adjuvant radiation therapy is used in an attempt to control the disease. Most intraoral mucoepidermoid carcinomas are classified as low-to-intermediate grade.

# INTRAOSSEOUS MUCOEPIDERMOID CARCINOMA

## Fig. 8.21

Intraosseous mucoepidermoid carcinoma is a type of mucoepidermoid carcinoma that develops centrally within bone. It usually develops in the posterior mandible of adults and may be associated with an impacted molar, giving the appearance of an odontogenic lesion such as a dentigerous cyst, an odontogenic keratocyst, or an ameloblastoma. Its radiographic appearance may be unilocular or multilocular, and it can occur in the anterior mandible and maxilla. Bone expansion may be present. Because of its association with impacted teeth, it has been postulated that these tumors arise from pluripotential odontogenic epithelium, such as a dentigerous cyst lining. Other possibilities include from actual minor salivary glands developmentally occurring within bone and from mucous glands of the sinus for maxillary tumors.

Treatment usually is en bloc resection. The prognosis generally is good, but recurrences do occur. Distant metastasis has been reported but is uncommon.

### Figure 8.19
**MUCOEPIDERMOID CARCINOMA**

Cystic-appearing mass of lateral soft palate and pterygomandibular raphe.

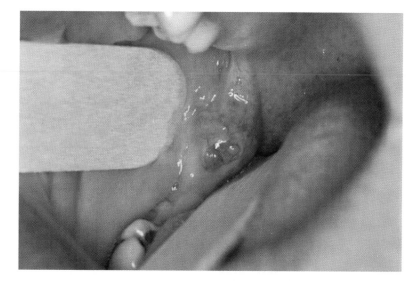

### Figure 8.20
**MUCOEPIDERMOID CARCINOMA**

Soft, blue-tinted mass of the hard palate. (Courtesy of Dr. James T. McClung, Jr.)

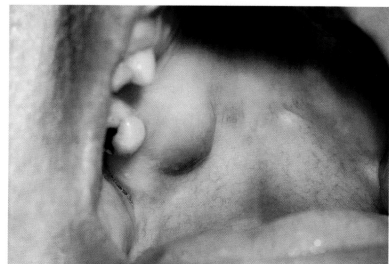

### Figure 8.21
**INTRAOSSEOUS MUCOEPIDERMOID CARCINOMA**

Multilocular radiolucency of the posterior mandible on the right side. (Courtesy of Dr. Joseph Finelli.)

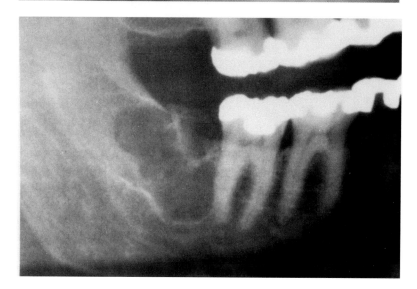

# POLYMORPHOUS LOW-GRADE ADENOCARCINOMA (LOBULAR CARCINOMA, TERMINAL DUCT CARCINOMA)

## Fig. 8.22

Polymorphous low-grade adenocarcinoma is a distinctive cancer of salivary gland origin first described in 1983. It is characterized microscopically by a proliferation of rather uniform cells that can form a variety of structural patterns. It is almost exclusively seen in minor salivary gland tissue, but it also can develop in the parotid and submandibular glands. The palate is the most common location, followed by the buccal mucosa and the lips. It exhibits a prominent female predilection, and it typically presents as a slow-growing mass in an adult.

Treatment is wide surgical excision. The prognosis is considered good, but recurrent disease is seen in about one-fourth of affected patients. Metastasis is uncommon but can occur years after initial therapy. Because of its recent history as a distinct entity, longer-term follow-up studies are needed to assess its true biologic behavior.

# ADENOID CYSTIC CARCINOMA (CYLINDROMA)

## Fig. 8.23

Adenoid cystic carcinoma is one of the more common salivary gland cancers. Microscopically, it is characterized by the formation of infiltrating tubular structures and islands of cells that form multiple cystic spaces within the individual nests. It infiltrates along perineural spaces, which allows the tumor to spread far beyond its site of origin without lymphatic or hematogenous involvement. It is distributed almost equally between minor salivary gland tissue and the parotid and submandibular glands, with the most common location in the mouth being the palate. These tumors typically are seen in middle-aged adults and exhibit a slight female predilection.

Adenoid cystic carcinoma usually presents as a slow-growing mass that may ulcerate in the oral cavity. Patients often complain of pain even before the swelling is of substantial size and before ulceration occurs. Palatal tumors also may be associated with paresthesia because of palatine nerve involvement. Parotid tumors may involve the facial nerve, and patients may complain of weakness or paralysis of muscles innervated by the facial nerve. Pain also may be present.

The most effective therapy for adenoid cystic carcinoma is a combination of radical surgery and radiation therapy. This carcinoma commonly recurs because of incomplete removal of nests of tumor far away from the primary site of the original tumor. The 5-year survival rate is good, but long-term survival is poor because of recurrences and distant metastasis that can appear many years after initial therapy. This tumor spreads by both perineural extension and hematogenous pathways, with distant metastasis often seen without lymph node involvement.

# ACINIC CELL CARCINOMA (ACINIC CELL ADENOCARCINOMA)

## Fig. 8.24

Acinic cell carcinoma is a cancer of salivary glands that microscopically exhibits acinar differentiation in contrast to most other salivary gland tumors in which ductal structures are formed by the neoplastic cells. It is seen most often in the parotid gland, and a small percentage of the tumors develop from minor salivary glands and the other major salivary glands. Intraoral tumors are observed most often in the upper lip and the buccal mucosa and present as slow-growing, nonspecific submucosal masses. Most tumors occur in adults, and they exhibit a predilection for females. Treatment is complete surgical removal. The tumor cells are radioresistant. The 5-year survival rate is high, but the long-term survival rate is moderate. Recurrences can develop years after initial therapy, and approximately 15% of patients develop metastasis, in some instances occurring years later.

### Figure 8.22
**POLYMORPHOUS LOW-GRADE ADENOCARCINOMA**
Large, firm swelling of the hard and soft palates.

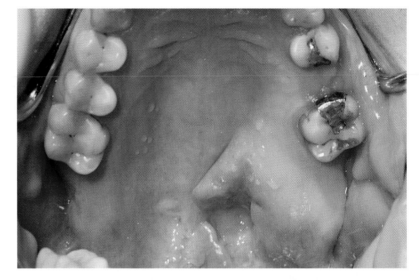

### Figure 8.23
**ADENOID CYSTIC CARCINOMA**
Large, raised mass of the entire palate.

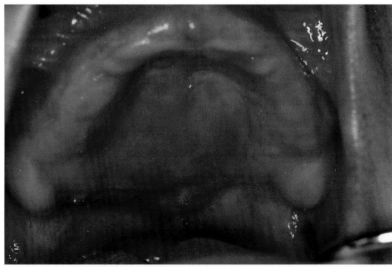

### Figure 8.24
**ACINIC CELL CARCINOMA**
Firm, discrete submucosal mass of the left upper lip in an elderly female.

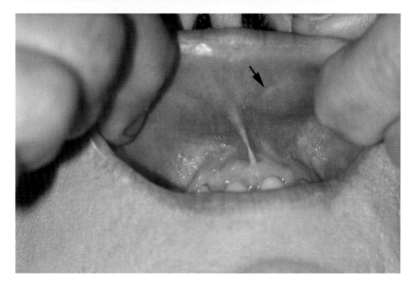

## MALIGNANT MIXED TUMOR

**Fig. 8.25**

Malignant mixed tumor is a cancer of salivary glands in which a component of a previously existing mixed tumor (pleomorphic adenoma) has undergone malignant transformation or a histopathologically benign pleomorphic adenoma has metastasized (metastasizing mixed tumor). Most represent carcinoma ex pleomorphic adenoma in which the epithelial component of a benign pleomorphic adenoma has undergone malignant transformation. In rare instances, both the epithelial and connective tissue components exhibit malignant changes. This variant is termed a "carcinosarcoma." It is believed that carcinosarcoma also may arise de novo.

Only a small percentage of salivary gland cancers are malignant mixed tumors, and they most often develop in the parotid gland. The palate is the most common intraoral site. The tumor most often is diagnosed in middle-aged or older adults, and it exhibits a slight female predilection.

The typical history is that of a previously existing mass that suddenly increases in size. The mass may be fixed to underlying tissue and exhibit surface ulceration. Patients often complain of pain. Those with parotid gland involvement may exhibit facial nerve palsy because of nerve invasion by the tumor. Treatment generally is surgical, but radiation therapy also may be used, depending on the extent of the neoplasm. Prognosis is variable. Patients with a minimally invasive component that is contained within the body of the tumor have a favorable prognosis. Patients who exhibit invasion of adjacent structures or metastasis have a poor prognosis.

## ADENOCARCINOMA, NOT OTHERWISE SPECIFIED

**Fig. 8.26**

This designation is given to a small percentage of malignant salivary gland tumors whose histopathologic appearance does not fit into any of the well-recognized types of salivary gland cancers. They typically occur in adults and exhibit a predilection for females. The parotid gland is the most common location, and the palate is the most common intraoral site. They present as an expanding mass with variable growth. Pain and paralysis may be present because of nerve involvement.

These tumors exhibit a wide range of biologic behavior, from locally invasive neoplasms to aggressive carcinomas that exhibit rapid growth and metastasis. Some of the neoplasms lack significant cellular alterations microscopically and are determined to be malignant by their infiltrating or invasive growth. These are termed "low-grade" or "well-differentiated" malignancies and usually are treated by wide, local excision. The prognosis of the low-grade tumors generally is good, but metastasis still is possible. Others may exhibit considerable variation in cellular morphology and are termed "high-grade" or "poorly differentiated" cancers. These are treated by more radical surgery often combined with adjuvant radiation therapy. The prognosis for the higher grade tumors is not good, and those patients with disseminated disease have a poor prognosis.

## NECROTIZING SIALOMETAPLASIA

**Fig. 8.27**

Necrotizing sialometaplasia is a benign, acute inflammatory reaction in which lobules of minor salivary gland undergo coagulative necrosis, with the adjacent salivary gland ducts exhibiting squamous metaplasia. It also occurs in other mucous glands that are present in the nasal cavity and larynx. Although the major salivary glands may be involved rarely, most cases arise in the minor salivary glands of the palate during adulthood. Most lesions appear as ulcers of varying size but also may present as submucosal swelling. Patients may complain of pain, swelling, fever, and not feeling well. Most lesions are unilateral, but bilateral palatal involvement can occur. Patients also may have recurrent episodes. There is a male:female ratio of 2:1.

Necrotizing sialometaplasia most likely results from vascular compromise (ischemia) of the arterial supply of the affected salivary glands. Various forms of trauma, such as direct contact and injection of local anesthetic agents, have been implicated. Although the disease typically is self-limiting and resolves spontaneously, healing may take weeks. The importance of the lesion is that it may mimic a true neoplasm clinically and may be mistaken for squamous cell carcinoma or mucoepidermoid carcinoma histopathologically.

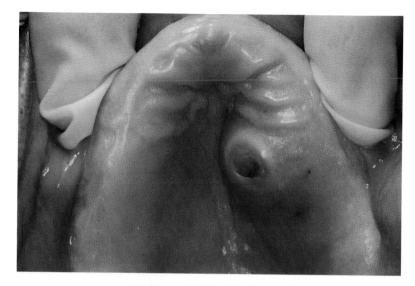

**Figure 8.25**
**CARCINOMA EX PLEOMORPHIC ADENOMA**
Ulcerated submucosal mass of the hard palate.

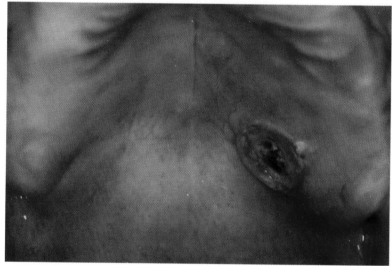

**Figure 8.26**
**ADENOCARCINOMA, NOT OTHERWISE SPECIFIED**
Ulcerated, raised mass of the palate.

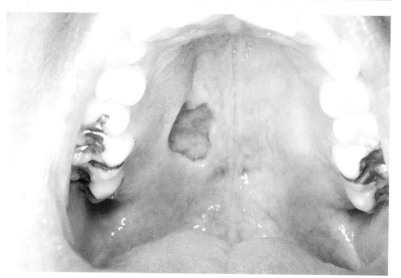

**Figure 8.27**
**NECROTIZING SIALOMETAPLASIA**
Painful ulceration of the palate of 2 weeks' duration.

### Mucocele, Ranula, Salivary Gland Duct Cyst

Bodner L, Tal H. Salivary gland cysts of the oral cavity: clinical observation and surgical management. Compendium 1991;12:150.

Cataldo E, Mosadomi A. Mucoceles of the oral mucous membrane. Arch Otolaryngol 1970;91:360.

Catone GA, Merrill RG, Henny FA. Sublingual gland mucus-escape phenomenon: treatment by excision of the sublingual gland. J Oral Surg 1969;27:774.

Danford M, Eveson JW, Flood TR. Papillary cystadenocarcinoma of the sublingual gland presenting as a ranula. Br J Oral Maxillofac Surg 1992;30:270.

de Visscher JGAM, van der Wal KGH, de Vogel PL. The plunging ranula: pathogenesis, diagnosis and management. J Craniomaxillofac Surg 1989;17:182.

Eversole LR. Oral sialocysts. Arch Otolaryngol Head Neck Surg. 1987;113:51.

Harrison JD. Salivary mucoceles. Oral Surg Oral Med Oral Pathol 1975;39:268.

Galloway RH, Gross PD, Thompson SH, et al. Pathogenesis and treatment of ranula: report of three cases. J Oral Maxillofac Surg 1989;47:299.

Ichimura K, Ohta Y, Tayama N. Surgical management of the plunging ranula: a review of seven cases. J Laryngol Otol 1996;110:554.

Jensen JL. Superficial mucoceles of the oral mucosa. Am J Dermatopathol 1990;12:88.

McClatchey KD, Appelblatt NH, Zarbo RJ, et al. Plunging ranula. Oral Surg Oral Med Oral Pathol 1984;57:408.

Mintz S, Barak S, Horowitz I. Carbon dioxide laser excision and vaporization of nonplunging ranulas: a comparison of two treatment protocols. J Oral Maxillofac Surg 1994;52:370.

Morton RP, Bartley JR. Simple sublingual ranulas: pathogenesis and management. J Otolaryngol 1995;24:253.

Praetorius F, Hammarstrom L. A new concept of the pathogenesis of oral mucous cysts based on a study of 200 cases. J Dent Assoc S Afr 1992;47:226.

Quick CA, Lowell SH. Ranula and sublingual salivary glands. Arch Otolaryngol 1977;103:397.

Southam JC. Retention mucoceles of the oral mucosa. J Oral Pathol. 1974;3:197.

Yamasoba T, Tayama N, Syoji M, et al. Clinicostatistical study of lower lip mucoceles. Head Neck 1990;12:316.

### Sjögren Syndrome

Alexander EL. Neurologic disease in Sjögren's syndrome: mononuclear inflammatory vasculopathy affecting central/peripheral nervous system and muscle: a clinical review and update of immunopathogenesis. Rheum Dis Clin North Am 1993;19:869.

Anaya JM, Ogawa N, Talal N. Sjögren's syndrome in childhood. J Rheumatol 1995;22:1152.

Atkinson JC, Fox PC. Sjögren's syndrome: oral and dental considerations. J Am Dent Assoc 1993;124:74.

Aziz KE, Montanaro A, McCluskey PJ, et al. Sjögren's syndrome: review with recent insights into immunopathogenesis. Aust N Z J Med 1992;22:671.

Daniels TE. Sjögren's syndrome: clinical spectrum and current diagnostic controversies. Adv Dent Res 1996;10:3.

Daniels TE, Fox PC. Salivary and oral components of Sjögren's syndrome. Rheum Dis Clin North Am 1992;18:571.

Foster HE, Gilroy JJ, Kelly CA, et al. The treatment of sicca features in Sjögren's Syndrome: a clinical review. Br J Rheumatol 1994;33:278.

Fox PC. Differentiation of dry mouth etiology. Adv Dent Res 1996;10:13.

Fox RI, Saito I. Criteria for diagnosis of Sjögren's syndrome. Rheum Dis Clin North Am 1994;20:391.

Santana V, Rose NR. Neoplastic lymphoproliferation in autoimmune disease: an updated review. Clin Immunol Immunopathol. 1992;63:205.

Wise CM, Woodruff RD. Minor salivary gland biopsies in patients investigated for primary Sjögren's syndrome: a review of 187 patients. J Rheumatol 1993;20:1515.

### Sialolithiasis

Arzoz K, Santiago A, Esnall F, et al. Endoscopic intracorporeal lithotripsy. J Oral Maxillofac Surg 1996;54:847.

Bodner L, Fliss DM. Parotid and submandibular calculi in children. Int J Pediatr Otorhinolaryngol 1995;31:35.

Ellies M, Laskawi R, Arglebe C, et al. Surgical management of nonneoplastic diseases of the submandibular gland: a follow-up study. Int J Oral Maxillofac Surg. 1996;25:285.

Ho V, Currie WJ, Walker A. Sialolithiasis of minor salivary glands. Br J Oral Maxillofac Surg 1992;30:273.

Jensen JL, Howell FV, Rick GM, et al. Minor salivary gland calculi: a clinicopathologic study of forty-seven new cases. Oral Surg Oral Med Oral Pathol 1979;47:44.

Levy DM, Remine WH, Devine KD. Salivary gland calculi: pain, swelling associated with eating. JAMA 1962;181:1115.

Lustmann J, Regev E, Melamed Y. Sialolithiasis: a survey on 245 patients and a review of the literature. Int J Oral Maxillofac Surg 1990;19:135.

Ottaviani F, Capaccio P, Campi M, et al. Extracorporeal electromagnetic shock-wave lithotripsy for salivary gland stones. Laryngoscope 1996;106:761.

Pullon PA, Miller AS. Sialolithiasis of accessory salivary glands: review of 55 cases. J Oral Surg 1972;30:832.

Yoshino N, Hosokawa A, Sasaki T, et al. Interventional radiology for the non-surgical removal of sialoliths. Dentomaxillofac Radiol 1996;25:242.

## Salivary Gland Neoplasms—General Considerations

Anderson JN Jr, Beenken SW, Crowe R, et al. Prognostic factors in minor salivary gland cancer. Head Neck 1995;17:480.

Batsakis JG. Salivary gland neoplasia: an outcome of modified morphogenesis and cytodifferentiation. Oral Surg Oral Med Oral Pathol 1980;49:229.

Beckhardt RN, Weber RS, Zane R, et al. Minor salivary gland tumors of the palate: clinical and pathologic correlates of outcome. Laryngoscope 1995;105:1155.

Callender DL, Frankenthaler RA, Luna MA, et al. Salivary gland neoplasms in children. Arch Otolaryngol Head Neck Surg 1992;118:472.

Chidzonga MM, Lopez Perez VM, Portilla Alvarez AL. A clinicopathologic study of parotid gland tumors. J Oral Maxillofac Surg 1994;52:1253.

Chou C, Zhu G, Luo M, et al. Carcinoma of the minor salivary glands: results of surgery and combined therapy. J Oral Maxillofac Surg. 1996;54:448.

Comoretto R, Barzan L. Benign parotid tumour enucleation: a reliable operation in selected cases. J Laryngol Otol. 1990;104:706.

Ellis GL, Auclair PL. Tumors of the salivary glands. Washington, DC: Armed Forces Institute of Pathology, 1995.

Ellis GL, Auclair PL, Gnepp DR. Surgical pathology of the salivary glands. Philadelphia: WB Saunders Co, 1991.

Main JHP, Orr JA, McGurk FM, et al. Salivary gland tumors: review of 643 cases. J Oral Pathol 1976;5:88.

Nagler RM, Laufer D. Tumors of the major and minor salivary glands: review of 25 years of experience. Anticancer Res 1997;17:701.

Neville BW, Damm DD, Weir JC, et al. Labial salivary gland tumors. Cancer 1988;61:2113.

Renehan A, Gleave EN, Hancock BD, et al. Long-term follow-up of over 1000 patients with salivary gland tumours treated in a single centre. Br J Surg 83:1750, 1996.

Seifert G, Donath K. Multiple tumours of the salivary glands: terminology and nomenclature. Eur J Cancer Oral Oncol 1996;32B:3.

Seifert G, Sobin LH. The World Health Organization's histological classification of salivary gland tumors. Cancer 1992;70:379.

Takahashi H, Fujita S, Tsuda N, et al. Intraoral minor salivary gland tumors: a demographic and histologic study of 200 cases. Tohoku J Exp Med 1990;161:111.

Waldron CA, El-Mofty SK, Gnepp DR. Tumors of the intraoral minor salivary glands: a demographic and histologic study of 426 cases. Oral Surg Oral Med Oral Pathol 1988;66:323.

## Pleomorphic Adenoma

Chau MNY, Radden BG. A clinical-pathologic study of 53 intraoral pleomorphic adenomas. Int J Oral Maxillofac Surg 1989;18:158.

Chidzonga MM, Lopez Perez VM, Portilla Alvarez AL. Pleomorphic adenoma of the salivary glands: clinicopathologic study of 206 cases in Zimbabwe. Oral Surg Oral Med Oral Pathol Oral Radiol Endod 1995;79:747.

Krolls SO, Boyers RC. Mixed tumors of salivary glands: long-term follow-up. Cancer 1972;30:276.

Krolls SO, Hicks JL. Mixed tumors of the lower lip. Oral Surg Oral Med Oral Pathol 1973;35:212.

Naeim F, Forsberg MI, Waisman J, et al. Mixed tumors of the salivary glands: growth pattern and recurrence. Arch Pathol Lab Med 1976;100:271.

Phillips PP, Olsen KD. Recurrent pleomorphic adenoma of the parotid gland: report of 126 cases and a review of the literature. Ann Otol Rhinol Laryngol 1995;104:100.

## Monomorphic Adenoma

Batsakis JG, Brannon RB, Sciubba JJ. Monomorphic adenomas of the major salivary glands: a histologic study of 96 tumors. Clin Otolaryngol 1981;6:129.

Batsakis JG, Luna MA, el-Naggar AK. Basaloid monomorphic adenomas. Ann Otol Rhinol Laryngol 1991;100:687.

Daley TD, Gardner DG, Smout MS. Canalicular adenoma: not a basal cell adenoma. Oral Surg Oral Med Oral Pathol 1984;57:181.

Dardick I, Lyfwyn A, Bourne AJ, et al. Trabecular and solid-cribriform types of basal cell adenoma. Oral Surg Oral Med Oral Pathol 1992;73:75.

Fantasia JE, Neville BW. Basal cell adenomas of the minor salivary glands. Oral Surg Oral Med Oral Pathol 1980;50:433.

Feinmesser M, Feinmesser R, Okon E, et al. A monomorphic adenoma of the minor salivary glands presenting at the base of the tongue: a case report and review of the literature. J Otolaryngol 1993;22:110.

Gardner DG, Daley TD. The use of the terms monomorphic adenoma, basal cell adenoma and canalicular adenoma as applied to salivary gland tumors. Oral Surg Oral Med Oral Pathol 1983;56:608.

Kratochvil F, Auclair P, Ellis G. Clinical features of 160 cases of basal cell adenoma and 121 cases of canalicular adenoma. Oral Surg Oral Med Oral Pathol 1990;70:605.

Mair IW, Stalsburg H. Basal cell adenomatosis of the minor salivary glands of the upper lip. Arch Otorhinolaryngol. 1988;245:191.

Maurizi M, Salvinelli F, Capelli A, et al. Monomorphic adenomas of the major salivary glands: clinicopathological study of 44 cases. J Laryngol Otol 1990;104:790.

Mintz GA, Abrams AM, Melrose RJ. Monomorphic adenomas of the major and minor salivary glands: report of twenty-one cases and review of the literature. Oral Surg Oral Med Oral Pathol 1982;53:375.

Nelson JF, Jacoway JR. Monomorphic adenoma (canalicular type). Cancer 1973;31:1511.

Pogrel MA. The intraoral basal cell adenoma. J Craniomaxillofac Surg 1987;15:372.

## Warthin's Tumor

Eveson JW, Cawson RA. Warthin's tumor (cystadenolymphoma) of salivary glands: a clinicopathologic investigation of 278 cases. Oral Surg Oral Med Oral Pathol 1086;61:256.

Fantasia JE, Miller AS. Papillary cystadenoma lymphomatosum arising in minor salivary glands. Oral Surg Oral Med Oral Pathol 1981;52:411.

Gallo O. New insights into the pathogenesis of Warthin's tumour. Eur J Cancer Oral Oncol 1995;31B:211.

Lam KH, Ho HC, Ho CM, et al. Multifocal nature of adenolymphoma of the parotid. Br J Surg 1994;81:1612.

Lefor AT, Ord RA. Multiple synchronous bilateral Warthin's tumors of the parotid glands with pleomorphic adenoma: case report and review of the literature. Oral Surg Oral Med Oral Pathol 1993;76:319.

Monk JS Jr, Church JS. Warthin's tumor: a high incidence and no sex predominance in central Pennsylvania. Arch Otolaryngol Head Neck Surg 1992;118:477.

Pinkston JA, Cole P. Cigarette smoking and Warthin's tumor. Am J Epidemiol 1996;144:183.

Skalova A, Michal M, Nathansky Z. Epidermoid carcinoma arising in Warthin's tumor: a case study. J Oral Pathol Med 1994;23:330.

Vories AA, Romirez SG. Warthin's tumor and cigarette smoking. South Med J 1997;90:416.

Yoo GH, Eisele DW, Askin FB, et al. Warthin's tumor: a 40-year experience at Johns Hopkins Hospital. Laryngoscope 1994;104:799.

## Mucoepidermoid Carcinoma

Accetta PA, Gary GF, Hunter RM, et al. Mucoepidermoid carcinoma of salivary glands. Arch Pathol Lab Med 1984;108:321.

Auclair PL, Goode RK, Ellis GL. Mucoepidermoid carcinoma of intraoral salivary glands: evaluation and application of grading criteria in 143 cases. Cancer 1992;15:2021.

Batsakis JG, Luna MA. Histopathologic grading of salivary gland neoplasms, I: mucoepidermoid carcinomas. Ann Otol Rhinol Laryngol 1990;99:835.

Evans HL. Mucoepidermoid carcinoma of salivary glands: a study of 69 cases with special attention to histologic grading. Am J Clin Pathol 1984;81:696.

Garden AS, el-Naggar AK, Morrison WH, et al. Postoperative radiotherapy for malignant tumors of the parotid gland. Int J Radiat Oncol Biol Phys 1997;37:79.

Hicks MJ, el-Naggar AK, Flaitz CM, et al. Histocytologic grading of mucoepidermoid carcinoma of major salivary glands in prognosis and survival: a clinicopathologic and flow cytometric investigation. Head Neck Surg 1995;17:89.

Nascimento AG, Amaral LP, Prado LA, et al. Mucoepidermoid carcinoma of salivary glands: a clinicopathologic study of 46 cases. Head Neck Surg 1986;8:409.

Olsen KD, Devine KD, Weiland LH. Mucoepidermoid carcinoma of the oral cavity. Otolaryngol Head Neck Surg 1981;89:783.

Parsons JT, Mendenhall WM, Stinger SP, et al. Management of minor salivary gland carcinomas. Int J Radiat Oncol Biol Phys 1996;35:443.

Plambeck K, Fredrich RE, Schmelzle R. Mucoepidermoid carcinoma of salivary gland origin: classification, clinical-pathological correlation, treatment results and long-term follow-up in 55 patients. J Craniomaxillofac Surg 1996;24:133.

Sadeghi A, Tran LM, Mark R, et al. Minor salivary gland tumors of the head and neck: treatment strategies and prognosis. Am J Clin Oncol 1993;16:3.

Saku T, Hayashi Y, Takahara O, et al. Salivary gland tumors among atomic bomb survivors, 1950-1987. Cancer 1997;79:1465.

Spiro RH, Huvos AG, Berk R, et al. Mucoepidermoid carcinoma of salivary gland origin: a clinicopathologic study of 367 cases. Am J Surg 1978;136:461.

Tran L, Sidrys J, Sadeghi A, et al. Salivary gland tumors of the oral cavity. Int J Radiat Oncol Biol Phys 1990;18:413.

## Intraosseous Mucoepidermoid Carcinoma

Brookstone MS, Huvos AG. Central salivary gland tumors of the maxilla and mandible: a clinicopathologic study of 11 cases with an analysis of the literature. J Oral Maxillofac Surg 1992;50:229.

Bruner JM, Batsakis JG. Salivary neoplasms of the jaw bones with particular reference to central mucoepidermoid carcinomas. Ann Otol Rhinol Laryngol 1991;100:954.

Eversole LR, Sabes WR, Rovin S. Aggressive growth and neoplastic potential of odontogenic cysts with special reference to central epidermoid and mucoepidermoid carcinoma. Cancer 1975;35:270.

Ezsias A, Sugar AW, Milling MA, et al. Central mucoepidermoid carcinoma in a child. J Oral Maxillofac Surg 1994;52:512.

Grubka JM, Wesley RK, Monaco F. Primary intraosseous mucoepidermoid carcinoma of the anterior part of the mandible. J Oral Maxillofac Surg 1983;41:389.

Lebsack JP, Marrogi AJ, Martin SA. Central mucoepidermoid carcinoma of the jaw with distant metastasis: a case report and review of the literature. J Oral Maxillofac Surg 1990;48:518.

Pincock JL, El-Mofty SK. Recurrence of cystic central mucoepidermoid tumor of the mandible: report of a case with 3 recurrences in 7 years. Int J Oral Surg 1985;14:81.

Sidoni AD, Errico P, Simoncelli C, et al. Central mucoepidermoid carcinoma of the mandible: report of a case treated 13 years after first radiographic demonstration. J Oral Maxillofac Surg 1996;54:1245.

Waldron CA, Koh GA. Central mucoepidermoid carcinoma of the jaws: report of four cases with analysis of the literature and discussion of the relationship to mucoepidermoid, sialodontogenic, and glandular odontogenic cysts. J Oral Maxillofac Surg 1990;48:871.

## Polymorphous Low-Grade Adenocarcinoma

Aberle AM, Abrams AM, Bowe R, et al. Lobular (polymorphous low-grade) carcinoma of minor salivary glands. Oral Surg Oral Med Oral Pathol 1985;60:387.

Batsakis JG, Pinkston GR, Luna MA, et al. Adenocarcinomas of the oral cavity: a clinicopathologic study of terminal duct carcinomas. J Laryngol Otol 1983;97:825.

Clayton JR, Pogrel MA, Regezi JA. Simultaneous multifocal polymorphous low-grade adenocarcinoma: report of two cases. Oral Surg Oral Med Oral Pathol Oral Radiol Endod 1995;80:71.

Colmenero CM, Patron M, Burgueno M, et al. Polymorphous low-grade adenocarcinoma of the oral cavity: a report of 14 cases. J Oral Maxillofac Surg 1992;50:595.

Evans HL, Batsakis JG. Polymorphous low-grade adenocarcinoma of minor salivary glands: a study of 14 cases of a distinctive neoplasm. Cancer 1984;53:935.

Freedman PD, Lumerman H. Lobular carcinoma of intraoral minor salivary gland origin: report of twelve cases. Oral Surg Oral Med Oral Pathol 1983;56:157.

Haba R, Kobayashi S, Miki H, et al. Polymorphous low-grade adenocarcinoma of submandibular gland origin. Acta Pathol Jpn 1993;43:774.

Merchant WJ, Cook MG, Eveson JW. Polymorphous low-grade adenocarcinoma of parotid gland. Br J Oral Maxillofac Surg 1996;34:328.

Thomas KM, Cumberworth VL, McEwan J. Orbital and skin metastases in a polymorphous low grade adenocarcinoma of the salivary gland. J Laryngol Otol 1995;109:1222.

Vincent SD, Hammond HL, Finkelstein MW. Clinical and therapeutic features of polymorphous low-grade adenocarcinoma. Oral Surg Oral Med Oral Pathol 1994;77:41.

## Adenoid Cystic Carcinoma

Ampil FL, Misra RP. Factors influencing survival of patients with adenoid cystic carcinoma of the salivary glands. J Oral Maxillofac Surg 1987;45:1005.

Batsakis JG, Luna MA, el-Naggar A. Histopathologic grading of salivary gland neoplasms, III: adenoid cystic carcinomas. Ann Otol Rhinol Laryngol 1990;99:1007.

Douglas JG, Laramore GE, Austin-Seymour M, et al. Neutron radiotherapy for adenoid cystic carcinoma of minor salivary glands. Int J Radiat Oncol Biol Phys 1996;36:87.

Garden AS, Weber RS, Morrison WH, et al. The influence of positive margins and nerve invasion in adenoid cystic carcinoma of the head and neck treated with surgery and radiation. Int J Radiat Oncol Biol Phys 1995;15:619.

Haddad A, Enepekides DJ, Manolidis S, et al. Adenoid cystic carcinoma of the head and neck: a clinicopathologic study of 37 cases. J Otolaryngol 1995;24:201.

McFall MR, Irvine GH, Eveson JW. Adenoid cystic carcinoma of the sublingual salivary gland in a 16-year-old female: report of a case and review of the literature. J Laryngol Otol 1997;111:485.

Silvester KC, Barnes S. Adenoid cystic carcinoma of the tongue presenting as a hypoglossal nerve palsy. Br J Oral Maxillofac Surg 1990;28:122.

Szanto PA, Luna MA, Tortoledo ME, et al. Histologic grading of adenoid cystic carcinoma of the salivary glands. Cancer 1984;54:1062.

van der Wal JE, Snow GB, van der Waal I. Intraoral adenoid cystic carcinoma: the presence of perineural spread in relation to site, size, local extension, and metastatic spread in 22 cases. Cancer 1990;66:2031.

Vrielinck LJG, Ostyn F, Van Damme B, et al. The significance of perineural spread in adenoid cystic carcinoma of the major and minor salivary glands. Int J Oral Maxillofac Surg 1988;17:190.

## Acinic Cell Carcinoma

Abrams AM, Melrose RJ. Acinic cell tumors of minor salivary gland origin. Oral Surg Oral Med Oral Pathol 1978;46:220.

Batsakis JG, Luna MA, el-Nagger AK. Histopathologic grading of salivary gland neoplasms, II: acinic cell carcinomas. Ann Otol Rhinol Laryngol 1990;99:929.

Chen S-Y, Brannon RB, Miller AS, et al. Acinic cell adenocarcinoma of minor salivary glands. Cancer 1978;42:678.

Ellis GL, Corio RL. Acinic cell adenocarcinoma: a clinicopathologic analysis of 294 cases. Cancer 1983;52:542.

Lewis JE, Olsen KD, Weiland LH. Acinic cell carcinoma: clinicopathologic review. Cancer 1991;67:172.

Zbaeren P, Lehmann W, Widgren S. Acinic cell carcinoma of minor salivary origin. J Larynogol Otol 1991;105:782.

## Malignant Mixed Tumor (Carcinoma ex Pleomorphic Adenoma)

Brandwein M, Huvos AG, Dardick I, et al. Noninvasive and minimally invasive carcinoma ex mixed tumor: a clinicopathologic and ploidy study of 12 patients with major salivary tumors of low (or no?) malignant potential. Oral Surg Oral Med Oral Pathol Oral Radiol Endod 1996;81:655.

Gnepp DR. Malignant mixed tumors of the salivary glands: a review. Pathol Annual 1993;28:279.

LiVolsi VA, Perzin KH. Malignant mixed tumors arising in salivary glands, I: carcinomas arising in benign mixed tumor: a clinicopathologic study. Cancer 1977;39:2209.

Qureshi AA, Gitelis S, Templeton AA, et al. "Benign" metastasizing pleomorphic adenoma: a case report and review of literature. Clin Orthop 1994;308:192.

Takeda Y. True malignant mixed tumor (carcinosarcoma) of palatal minor salivary gland origin. Ann Dent 1991;50:33.

Talmi YP, Halpren M, Finkelstein Y, et al. True malignant mixed tumour of the parotid gland. J Laryngol Otol 1990;104:360.

Tortoledo ME, Luna MA, Batsakis JG. Carcinoma ex pleomorphic adenoma and malignant mixed tumors. Arch Otolaryngol 1984;110:172.

Yoshihara T, Tanaka M, Itoh M, et al. Carcinoma ex pleomorphic adenoma of the soft palate. J Laryngol Otol 1995;109:240.

### Adenocarcinoma, Not Otherwise Specified

Auclair PL, Ellis GL. Adenocarcinoma, not otherwise specified. In: Ellis GL, Auclair PL, Gnepp DR, eds. Surgical pathology of the salivary glands. Philadelphia: WB Saunders, 1991:318.

Foote FW Jr, Frazell EL. Tumors of the major salivary glands. Cancer 1953;6:1065.

Spiro RH, Huvos AG, Strong EW. Adenocarcinoma of salivary origin: clinicopathologic study of 204 patients. Am J Surg 1982;144:423.

Tran L, Sadeghi A, Hanson D, et al. Major salivary gland tumors: treatment results and prognostic factors. Laryngoscope 1986;96:1139.

### Necrotizing Sialometaplasia

Abrams AM, Melrose RJ, Howell FV. Necrotizing sialometaplasia: a disease simulating malignancy. Cancer 1973;32:130.

Brannon RB, Fowler CB, Hartman KS. Necrotizing sialometaplasia: a clinicopathologic study of sixty-nine cases and review of the literature. Oral Surg Oral Med Oral Pathol 1991;72:317.

Imbery TA, Edwards PA. Necrotizing sialometaplasia: literature review and case reports. J Am Dent Assoc 1996;127:1087.

Rossie KM, Allen CM, Burns RA. Necrotizing sialometaplasia: a case with metachronous lesions. J Oral Maxillofac Surg 1986;44:1006.

Shigematsu H, Shigematsu Y, Noguchi Y, et al. Experimental study on necrotizing sialometaplasia of the palate in rats. Int J Oral Maxillofac Surg 1996;25:239.

Sneige N, Batsakis JG. Necrotizing sialometaplasia. Ann Otol Rhinol Laryngol 1992;101:282.

Wenig BM. Necrotizing sialometaplasia of the larynx: a report of two cases and a review of the literature. Am J Clin Pathol 1995;103:609.

# chapter 9
## SOFT-TISSUE TUMORS

# FIBROMA (IRRITATION FIBROMA, TRAUMATIC FIBROMA, FIBROUS NODULE, FOCAL FIBROUS HYPERPLASIA)

**Figs. 9.1 and 9.2**

The fibroma is the most common soft tissue tumor of the oral cavity. In most cases, it is doubtful that it represents a true neoplasm, but rather a reactive hyperplasia of the fibrous connective tissue in response to local irritation or trauma. The fibroma usually presents as a well-defined, smooth-surfaced pink nodule that may be sessile or pedunculated. Most fibromas are less than 2 cm in diameter, but sometimes they become considerably larger. They are seen more frequently in adults than in children. Fibromas are most commonly located on the buccal mucosa along the bite line, presumably arising as a result of irritation from the teeth. The labial mucosa, gingiva, and tongue are also common sites. Fibromas are typically slow-growing and asymptomatic, unless secondarily traumatized. Treatment consists of local surgical excision; the lesion rarely recurs.

# GIANT CELL FIBROMA

**Fig. 9.3**

The giant cell fibroma is a fibrous connective tissue tumor that appears to be a distinct entity, different from the typical fibroma. It derives its name from the histopathologic presence of large, stellate fibroblasts, which occasionally are multinucleated. Compared with the irritation fibroma, the giant cell fibroma occurs at a younger average age: nearly 60% are seen in the first three decades of life. Also, the most common location is the gingiva, with the tongue, palate, and buccal mucosa being less frequent sites. The lesions are usually less than 1 cm in diameter and often exhibit a rough surface so that, clinically, they may be mistaken for papillomas. Giant cell fibromas are treated by conservative surgical excision; recurrence is rare.

**Figure 9.1**
**FIBROMA**
Pink nodular mass of the buccal mucosa.

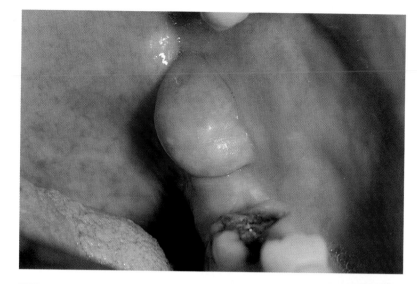

**Figure 9.2**
**FIBROMA**
Smooth-surfaced tongue nodule.

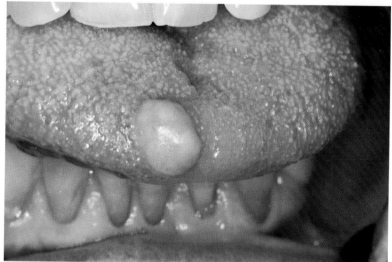

**Figure 9.3**
**GIANT CELL FIBROMA**
Three-year-old black male with gingival nodule exhibiting a papillary surface.

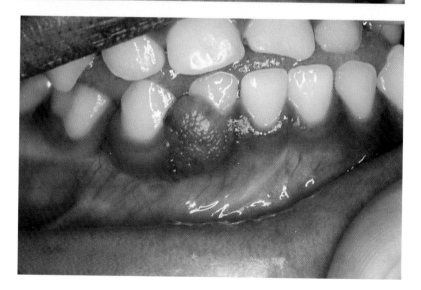

# EPULIS FISSURATUM (INFLAMMATORY FIBROUS HYPERPLASIA, DENTURE INJURY TUMOR, DENTURE EPULIS)

## Figs. 9.4, 9.5, and 9.6

The epulis fissuratum is a reactive hyperplasia of fibrous connective tissue and epithelium, occurring in the alveolar vestibule in association with long-standing irritation from a poorly fitting denture. It is characterized by the growth of a single or multiple folds of redundant tissue, with the denture flange often fitting into the depth of one of the folds. Lesions are much more common in the anterior areas and occur more frequently on the facial aspect of the alveolar ridge than on the lingual aspect. Women are affected more often than men. The epulis fissuratum is often asymptomatic, although it may become tender if ulceration occurs at the base of the tissue fold. Treatment consists of surgical removal of the excess tissue, followed by construction of new dentures. With a well-fitting denture, the lesion should not recur.

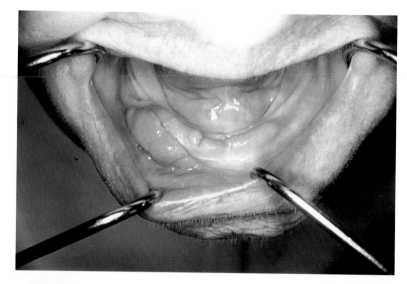

**Figure 9.4**
**EPULIS FISSURATUM**
Redundant fold of tissue in the mandibular vestibule. (Courtesy of Dr. E.R. Costich.)

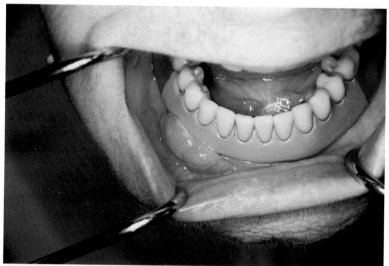

**Figure 9.5**
**EPULIS FISSURATUM**
Appearance of lesion in Figure 9.4 with denture in place. (Courtesy of Dr. E.R. Costich.)

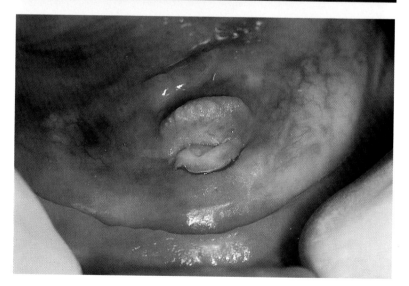

**Figure 9.6**
**EPULIS FISSURATUM**
Hyperplastic tissue in the floor of the mouth.

## LEAFLIKE DENTURE FIBROMA (FIBROEPITHELIAL POLYP)

**Fig. 9.7**

In addition to the epulis fissuratum, another variant of fibrous hyperplasia that may occur in association with an ill-fitting maxillary denture is the leaflike denture fibroma. This distinctive lesion develops as a flattened pink mass that is attached to the hard palate by a narrow stalk. The edges of the lesion often have a lobulated or serrated appearance that resembles a leaf. The mass usually lies closely applied to the palate within a cupped-out depression. However, the edge of the lesion can be easily lifted up with a probe, revealing its pedunculated attachment. Treatment consists of surgical removal before construction of the new denture.

## INFLAMMATORY PAPILLARY HYPERPLASIA

**Figs. 9.8 and 9.9**

Inflammatory papillary hyperplasia is a benign proliferation of oral mucosa, usually associated with wearing of a partial or complete denture 24 hours a day. It usually develops on the palate but will occasionally develop on alveolar ridge mucosa or on top of an epulis fissuratum. Clinically, it is characterized by multiple, broad-based papillary projections that closely approximate one another. The lesion may be normal colored or erythematous; erythematous lesions indicate the possibility of secondary candidiasis. On rare occasions, the condition may occur on the palate of a patient without a denture, especially if the individual is a mouth-breather or has a high palatal vault. Histopathologically, the lesion may exhibit pseudocarcinomatous hyperplasia and, on occasion, has been misdiagnosed as squamous cell carcinoma. Partial regression of the lesion may take place if the patient discontinues wearing the denture for a short period of time. Mild cases may improve somewhat with the use of antifungal agents accompanied by fabrication of a new denture. Surgical stripping, electrocautery, or laser excision may be used in severe cases.

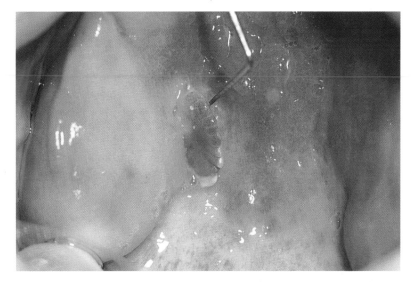

▶ **Figure 9.7**
**LEAFLIKE DENTURE FIBROMA**
Flattened mass of hyperplastic tissue on the hard palate beneath a denture.

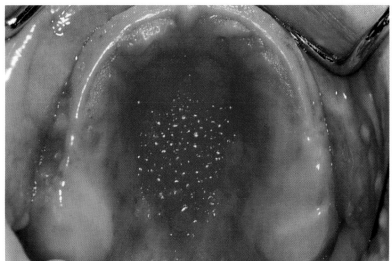

▶ **Figure 9.8**
**INFLAMMATORY PAPILLARY HYPERPLASIA**
Palatal mucosa forming numerous papillary projections with erythematous changes.

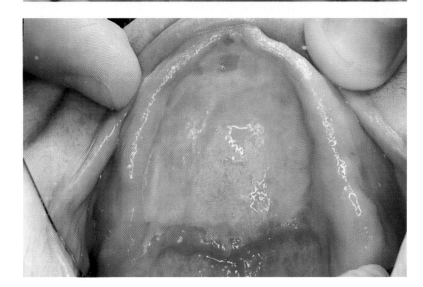

▶ **Figure 9.9**
**INFLAMMATORY PAPILLARY HYPERPLASIA**
Skin graft of the entire hard palate in a patient who had received wide surgical excision and bone removal for inflammatory papillary hyperplasia misdiagnosed as squamous cell carcinoma.

## AGGRESSIVE FIBROMATOSIS

**Fig. 9.10**

Fibromatoses are a diverse group of locally aggressive fibrous proliferations that occupy a pathologic gray zone between benign and malignant tumors. Aggressive fibromatosis of the oral cavity is a rare condition, usually encountered in children and young adults. The lesion presents as an infiltrative mass that may exhibit either slow or rapid growth. It most commonly involves the soft tissues surrounding the mandible, often in association with underlying bone destruction. The surface may be ulcerated, but the lesion is usually relatively painless. Treatment consists of wide local excision including a generous margin of clinically normal tissue. Local recurrence is not uncommon, but metastasis does not occur. In rare cases, spontaneous regression of the tumor has been reported.

## FIBROSARCOMA

**Fig. 9.11**

The fibrosarcoma is a malignant neoplasm of fibrous connective tissue origin that is uncommon in the oral cavity. It may occur at any age, but is most common in young and middle-aged adults. It presents clinically as an infiltrative tumor mass that may be rapid or slow in its growth. The tumor may arise in the soft tissues or as a primary intrabony neoplasm. Some examples develop in patients with a history of radiation therapy to the head and neck. Histopathologic distinction from aggressive fibromatosis may be difficult in many cases. Treatment consists of wide local excision. Prognosis depends on the size, location, and histopathologic grade of the tumor. The overall 5-year survival rate ranges from 40 to 70%; intrabony tumors have a worse prognosis than peripheral tumors.

## LIPOMA

**Fig. 9.12**

The lipoma is a benign tumor of fat that is common in the subcutaneous tissues but relatively uncommon in the oral cavity. Although the lipoma may occur almost anywhere in the mouth, the buccal mucosa is the most common location, followed by the tongue. The lipoma is most common in adults, usually presenting as a soft nodular mass that may be sessile or pedunculated. The tumor often appears yellow, unless it is a deep-seated mass. Multiple subcutaneous tumors occur in some patients. Treatment consists of surgical removal; recurrence is rare.

### ▶ Figure 9.10
### AGGRESSIVE FIBROMATOSIS

Rapidly growing mass of the left mandibular retromolar area. (Courtesy of B. Rodu, D.R. Weathers, W.G. Campbell, Jr. Aggressive fibromatosis involving the paramandibular soft tissues. Oral Surg Oral Med Oral Pathol 1981;52:395)

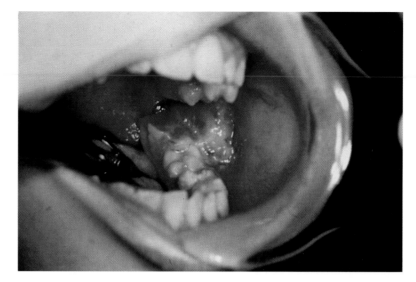

### ▶ Figure 9.11
### FIBROSARCOMA

Mass of the right mandibular retromolar area. (Courtesy of Dr. Lindsey R. Douglas.)

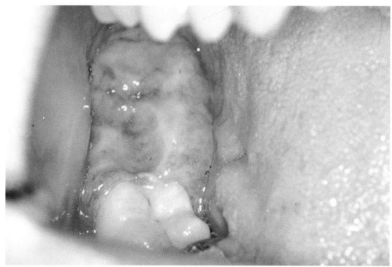

### ▶ Figure 9.12
### LIPOMA

Nodular mass of the buccal mucosa.

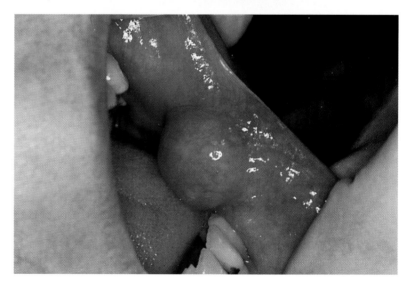

## Figs. 9.13, 9.14, and 9.15

The pyogenic granuloma is a relatively common reactive, tumorlike growth of the oral cavity that occurs as a result of local irritation. It may occur at any age but seems to be most common in teenagers and young adults. Pyogenic granulomas can develop almost anywhere in the oral cavity, but the gingiva is the most common site. Clinically, the pyogenic granuloma presents as a pedunculated or sessile mass ranging in size from a few millimeters to several centimeters in some cases. The mass is characteristically red and highly vascular, showing a tendency to bleed in some cases. The epithelial surface is usually ulcerated, but the lesion is typically not painful. Sometimes, the mass exhibits rapid growth, which may be clinically alarming.

The pyogenic granuloma is more common in females than in males, especially during pregnancy, presumably because of heightened tissue responsiveness from hormonal alterations. It has sometimes been termed a "pregnancy tumor" or "granuloma gravidarum" but is clinically and histopathologically identical to lesions in nonpregnant individuals.

Treatment for the pyogenic granuloma consists of local surgical excision. For gingival lesions, it is advisable to excise the lesion down to the periosteum and to scale the adjacent teeth to remove any calculus and plaque that may be a source of irritation. Recurrence is occasionally seen. If not removed, some pyogenic granulomas will eventually undergo fibrous maturation and resemble a fibroma. For pregnant women, it is often advisable to wait until parturition before surgical removal because of a greater tendency for recurrence during pregnancy. In some cases, the lesion will regress spontaneously after the patient has given birth.

**Figure 9.13**
**PYOGENIC GRANULOMA**
Ulcerated gingival mass.

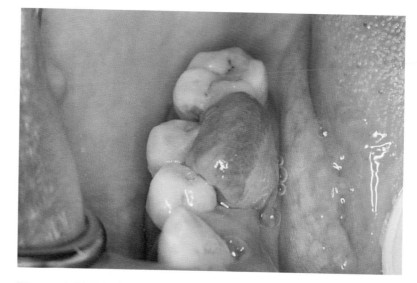

**Figure 9.14**
**PYOGENIC GRANULOMA**
Hemorrhagic, ulcerated gingival mass in a
pregnant woman.

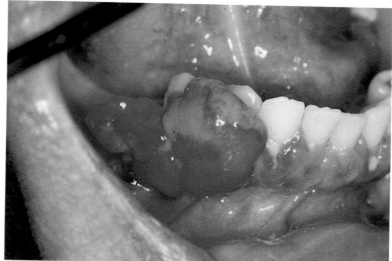

**Figure 9.15**
**PYOGENIC GRANULOMA**
Ulcerated mass on the dorsum of the
tongue.

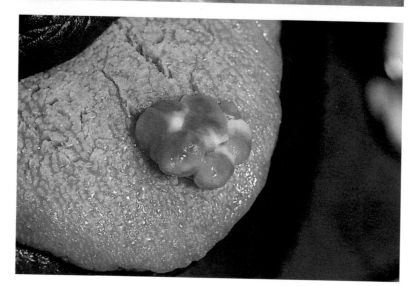

## PERIPHERAL GIANT CELL GRANULOMA

**Fig. 9.16**

The peripheral giant cell granuloma is a tumorlike growth of the gingiva or alveolar ridge that is apparently the soft-tissue counterpart of the central giant cell granuloma. Clinically, it is similar to the pyogenic granuloma, presenting as a sessile or pedunculated mass, often with an ulcerated surface. It is usually red but frequently exhibits a somewhat deeper bluish-purple hue compared with the pyogenic granuloma. The peripheral giant cell granuloma may occur at any age, but it is most common in young and middle-aged adults. Females are affected more frequently than males, and the lesion is more common in the mandible than in the maxilla. Superficial alveolar bone erosion may occur. Treatment consists of surgical excision down to the underlying bone, along with scaling of the adjacent teeth to remove any source of irritation and to minimize the chance of recurrence. Approximately 10% of cases are reported to recur, probably because of incomplete removal.

## PERIPHERAL OSSIFYING FIBROMA

**Fig. 9.17**

The peripheral ossifying fibroma is a relatively common tumorlike growth of the gingiva that may be reactive rather than neoplastic in nature. It is characterized by a proliferation of fibrous connective tissue arising from the periodontal ligament, associated with the formation of bone, dystrophic calcification, or a cementumlike product. The peripheral ossifying fibroma usually occurs in teenagers and young adults but can be seen at any age. Females are affected more frequently than males. Lesions may occur on either the maxillary or mandibular gingiva and are most common in the incisor/cuspid region. The peripheral ossifying fibroma typically presents as a well-circumscribed nodular mass that may have a smooth, pink surface or may be ulcerated. Treatment consists of surgical excision down to the underlying bone, and the adjacent teeth should be scaled to remove any source of irritation that may stimulate redevelopment of the lesion. Recurrence is seen in 16 to 20% of reported cases, probably because of incomplete removal.

## OSSEOUS CHORISTOMA

**Fig. 9.18**

A choristoma is a tumorlike mass of histologically normal tissue occurring in an abnormal location. Choristomas within the oral cavity are rare; the most common location is the posterior dorsum of the tongue in the region of the foramen cecum and circumvallate papillae. The most common types are osseous, cartilaginous, and mixed osteocartilaginous choristomas. Clinically, the lesion presents as a sessile or pedunculated mass that may produce dysphagia or gagging. Treatment consists of surgical removal, and recurrence should not be expected.

### Figure 9.16
**PERIPHERAL GIANT CELL GRANULOMA**
Ulcerated blue-purple gingival mass.

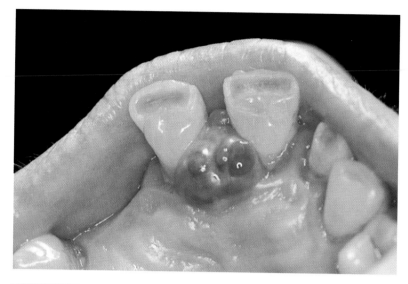

### Figure 9.17
**PERIPHERAL OSSIFYING FIBROMA**
Ulcerated gingival nodule.

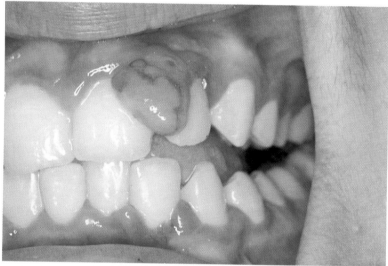

### Figure 9.18
**OSSEOUS CHORISTOMA**
Pedunculated nodule of the posterior
dorsum of the tongue.

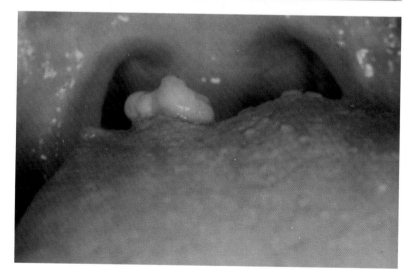

# HEMANGIOMA

### Figs. 9.19 and 9.20

The hemangioma is a relatively common benign tumor of blood vessels. In some cases they are congenital, presenting on the skin as a so-called "birthmark." Other cases develop during childhood or later in life. Many investigators prefer to consider the hemangioma, especially the congenital variety, a hamartoma rather than a true neoplasm. The head and neck area is the most common site for hemangiomas; more than half of all cases are seen there. Females are affected more frequently than males. Oral tumors can occur at any site, presenting as a flat or raised lesion appearing blue to purple or red. They may range in size from small lesions less than 1 cm in diameter to rare massive lesions that may produce severe disfigurement and be life-threatening. Hemangiomas are often asymptomatic but may exhibit hemorrhage when traumatized. Treatment depends on the individual case. Many congenital tumors may exhibit rapid growth during the first year of life and then gradually involute as the child grows older so that no therapy is required. Systemic high-dose corticosteroids are used for childhood hemangiomas that demonstrate significant facial distortion, major ulceration, recurrent infection, or obstruction of respiratory, visual, or auditory function. Tumors that are unresponsive to corticosteroid treatment can be treated with interferon alpha. Other hemangiomas may have to be surgically removed or debulked. Large tumors may be embolized or injected with sclerosing agents to induce fibrosis and shrinkage.

# KAPOSI'S SARCOMA

### Fig. 9.21

Kaposi's sarcoma is an unusual malignant vascular tumor that is currently believed to be caused by a strain of human herpesvirus known as KSHV/HHV-8 (Kaposi's sarcoma–associated human herpesvirus). Four clinical presentations of this tumor are recognized: classic, endemic (African), acquired immunodeficiency disease (AIDS)–related, and iatrogenic. Classic Kaposi's sarcoma primarily affects older men of Mediterranean origin, beginning as multiple blue-red tumors on the lower extremities that slowly enlarge and spread proximally. Oral involvement is uncommon. The prognosis, although variable, is generally good because of the slow progression of the disease, although many patients die from lymphoreticular neoplasms that are often associated with this tumor. Before the advent of the AIDS epidemic, Kaposi's sarcoma was rare in most of the world but common in central Africa, where it accounted for up to 9% of all malignancies. African and AIDS-associated Kaposi's sarcoma (see Figures 4.64 and 4.65) tend to occur in younger persons. It is associated with a more aggressive clinical course and a poorer prognosis, with a greater tendency for internal organ and lymph node involvement. Iatrogenic Kaposi's sarcoma most often occurs in recipients of organ transplants and has been reported in 0.4% of renal transplant patients. It is probably related to the patient's immunosuppressive therapy. Remission of the tumors can frequently be accomplished by reduction or discontinuation of the patient's immunosuppressive medications.

**Figure 9.19**
**HEMANGIOMA**
Massive purple tumor of the tongue.

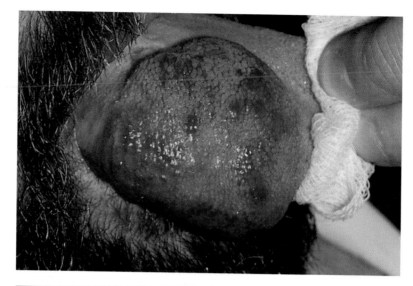

**Figure 9.20**
**HEMANGIOMA**
Diffuse blue-purple lesion of soft palate.

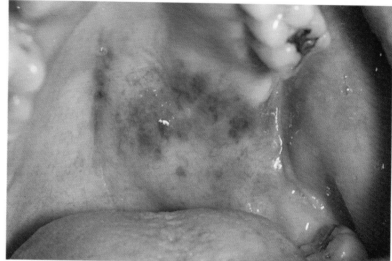

**Figure 9.21**
**KAPOSI'S SARCOMA**
Generalized involvement of the edentulous maxillary alveolar mucosa in a renal transplant patient who died from iatrogenic Kaposi's sarcoma.

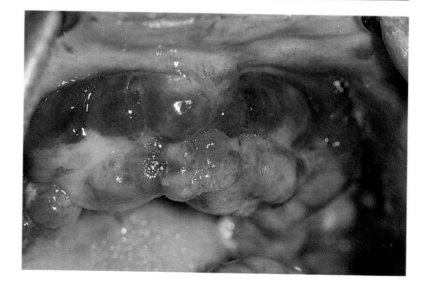

SOFT-TISSUE TUMORS

## LYMPHANGIOMA

**Fig. 9.22**

The lymphangioma is a benign tumor of lymphatic vessels. The majority of cases are congenital or arise during early childhood, suggesting that the lesion represents a hamartoma rather than a true neoplasm. Like the hemangioma, the head and neck area is the most common location for the lymphangioma. The anterior two-thirds of the tongue is the most common oral site, often resulting in macroglossia. Superficial tumors usually exhibit a pebbly surface resembling a cluster of amber translucent, grapelike vesicles; deeper tumors present as a soft, ill-defined mass. Trauma or infection may produce episodes of rapid, massive engorgement. Treatment most often consists of surgical excision, but the diffuse infiltrative nature of the tumor makes recurrence common. If total removal is not possible in a large tumor, surgical debulking may be performed. Some clinicians do not recommend treatment for nonenlarging lymphangiomas that do not interfere with normal function. Unfortunately, lymphangiomas do not respond to sclerosing agents as do hemangiomas. Recently, however, some success has been reported using intralesional injections of OK-432, a lyophilized mixture of a low-virulent strain of *Streptococcus pyogenes* with penicillin G.

## CYSTIC HYGROMA

**Figs. 9.23 and 9.24**

The cystic hygroma is a variety of lymphangioma most commonly occurring in the neck and characterized by large, deeply located cystlike lymphatic vessels. Extension of the tumor upward to involve the oral cavity is not uncommon. Respiratory difficulties and dysphagia may occur in deep-seated tumors; on rare occasions death may occur from edema of the tongue and cervical tissues producing airway obstruction. Treatment is surgical removal, which should be as complete as possible without sacrificing vital structures or cosmetically valuable tissues. The tumor may recur, but the rate of recurrence is lower than that for solely oral tumors composed of smaller lymphatic vessels. Intralesional injection of OK-432 also has been used with success.

► **Figure 9.22**
**LYMPHANGIOMA**
Pebbly mass of the right lateral tongue.

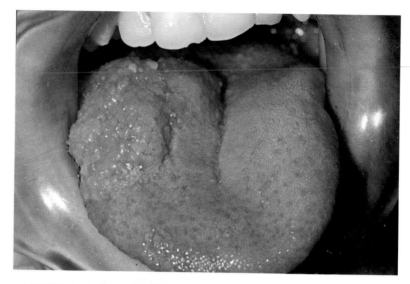

► **Figure 9.23**
**CYSTIC HYGROMA**
Soft, fluctuant mass involving the neck and submandibular region.

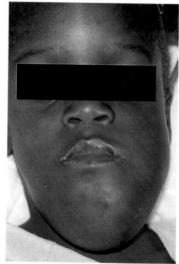

► **Figure 9.24**
**CYSTIC HYGROMA**
Same patient as in Figure 9.23 showing intraoral extension of the tumor with elevation of the tongue.

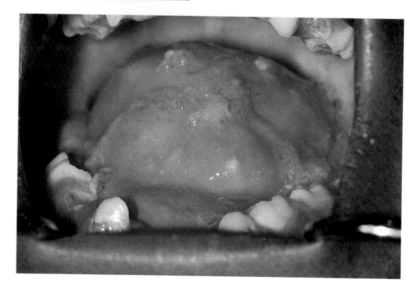

## STURGE-WEBER ANGIOMATOSIS (ENCEPHALOTRIGEMINAL ANGIOMATOSIS, STURGE-WEBER SYNDROME)

**Figs. 9.25, 9.26, and 9.27**

Sturge-Weber angiomatosis is a congenital anomaly characterized by hemangiomatosis involving the facial skin, oral mucosa, eyes, and meninges. The condition is typically unilateral, with skin and mucosal lesions following the distribution of one or more divisions of the trigeminal nerve. Occasionally, the patient will have bilateral involvement. The cutaneous lesion is usually flat and pink to purplish-red, often referred to as a "port-wine nevus" or "nevus flammeus." However, only slightly more than 10% of patients with facial port-wine nevi have Sturge-Weber angiomatosis; unless the lesion involves the distribution of the ophthalmic branch of the trigeminal nerve, the patient is typically not at risk for the full condition. These angiomatous skin lesions can be treated using flashlamp-pulsed dye lasers.

The meningeal angiomatosis is most common in the temporal and occipital regions and may be associated with cerebral cortical atrophy, seizures, mental retardation, and contralateral hemiplegia. Gyriform intracranial calcifications resembling a tram-line or railroad tracks may be seen. Neurosurgical removal of angiomatous meningeal lesions or hemispherectomy may be necessary in some cases. Ocular lesions are often associated with the development of glaucoma.

Oral involvement is often similar to that of the cutaneous lesion, presenting as a flat, bluish-red hypervascularity of the ipsilateral mucosa. In some instances, the gingiva may exhibit slight vascular hyperplasia, or massive hemangiomatous or pyogenic granuloma-like areas of enlargement. This gingival hyperplasia may be a result of the increased vascular component, phenytoin therapy used to control epileptic seizures, or both. Underlying alveolar bone destruction also has been reported in rare instances. Great care must be exercised in performing oral surgical or periodontal procedures because severe hemorrhage may be encountered.

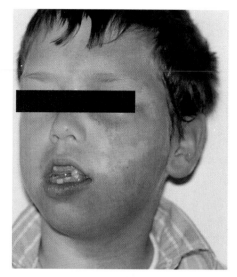

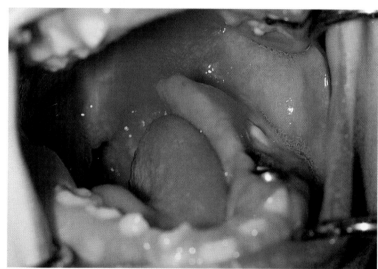

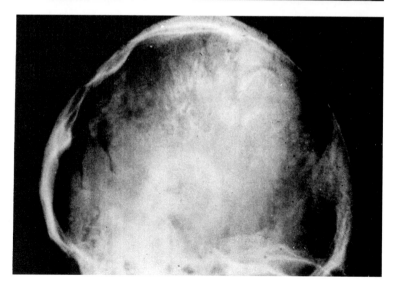

## TRAUMATIC NEUROMA (AMPUTATION NEUROMA)

**Fig. 9.28**

The traumatic neuroma is not a true neoplasm but a reactive hyperplasia of nerve elements following damage or severance of a nerve bundle. Once a nerve has been damaged or sectioned, the distal portion of the bundle undergoes degeneration, and the proximal nerve axons attempt to regenerate along the axis cylinders and reestablish innervation. If these sprouting nerve elements encounter scar tissue or otherwise cannot reestablish innervation, a tumorlike mass of disorganized nerve and scar tissue may develop at the site of injury. Oral traumatic neuromas typically present as small, smooth-surfaced, pink nodules that are frequently, but not always, painful. The mental foramen is the most common location, presumably arising from damage to the mental nerve during tooth extraction or from a mandibular denture. Treatment consists of surgical removal; recurrence is uncommon.

## NEURILEMOMA (SCHWANNOMA)

**Fig. 9.29**

The neurilemoma is a benign tumor of Schwann cell origin that is uncommon in the oral cavity. It typically presents as a solitary, slow-growing, encapsulated nodular mass that is usually painless, although pain or tenderness may occur in some instances. The tongue is the most common oral location, but the tumor can occur almost anywhere in the oral cavity. Rare intrabony tumors of the jaws have been reported, usually in the mandible. Occasionally, neurilemomas may be seen in patients with neurofibromatosis. Treatment consists of surgical removal; recurrence is rare.

## NEUROFIBROMA

**Fig. 9.30**

The neurofibroma is a relatively common, benign tumor of nerve origin that contains Schwann cells, perineural cells, and neurites. It may occur as a solitary neoplasm or in association with neurofibromatosis. The solitary oral neurofibroma is typically a painless, slow-growing, soft nodular mass that is usually nonulcerated and similar in color to the adjacent mucosa. Unlike the neurilemoma, the neurofibroma is usually nonencapsulated. Oral tumors may occur at almost any site and have even rarely been reported within bone (see Figure 11.35). Treatment for the solitary neurofibroma consists of local surgical excision. Further clinical evaluation to rule out neurofibromatosis should be performed.

**Figure 9.28**
**TRAUMATIC NEUROMA**
Small nodule on the upper lip.

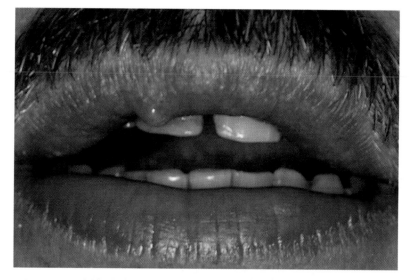

**Figure 9.29**
**NEURILEMOMA**
Smooth-surfaced mass in the floor of the
mouth. (Courtesy of Dr. Art A. Gonty.)

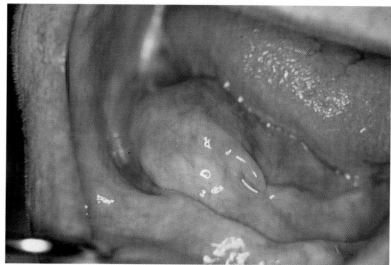

**Figure 9.30**
**NEUROFIBROMA**
Nodular mass of the ventral tongue.

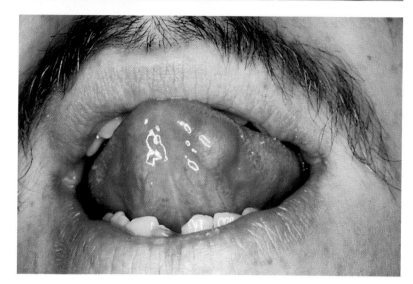

# NEUROFIBROMATOSIS (VON RECKLINGHAUSEN DISEASE OF THE SKIN)

## Figs. 9.31, 9.32, 9.33, and 9.34

Neurofibromatosis refers to a group of genetic disorders that are characterized by the development of multiple neural tumors, especially neurofibromas. Although at least eight forms of neurofibromatosis have been described, the most common form of the disease is neurofibromatosis type I (von Recklinghausen disease of the skin), which accounts for 85 to 90% of cases. Type I neurofibromatosis is inherited as an autosomal-dominant trait and is one of the most common hereditary diseases, occurring in 1 of approximately every 3000 births. About half of all affected individuals have no family history of the disorder and therefore apparently represent new mutations. The discussion here is limited to type I neurofibromatosis.

One of the earliest clinical manifestations of neurofibromatosis is the presence of flat, yellow-brown skin lesions known as "café au lait" spots. These spots are usually evident within the first few years of life, beginning as freckle-like areas that gradually become larger. They are more common in unexposed areas of the body. A characteristic site is the axilla, where multiple spots may result in axillary freckling, or Crowe's sign. Café au lait spots are present in more than 90% of patients with neurofibromatosis, and the presence of six or more spots greater than 1.5 cm in diameter is considered pathognomonic. Another characteristic clinical sign is the presence of small pigmented spots on the iris, which are known as "Lisch nodules."

Neurofibromas usually begin to appear during childhood and adolescence, after the appearance of the café au lait spots. These tumors are usually slow growing and may occur in almost any location. A wide clinical variation is seen; some patients exhibit few neurofibromas, others are covered with hundreds of tumors. The tumors seem to be sensitive to hormonal influence because an accelerated growth rate during puberty and pregnancy often occurs. Clinically, these tumors may present as discrete soft nodules or as larger, diffuse, pendulous masses. Unilateral involvement may rarely be seen.

Skeletal abnormalities are not uncommon, including kyphoscoliosis, macrocephaly, craniofacial asymmetry, central bone tumors, and bony erosion from adjacent tumors. Other neural tumors, including pheochromocytomas, may be seen. Mental deficiency is seen in a small percentage of patients.

Early reports suggested that oral lesions could be expected in 4 to 7% of cases of neurofibromatosis. However, more recent studies have suggested that oral lesions may be found in 72 to 92% of cases if a detailed clinical and radiographic examination is performed. Actual intraoral neurofibromas are seen in only about 25% of affected patients. Other oral lesions include enlargement of the fungiform papillae of the tongue, enlargement of the mandibular canal, occlusal plane distortion, and impacted teeth.

No effective treatment exists for neurofibromatosis, although surgery may be performed for tumors that are particularly large or painful or that involve vital structures. A feared complication is malignant transformation of one of the tumors, which is estimated to occur in about 5% of cases.

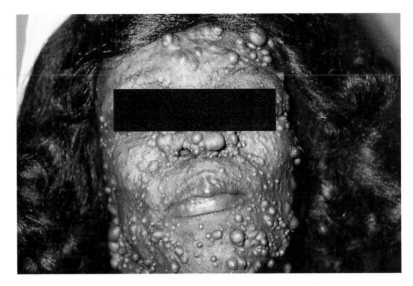

▶ **Figure 9.31**
**NEUROFIBROMATOSIS**
Multiple neurofibromas of the skin.

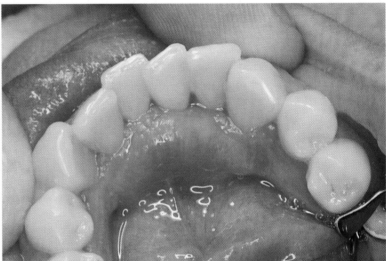

▶ **Figure 9.32**
**NEUROFIBROMATOSIS**
Neurofibroma of the anterior lingual
mucosa.

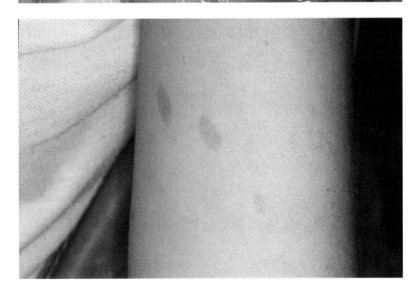

▶ **Figure 9.33**
**NEUROFIBROMATOSIS**
Café au lait pigmentation.

## MALIGNANT SCHWANNOMA (NEUROFIBROSARCOMA)

### Figs. 9.35 and 9.36

The malignant schwannoma is the principal sarcoma of peripheral nerve origin, but it rarely occurs in the oral cavity. The tumor is most common in young adults, presenting as a mass that may exhibit slow or rapid growth. Associated pain and paresthesia may be present. About half of the cases arise in patients with neurofibromatosis from malignant transformation of one of the tumors. Males with neurofibromatosis are more likely than females to exhibit such malignant change. Sarcomatous transformation is more likely to occur in a deep-seated tumor, and it often arises along a major nerve trunk.

Treatment for the malignant schwannoma consists primarily of radical surgical removal, possibly with adjuvant radiation therapy or chemotherapy. Many patients develop local recurrence or distant metastases. The prognosis for individuals with neurofibromatosis is poor; the long-term survival rate is around 10 to 15%. Patients without neurofibromatosis fare better, with a survival rate in the 30 to 50% range.

► **Figure 9.34**
**NEUROFIBROMATOSIS**
Axillary freckling.

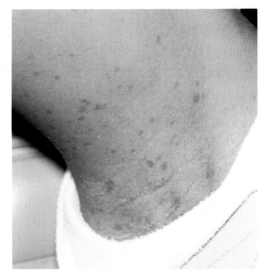

► **Figure 9.35**
**MALIGNANT SCHWANNOMA**
Rapidly growing tumor in a patient with
neurofibromatosis.

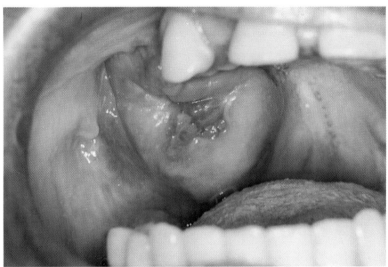

► **Figure 9.36**
**MALIGNANT SCHWANNOMA**
Computed tomographic scan of lesion
shown in Figure 9.35.

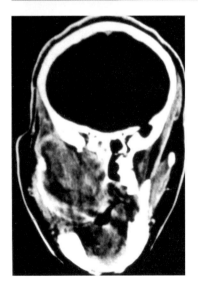

## Figs. 9.37, 9.38, and 9.39

The multiple endocrine neoplasia (MEN) syndromes are a family of rare autosomal-dominant disorders that are characterized by the development of multiple tumors or hyperplasias of neuroendocrine origin. The discussion here is limited to MEN type 2B because of its important oral and maxillofacial findings. This condition is characterized by (1) multiple mucosal neuromas, (2) adrenal pheochromocytomas, (3) medullary thyroid carcinoma, and (4) a Marfanoid body build with muscle wasting of the extremities.

The mucosal neuromas are created by marked hyperplasia of nerve bundles and may be present at birth or develop during early childhood. Multiple nodules may be seen on the anterior third of the tongue, bilaterally at the commissures, and along the lips, which are often thick and protuberant. Similar neuromas may occur along the eyelids and at other mucosal sites. Pheochromocytomas, which may be bilateral, are seen in about half of all patients and usually develop during the second and third decades of life. These catecholamine-producing adrenal tumors can produce a variety of clinical symptoms, including hypertension, weakness, heart palpitations, dizziness, headaches, sweating, and diarrhea.

The most serious manifestation of MEN type 2B is the development of medullary carcinoma of the thyroid gland, which most commonly occurs in the late teens and early twenties but can develop as early as the first year of life. This tumor arises from the parafollicular "C" cells of the thyroid, which are responsible for calcitonin production. These medullary thyroid carcinomas have a high prevalence of metastasis and are the most common cause of death in patients with this disorder.

Individuals with MEN 2B can now be identified via genetic testing for the presence of mutations in the *RET* protooncogene. Good prognosis depends on early diagnosis and prophylactic thyroidectomy to prevent the evolution of medullary thyroid carcinoma, which develops in 100% of affected individuals. Even when thyroidectomy is performed at an early age, evidence of the development of this tumor is frequently found. Therefore, some authorities have recommended performing this surgery as early as the first year of life. Serum calcitonin levels can be monitored to evaluate for the presence of recurrent or metastatic tumor. Urinary catecholamine excretion also can be used to evaluate for the presence of pheochromocytomas.

### Figure 9.37
**MULTIPLE ENDOCRINE NEOPLASIA TYPE 2B**
Multiple neuromas of the anterior tongue. Patient presented in a hypertensive crisis from an adrenal pheochromocytoma.

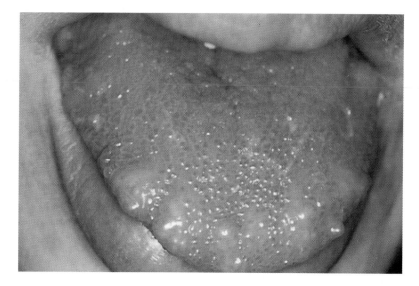

### Figure 9.38
**MULTIPLE ENDOCRINE NEOPLASIA TYPE 2B**
Same patient as in Figure 9.37 with bilateral neuromas at the commissures.

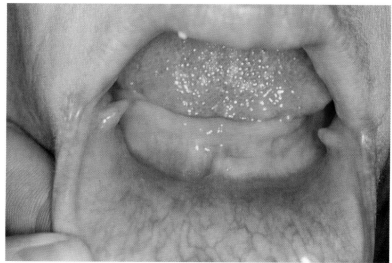

### Figure 9.39
**MULTIPLE ENDOCRINE NEOPLASIA TYPE 2B**
Conjunctival neuroma in a patient with oral mucosal neuromas and medullary thyroid carcinoma.

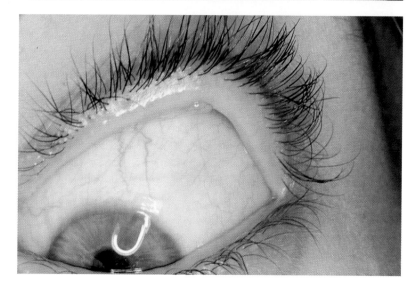

# MELANOTIC NEUROECTODERMAL TUMOR OF INFANCY

**Figs. 9.40 and 9.41**

The melanotic neuroectodermal tumor of infancy is a rare neoplasm that primarily occurs in the anterior maxilla, but it also may arise in other locations, including the mandible. Convincing evidence, including elevated urinary vanillylmandelic acid levels in many patients, indicates that the tumor is of neural crest origin, although previous theories considered a possible odontogenic or germ cell origin. Most cases have occurred in infants younger than 9 months of age, in whom the lesions present as a rapidly growing, nonulcerated mass of the anterior maxillary alveolar ridge. The tumor is frequently pigmented because of the presence of melanin-containing cells. Underlying bone destruction with displacement of the primary teeth is common. Despite its rapid growth and locally destructive clinical nature, the lesion is usually benign. Treatment typically consists of conservative surgical excision; recurrence is seen in 10 to 15% of cases. However, some reported cases have acted in a malignant fashion, resulting in metastasis and death.

# GRANULAR CELL TUMOR

**Fig. 9.42**

The granular cell tumor is a relatively uncommon neoplasm that shows a predilection for the oral cavity, especially the tongue. Formerly called the granular cell myoblastoma because of its suspected skeletal muscle origin, most investigators now believe it arises from either the Schwann cell or an undifferentiated mesenchymal cell. The tumor typically presents as a slow-growing, nonulcerated nodular mass that is usually pink but sometimes may appear yellow. It is most common in young and middle-aged adults and is twice as common in women as in men. Multiple granular cell tumors occasionally may occur. Treatment consists of local surgical excision; recurrence is uncommon. Microscopically, this benign tumor is often associated with pseudoepitheliomatous hyperplasia of the overlying epithelium, and it is important that the pathologist not mistake this for squamous cell carcinoma.

### Figure 9.40
**MELANOTIC NEUROECTODERMAL TUMOR OF INFANCY**

Swelling of the anterior maxillary alveolar ridge. (Courtesy of Drs. H. Tom Daniel and Len W. Morrow.)

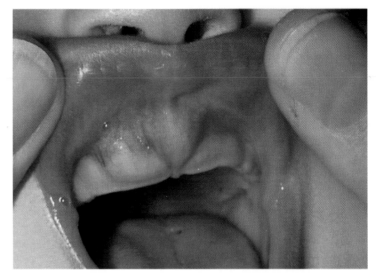

### Figure 9.41
**MELANOTIC NEUROECTODERMAL TUMOR OF INFANCY**

Radiograph of the patient depicted in Figure 9.40 demonstrating bone destruction and displacement of unerupted teeth.

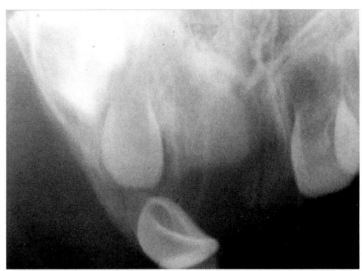

### Figure 9.42
**GRANULAR CELL TUMOR**

Sessile nodule of the tongue.

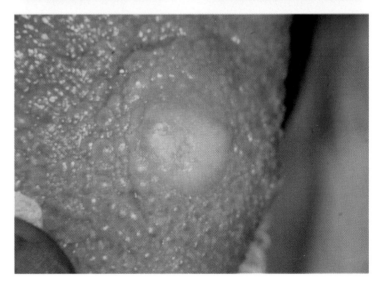

## CONGENITAL EPULIS (CONGENITAL EPULIS OF THE NEWBORN)

**Fig. 9.43**

The congenital epulis is a rare benign tumor of uncertain histogenesis that occurs on the alveolar ridge of newborn infants. It bears some histopathologic resemblance to the granular cell tumor, but seems to be a separate entity. Nearly 90% of reported cases have been in females. It is twice as common on the maxillary ridge as on the mandibular ridge. The tumor is more common along the anterior portion of the alveolar ridge, typically presenting as a pedunculated, smooth-surfaced mass. Multiple tumors develop in 10% of cases. The lesions range in size from a few millimeters to large tumors greater than several centimeters in diameter that may interfere with feeding or breathing. Treatment usually consists of surgical excision, although spontaneous regression has been reported in a few cases.

## ANGIOMYOMA (VASCULAR LEIOMYOMA)

**Fig. 9.44**

Leiomyomas, benign tumors of smooth muscle origin, are rare in the oral cavity. Most cases probably arise from smooth muscle in the walls of blood vessels. The most common type of oral leiomyoma is the angiomyoma, or vascular leiomyoma, which is composed of a combination of blood vessels and surrounding smooth muscle. Solid leiomyomas also may occur. Oral leiomyomas may develop at any site, with the lips, tongue, palate, and buccal mucosa being the most common locations. The tumor is more common in adults, typically presenting as a slow-growing, nonulcerated nodular mass. Angiomyomas often appear blue because of their vascular content. Treatment consists of surgical excision; recurrence is rare.

## RHABDOMYOMA

**Fig. 9.45**

Benign tumors of skeletal muscle origin, or rhabdomyomas, are extremely rare. Excluding examples of cardiac rhabdomyoma, however, these tumors show a striking predilection for the head and neck region. These extracardiac rhabdomyomas can be divided into adult and fetal varieties, based on their microscopic appearance. Adult rhabdomyomas occur primarily in middle-aged and older patients, with about 70% of cases seen in men. They are most common in the pharynx, larynx, and oral cavity and may grow to considerable size before discovery. Laryngeal and pharyngeal tumors may produce airway obstruction. Multiple tumors are not unusual. Fetal rhabdomyomas usually occur in young children and are most common on the face and preauricular region. Treatment for both varieties consists of local surgical excision; recurrence is uncommon.

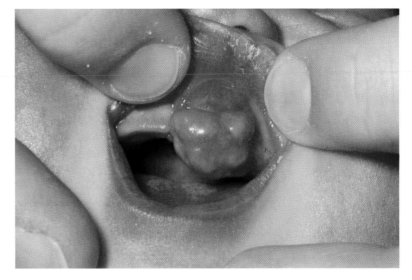

**Figure 9.43**
**CONGENITAL EPULIS**
Lobulated mass of the anterior maxillary alveolar ridge.

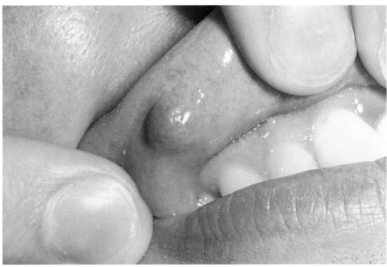

**Figure 9.44**
**ANGIOMYOMA**
Blue pigmented nodule of the upper lip.

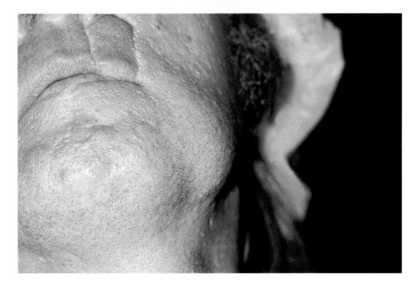

**Figure 9.45**
**RHABDOMYOMA**
Mass in the left cheek.

## Figs. 9.46, 9.47, and 9.48

Malignant skeletal muscle tumors, or rhabdomyosarcomas, are the most common soft-tissue sarcomas in children. The head and neck is the most common site for pediatric rhabdomyosarcomas, accounting for 40% of childhood cases. Rhabdomyosarcomas also may occur in young adults, but they are rare after the age of 45 years. The head and neck is a much less common site for adult cases. Several histopathologic subtypes of this tumor are recognized; the embryonal rhabdomyosarcoma is the most common in the head and neck.

In the head and neck region, the orbit is the most common site for rhabdomyosarcoma, followed by the nasal cavity and nasopharynx. The palate is the most common intraoral location. The tumor generally presents as an infiltrative mass that may exhibit rapid growth. Associated pain and underlying bone destruction may also be seen. Treatment usually involves a combination of surgery, radiation, and chemotherapy. Death may result from local recurrence or distant metastases, but the prognosis for rhabdomyosarcoma has greatly improved in recent years with the use of multimodal therapy. The 5-year survival rate in children ranges from 45 to 63%. However, the prognosis in adults is significantly lower, with survival ranging from 8 to 32%.

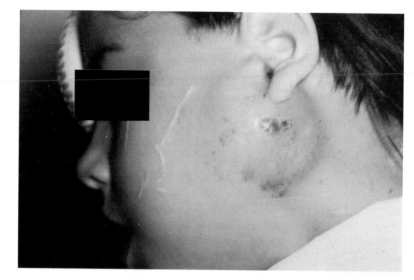

► **Figure 9.47**
**RHABDOMYOSARCOMA**
Same patient as shown in Figure 9.46
with intraoral extension of the tumor
involving the lateral soft palate.

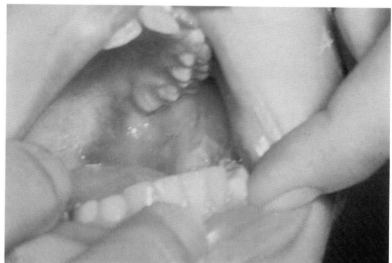

► **Figure 9.48**
**RHABDOMYOSARCOMA**
Bone destruction of the mandibular ramus
and displacement of the permanent
second molar in same patient as shown
in Figures 9.46 and 9.47.

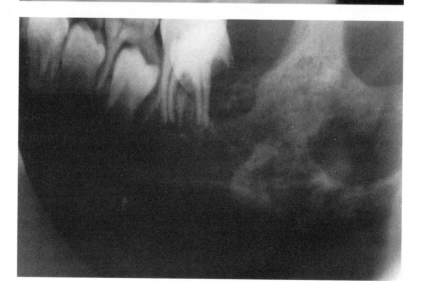

### Fibroma and Giant Cell Fibroma

Bouquot JE, Gundlach KKH. Oral exophytic lesions in 23,616 white Americans over 35 years of age. Oral Surg Oral Med Oral Pathol 1986;62:284.

Houston GD. The giant cell fibroma: a review of 464 cases. Oral Surg Oral Med Oral Pathol 1982;53:582.

Savage NW, Monsour PA. Oral fibrous hyperplasias and the giant cell fibroma. Aust Dent J 1985;30:405.

Weathers DR, Callihan MD. Giant-cell fibroma. Oral Surg Oral Med Oral Pathol 1974;37:374.

### Epulis Fissuratum and Leaflike Denture Fibroma

Buchner A, Begleiter A, Hansen LS. The predominance of epulis fissuratum in females. Quintessence Int 1984;15:699.

Cutright DE. The histopathologic findings in 583 cases of epulis fissuratum. Oral Surg Oral Med Oral Pathol 1974;37:401.

Sasai H, Yamamoto H, Matsumoto T, et al. A clinicopathological study of so-called denture fibroma. J Nihon Univ Sch Dent 1990;32:204.

### Inflammatory Papillary Hyperplasia

Bhaskar SN, Beasley JD, Cutright DE. Inflammatory papillary hyperplasia: report of 341 cases. J Am Dent Assoc 1970;81:949.

Dorey JL, Blasberg B, MacEntee MI, et al. Oral mucosal disorders in denture wearers. J Prosthet Dent 1985;53:210.

Ettinger RL. The etiology of inflammatory papillary hyperplasia. J Prosthet Dent 1975;34:254.

Monaco JG, Pickett AB. The role of Candida in inflammatory papillary hyperplasia. J Prosthet Dent 1981;45:470.

Salonen MAM, Raustia AM, Oikarinen KS. Effect of treatment of palatal inflammatory papillary hyperplasia with local and systemic antifungal agents accompanied by renewal of complete dentures. Acta Odontol Scand 1996;54:87.

### Aggressive Fibromatosis

Carr RJ, Zaki GA, Leader MB, et al. Infantile fibromatosis with involvement of the mandible. Br J Oral Maxillofac Surg 1992;30:257.

Fowler CB, Hartman KS, Brannon RB. Fibromatosis of the oral and paraoral region. Oral Surg Oral Med Oral Pathol 1994;77:373.

Rodu B, Weathers DR, Campbell WG Jr. Aggressive fibromatosis involving the paramandibular soft tissues. Oral Surg Oral Med Oral Pathol 1981;52:395.

Vally IM, Altini M. Fibromatoses of the oral and paraoral soft tissues and jaws: review of the literature and report of 12 new cases. Oral Surg Oral Med Oral Pathol 1990;69:191.

### Fibrosarcoma

Frankenthaler R, Ayala AG, Hartwick RW, et al. Fibrosarcoma of the head and neck. Laryngoscope 1990;100:799.

Greager JA, Reichard K, Campana JP, et al. Fibrosarcoma of the head and neck. Am J Surg 1994;167:437.

Mark RJ, Sercarz JA, Tran L, et al. Fibrosarcoma of the head and neck: the UCLA experience. Arch Otolaryngol Head Neck Surg 1991;117:396.

### Lipoma

de Visscher JGAM. Lipomas and fibrolipomas of the oral cavity. J Maxillofac Surg 1982;10:177.

Greer RO, Richardson JF. The nature of lipomas and their significance in the oral cavity: a review and report of cases. Oral Surg Oral Med Oral Pathol 1973;36:551.

Pélissier A, Sawaf MH, Shabana A-HM. Infiltrating (intramuscular) benign lipoma of the head and neck. J Oral Maxillofac Surg 1991;49:1231.

### Pyogenic Granuloma

Bhaskar SN, Jacoway JR. Pyogenic granuloma: clinical features, incidence, histology, and result of treatment: report of 242 cases. J Oral Surg 1966;24:391.

Daley TD, Nartey NO, Wysocki GP. Pregnancy tumor: an analysis. Oral Surg Oral Med Oral Pathol 1991;72:196.

Kerr DA. Granuloma pyogenicum. Oral Surg Oral Med Oral Pathol 1951;4:158.

Papageorge MB, Doku HC. An exaggerated response of intra-oral pyogenic granuloma during puberty. J Clin Pediat Dent 1992;16:213.

Vilmann A, Vilmann P, Vilmann H. Pyogenic granuloma: evaluation of oral conditions. Br J Oral Maxillofac Surg 1986;24:376.

## Peripheral Giant Cell Granuloma

Giansanti JS, Waldron CA. Peripheral giant cell granuloma: review of 720 cases. J Oral Surg 1969;27:787.

Katsikeris N, Kakarantza-Angelopoulos E, Angelopoulos AP. Peripheral giant cell granuloma: clinicopathologic study of 224 new cases and review of 956 reported cases. Int J Oral Maxillofac Surg 1988;17:94.

## Peripheral Ossifying Fibroma

Buchner A, Hansen LS. The histomorphologic spectrum of peripheral ossifying fibroma. Oral Surg Oral Med Oral Pathol 1987;63:452.

Kendrick F, Waggoner WF. Managing a peripheral ossifying fibroma. J Dent Child 1996;63:135.

Kenney JN, Kaugars GE, Abbey LM. Comparison between the peripheral ossifying fibroma and perpheral odontogenic fibroma. J Oral Maxillofac Surg 1989;47:378.

Poon C-K, Kwan P-C, Chao S-Y. Giant peripheral ossifying fibroma of the maxilla: report of a case. J Oral Maxillofac Surg 1995;53:695.

Zain RB, Fei YJ. Fibrous lesions of the gingiva: a histomorphologic analysis of 204 cases. Oral Surg Oral Med Oral Pathol 1990;70:466.

## Osseous and Cartilaginous Choristomas

Chou L, Hansen LS, Daniels TE. Choristomas of the oral cavity: a review. Oral Surg Oral Med Oral Pathol 1991;72:584.

Krolls SO, Jacoway JR, Alexander WN. Osseous choristomas (osteomas) of intraoral soft tissues. Oral Surg Oral Med Oral Pathol 1971;32:588.

Tohill MJ, Green JG, Cohen DM. Intraoral osseous and cartilaginous choristomas: report of three cases and review of the literature. Oral Surg Oral Med Oral Pathol 1987;63:506.

Ünal T, Ertürk S. Cartilaginous choristoma of the gingiva: report of two cases: review of the literature of both gingival choristomas and intraoral chondromas. Ann Dent 1994;53:19.

## Hemangioma

Fishman SJ, Mulliken JB. Hemangiomas and vascular malformations of infancy and childhood. Pediatr Clin North Am 1993;40:1177.

Kaban LB, Mulliken JB. Vascular anomalies of the maxillofacial region. J Oral Maxillofac Surg 1986;44:203.

Kane WJ, Morris S, Jackson IT, et al. Significant hemangiomas and vascular malformations of the head and neck: clinical management and treatment outcomes. Ann Plast Surg 1995;35:133.

Silverman RA. Hemangiomas and vascular malformations. Pediatr Clin North Am 1991;38:811.

Soumekh B, Adams GL, Shapiro RS. Treatment of head and neck hemangiomas with recombinant interferon alpha 2B. Ann Otol Rhinol Laryngol 1996;105:201.

## Kaposi's Sarcoma

Farman AG, Uys PB. Oral Kaposi's sarcoma. Oral Surg Oral Med Oral Pathol 1975;39:288.

Flaitz CM, Jin Y-T, Hicks MJ, et al. Kaposi's sarcoma-associated herpesvirus-like DNA sequences (KSHV/HHV-8) in oral AIDS-Kaposi's sarcoma: a PCR and clinicopathologic study. Oral Surg Oral Med Oral Pathol Oral Radiol Endod 1997;83:259.

Friedman-Kien AE, Saltzman BR. Clinical manifestations of classical, endemic African, and epidemic AIDS-associated Kaposi's sarcoma. J Am Acad Dermatol 1990;22:1237.

Qunibi WY, Barri Y, Alfurayh O, et al. Kaposi's sarcoma in renal transplant recipients: a report on 26 cases from a single institution. Transplant Proc 1993;25:1402.

Stein ME, Spencer D, Ruff P, et al. Endemic African Kaposi's sarcoma: clinical and therapeutic implications: 10-year experience in the Johannesburg Hospital (1980–1990). Oncology 1994;51:63.

## Lymphangioma and Cystic Hygroma

Farman AG, Katz J, Eloff J, et al. Mandibulo-facial aspects of the cervical cystic lymphangioma (cystic hygroma). Br J Oral Surg 1978;16:125.

Goldberg MH, Nemarich AN, Danielson P. Lymphangioma of the tongue: medical and surgical therapy. J Oral Surg 1977;35:841.

Ogita S, Tsuto T, Nakamura K, et al. OK-432 therapy in 64 patients with lymphangioma. J Pediatr Surg 1994;29:784.

Osborne TE, Levin LS, Tilghman DM, et al. Surgical correction of mandibulofacial deformities secondary to large cervical cystic hygromas. J Oral Maxillofac Surg 1987;45:1015.

Ricciardelli EJ, Richardson MA. Cervicofacial cystic hygroma: patterns of recurrence and management of the difficult case. Arch Otolaryngol Head Neck Surg 1991;117:546.

## Sturge-Weber Angiomatosis

Pascual-Castroviejo I, Díaz-Gonzalez C, García-Melian RM, et al. Sturge-Weber syndrome: study of 40 patients. Pediatr Neurol 1993;9:283.

Sujansky E, Conradi S. Outcome of Sturge-Weber syndrome in 52 adults. Am J Med Genet 1995;57:35.

Wilson S, Venzel JM, Miller R. Angiography, gingival hyperplasia and Sturge-Weber syndrome: report of case. ASDC J Dent Child. 1986;53:283.

Yukna RA, Cassingham RJ, Carr RF. Periodontal manifestations and treatment in a case of Sturge-Weber syndrome. Oral Surg Oral Med Oral Pathol 1979;47:408.

## Traumatic Neuroma

Peszkowski MJ, Larsson, Å. Extraosseous and intraosseous oral traumatic neuromas and their association with tooth extraction. J Oral Maxillofac Surg 1990;48:963.

Sist TC Jr, Greene GW. Traumatic neuroma of the oral cavity: report of thirty-one new cases and review of the literature. Oral Surg Oral Med Oral Pathol 1981;51:394.

## Neurilemoma and Neurofibroma

Ellis GL, Abrams AM, Melrose RJ. Intraosseous benign neural sheath neoplasms of the jaws: report of seven new cases and review of the literature. Oral Surg Oral Med Oral Pathol 1977;44:731.

Griffith BH, Lewis VL, McKinney P. Neurofibromas of the head and neck. Surg Gynecol Obstet 1985;160:534.

Hatziotis JC, Asprides H. Neurilemoma (schwannoma) of the oral cavity. Oral Surg Oral Med Oral Pathol 1967;24:510.

Williams HK, Cannell H, Silvester K, et al. Neurilemoma of the head and neck. Br J Oral Maxillofac Surg 1993;31:32.

Wright BA, Jackson D. Neural tumors of the oral cavity. Oral Surg Oral Med Oral Pathol 1980;49:509.

## Neurofibromatosis

D'Ambrosio JA, Langlais RP, Young RS. Jaw and skull changes in neurofibromatosis. Oral Surg Oral Med Oral Pathol 1988;66:391.

Geist JR, Gander DL, Stefanac SJ. Oral manifestations of neurofibromatosis types I and II. Oral Surg Oral Med Oral Pathol 1992;73:376.

Goldberg NS. Neurofibromatosis (von Recklinghausen's disease). In: Demis DJ, ed. Clinical dermatology. Hagerstown, Md: Harper & Row, 1993.

Lee L, Yan Y-H, Pharoah MJ. Radiographic features of the mandible in neurofibromatosis: a report of 10 cases and review of the literature. Oral Surg Oral Med Oral Pathol Oral Radiol Endod 1996;81:361.

Shapiro SD, Abramovich K, Van Dis ML, et al. Neurofibromatosis: oral and radiographic manifestations. Oral Surg Oral Med Oral Pathol 1984;58:493.

## Malignant Schwannoma (Neurofibrosarcoma)

Bailet JW, Abemayor E, Andrews JC, et al. Malignant nerve sheath tumors of the head and neck: a combined experience from two university hospitals. Laryngoscope 1991;101:1044.

DiCerbo M, Sciubba JJ, Sordill WC, et al. Malignant schwannoma of the palate: a case report and review of the literature. J Oral Maxillofac Surg 1992;50:1217.

Ducatman BS, Scheithauer BW, Piepgras DG, et al. Malignant peripheral nerve sheath tumors: a clinicopathologic study of 120 cases. Cancer 1986;57:2006.

Neville BW, Hann J, Narang R, et al. Oral neurofibrosarcoma associated with neurofibromatosis type I. Oral Surg Oral Med Oral Pathol 1991;72:456.

## Multiple Endocrine Neoplasia Type 2B

Ledger GA, Khosla S, Lindor NM, et al. Genetic testing in the diagnosis and management of multiple endocrine neoplasia type II. Ann Intern Med 1995;122:118.

O'Riordain DS, O'Brien T, Crotty TB, et al. Multiple endocrine neoplasia type 2B: more than an endocrine disorder. Surgery 1995;118:936.

Skinner MA, DeBenedetti MK, Moley JF, et al. Medullary thyroid carcinoma in children with multiple endocrine neoplasia types 2A and 2B. J Pediatr Surg 1996;31:177.

Vasen HFA, van der Feltz M, Raue F, et al. The natural course of multiple endocrine neoplasia type IIb: a study of 18 cases. Arch Intern Med 1992;152:1250.

## Melanotic Neuroectodermal Tumor of Infancy

Hupp JR, Topazian RG, Krutchkoff DJ. The melanotic neuroectodermal tumor of infancy: report of two cases and review of the literature. Int J Oral Surg 1981;10:432.

Kapadia SB, Frisman DM, Hitchcock CL, et al. Melanotic neuroectodermal tumor of infancy: clinicopathological, immunohistochemical, and flow cytometric study. Am J Surg Pathol 1993;17:566.

Mosby EL, Lowe MW, Cobb CM, et al. Melanotic neuroectodermal tumor of infancy: review of the literature and report of a case. J Oral Maxillofac Surg 1992;50:886.

## Granular Cell Tumor

Collins BM, Jones AC. Multiple granular cell tumors of the oral cavity: report of a case and review of the literature. J Oral Maxillofac Surg 1995;53:707.

Fliss DM, Puterman M, Zirkin H, et al. Granular cell lesions in head and neck: a clinicopathological study. J Surg Oncol 1989;42:154.

Mirchandani R, Sciubba JJ, Mir R. Granular cell lesions of the jaws and oral cavity: a clinicopathologic, immunohistochemical, and ultrastructural study. J Oral Maxillofac Surg 1989;47:1248.

Stewart CM, Watson RE, Eversole LR, et al. Oral granular cell tumors: a clinicopathologic and immunocytochemical study. Oral Surg Oral Med Oral Pathol 1988;65:427.

## Congenital Epulis of the Newborn

Damm DD, Cibull ML, Geissler RH, et al. Investigation into the histogenesis of congenital epulis of the newborn. Oral Surg Oral Med Oral Pathol 1993;76:205.

Lack EE, Worsham GF, Callihan MD, et al. Gingival granular cell tumors of the newborn (congenital "epulis"): a clinical and pathologic study of 21 patients. Am J Surg Pathol 1981;5:37.

## Angiomyoma

Damm DD, Neville BW. Oral leiomyomas. Oral Surg Oral Med Oral Pathol 1979;47:343.

Epivatianos A, Trigonidis G, Papanayotou P. Vascular leiomyoma of the oral cavity. J Oral Maxillofac Surg 1985;43:377.

Katou F, Andoh N, Motegi K, et al. Leiomyoma of the mandible: a rapid growing case with immunohistochemical and electron microscopic observations. Oral Surg Oral Med Oral Pathol Oral Radiol Endod 1997;84:45.

Svane TJ, Smith BR, Cosentino BJ, et al. Oral leiomyomas. Review of the literature and report of a case of palatal angioleiomyoma. J Periodontol 1986;57:433.

## Rhabdomyoma

Cleveland DB, Chen S-Y, Allen CM, et al. Adult rhabdomyoma: a light microscopic, ultrastructural, virologic, and immunologic analysis. Oral Surg Oral Med Oral Pathol 1994;77:147.

Corio RL, Lewis DM. Intraoral rhabdomyomas. Oral Surg Oral Med Oral Pathol 1979;48:525.

Kapadia SB, Meis JM, Frisman DM, et al. Adult rhabdomyoma of the head and neck: a clinicopathologic and immunophenotypic study. Hum Pathol 1993;24:608.

Kapadia SB, Meis JM, Frisman DM, et al. Fetal rhabdomyoma of the head and neck: a clinicopathologic and immunophenotypic study. Hum Pathol 1993;24:754.

## Rhabdomyosarcoma

Bras J, Batsakis JG, Luna MA. Rhabdomyosarcoma of the oral soft tissues. Oral Surg Oral Med Oral Pathol 1987;64:585.

Callender TA, Weber RS, Janjan N, et al. Rhabdomyosarcoma of the nose and paranasal sinuses in adults and children. Otolaryngol Head Neck Surg 1995;112:252.

Coene IMJH, Schouwenburg PF, Voûte PA, et al. Rhabdomyosarcoma of the head and neck in children. Clin Otolaryngol 1992;17:291.

Kaste SC, Hopkins KP, Bowman LC. Dental abnormalities in long-term survivors of head and neck rhabdomyosarcoma. Med Pediatr Oncol 1995;25:96.

Lyos AT, Goepfert H, Luna MA, et al. Soft tissue sarcoma of the head and neck in children and adolescents. Cancer 1996;77:193.

Nayar RC, Prudhomme F, Parise O Jr. Rhabdomyosarcoma of the head and neck in adults: a study of 26 patients. Laryngoscope 1993;103:1362.

# chapter 10
# LYMPHORETICULAR AND HEMATOPOIETIC DISEASES

## HEMOPHILIA

### Fig. 10.1

Hemophilia refers to a group of bleeding disorders that are caused by a hereditary deficiency of one of the clotting factors in the blood. The best known of these diseases are hemophilia A (classic hemophilia) and hemophilia B (Christmas disease), which are X-linked recessive disorders caused by a deficiency of Factor VIII and Factor IX, respectively. Because these conditions are X-linked recessive, females are typically only carriers of the disorders, which are then expressed in affected males in the family. Hemophiliacs are prone to severe, uncontrollable blood loss from any type of laceration or trauma, including surgical excisions, simple extractions, and periodontal scaling. Therefore, consultation with the patient's physician is mandatory before undergoing any dental or oral surgical procedure that may induce bleeding. If necessary, the missing clotting factor can be administered to the patient, plus epsilon-aminocaproic acid (EACA, an antifibrinolytic agent) can be used. Unfortunately, many hemophiliacs became infected with the human immunodeficiency virus when they received transfusions of concentrated clotting factors in the early 1980s. However, this risk has been eliminated with today's techniques, including purified factor concentrates and recombinant DNA technology.

## THROMBOCYTOPENIA

### Figs. 10.2 and 10.3

Thrombocytopenia, or platelet deficiency, is a hemorrhagic disorder that may occur secondarily in a wide variety of conditions, or it may appear as a primary disease, probably of autoimmune origin, called "idiopathic thrombocytopenic purpura" (ITP). Acute ITP most commonly occurs in children and frequently follows an acute viral illness. It is usually a self-limiting disease of several days' to several months' duration, with full recovery and no further problems. On the other hand, chronic ITP is more common in adults, often exhibiting multiple remissions and exacerbations. Secondary causes of thrombocytopenia include marrow-suppressive drug therapy, abnormal drug reactions, marrow infiltration by tumor cells, systemic lupus erythematosus, and various infections.

Clinically, petechial and ecchymotic skin lesions may occur, as may epistaxis, hematuria, gastrointestinal tract bleeding, and intracranial hemorrhage. Oral manifestations include gingival bleeding, submucosal hemorrhage, and excessive bleeding following tooth extraction or surgery. Treatment for thrombocytopenia may include systemic corticosteroid therapy, platelet transfusions, and splenectomy. Control of secondary thrombocytopenia also must include management of the underlying cause. In one rare form of platelet deficiency known as "thrombotic thrombocytopenic purpura," gingival biopsy has been used as a diagnostic aid to demonstrate the presence of intravascular platelet thrombi.

### Figure 10.1
### HEMOPHILIA
Persistent gingival bleeding following dental prophylaxis in a patient with hemophilia B. The patient also has Dilantin hyperplasia of the gingiva.

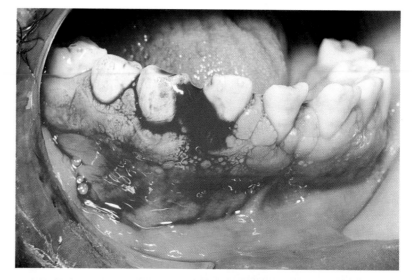

### Figure 10.2
### IDIOPATHIC THROMBOCYTOPENIC PURPURA
Gingival hemorrhage.

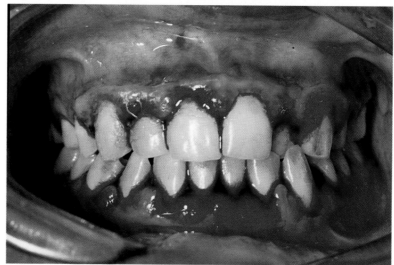

### Figure 10.3
### IDIOPATHIC THROMBOCYTOPENIC PURPURA
Palatal ecchymosis.

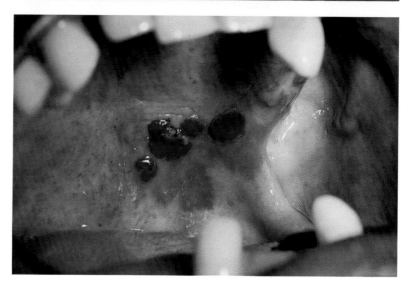

## Figs. 10.4, 10.5, and 10.6

Megaloblastic anemia is characterized by a reduction in the number of red blood cells combined with abnormal enlargement of proliferating marrow cells. Most megaloblastic anemias arise from a deficiency of vitamin B12 (cobalamin) or folic acid. In pernicious anemia, vitamin B12 deficiency is caused by autoimmune-mediated atrophy of the gastric mucosa, with failure to produce intrinsic factor necessary for vitamin B12 absorption. Other causes of vitamin B12 and folic acid deficiency include improper diet, impaired intestinal absorption, gastric or intestinal resection, and gastric bypass or stapling procedures for obesity.

Clinical manifestations of megaloblastic anemia include pallor, weakness, fatigue, shortness of breath, headache, palpitations, and syncope. Neurologic symptoms may occur, such as paresthesia of the extremities, unsteadiness of gait, and loss of vibratory and positional sense. Oral features include atrophy and burning of the tongue, with loss of papillae sometimes imparting a "beefy red" appearance. Atrophic, erythematous lesions also may be seen on other oral mucosal surfaces. Treatment usually consists of appropriate vitamin supplementation; in vitamin B12 deficiency, parenteral administration is necessary in most cases.

### ▶ Figure 10.4
### PERNICIOUS ANEMIA
Erythema and atrophy of the dorsal tongue.

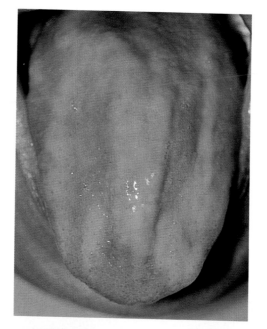

### ▶ Figure 10.5
### MEGALOBLASTIC ANEMIA
Burning macular, erythematous mucosal lesions in a patient with vitamin B12 deficiency secondary to gastric bypass for obesity. (Courtesy of Drummond JF, White DK, Damm, DD. Megaloblastic anemia with oral lesions: a consequence of gastric bypass surgery. Oral Surg Oral Med Oral Pathol 1985;59:149.)

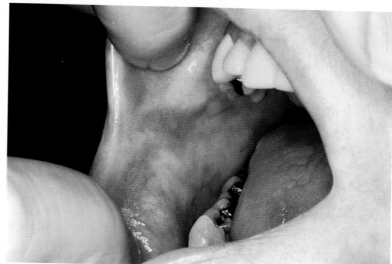

### ▶ Figure 10.6
### MEGALOBLASTIC ANEMIA
Resolution of lesions in Figure 10.5 following vitamin B12 injections. (Courtesy of Drummond JF, White DK, Damm DD. Megaloblastic anemia with oral lesions: a consequence of gastric bypass surgery. Oral Surg Oral Med Oral Pathol 1985;59:149.)

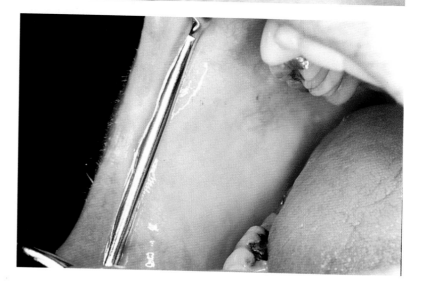

## PLUMMER-VINSON SYNDROME (PATERSON-KELLY SYNDROME, SIDEROPENIC DYSPHAGIA)

**Fig. 10.7**

Plummer-Vinson syndrome consists of iron-deficiency anemia with associated dysphagia caused by the development of webs or strictures in the lower part of the hypopharynx or the upper part of the esophagus. The condition is seen almost exclusively in middle-aged women but is uncommon today because of improved nutrition. Patients with Plummer-Vinson syndrome usually present with a hypochromic, microcytic anemia with resultant pallor of the skin and atrophy of the mucous membranes. Atrophy of the tongue papillae may lead to a smooth, red, painful glossitis. Angular cheilitis also is frequently seen. The condition is significant in that patients exhibit a significantly increased prevalence of carcinoma of the esophagus, hypopharynx, and oral cavity.

## NEUTROPENIA

**Figs. 10.8 and 10.9**

Neutropenia refers to a marked reduction of circulating neutrophils in the blood. It may be congenital or hereditary, a result of marrow infiltration by tumor cells, or caused by radiation, cytotoxic drugs, or an abnormal response to a variety of noncytotoxic drugs. Neutropenia also may be a consequence of a variety of viral or bacterial infections. Cyclic neutropenia is an interesting variant in which there are periodic severe reductions in neutrophil counts accompanied by clinical manifestations of infection. Although variable, these episodes of severe neutropenia occur about every 3 weeks, although the neutrophil counts are still generally low during asymptomatic periods.

Neutropenia is characterized clinically by generalized constitutional symptoms including fever, malaise, weakness, and sore throat, plus increased susceptibility to a variety of infections. Oral manifestations include gingivitis, severe periodontal bone destruction, and necrotizing ulcers that may resemble aphthous stomatitis. Management of neutropenia includes prompt diagnosis and aggressive treatment of secondary infections, plus correction of any underlying cause, if possible. Steroid therapy and white blood cell transfusions are sometimes used. Recombinant human granulocyte colony-stimulating factor, a cytokine that stimulates growth and differentiation of neutrophils, has recently shown great promise in the management of patients with neutropenia. Meticulous oral hygiene and periodontal care are needed for oral lesions.

### Figure 10.7
### PLUMMER-VINSON SYNDROME
Erythema of tongue with atrophy of filiform papillae.

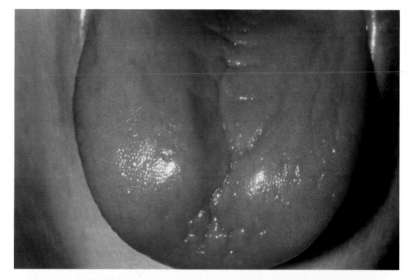

### Figure 10.8
### NEUTROPENIA
Hyperplastic gingivitis.

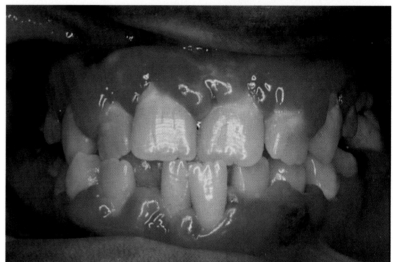

### Figure 10.9
### CYCLIC NEUTROPENIA
Severe periodontal bone destruction in a child.

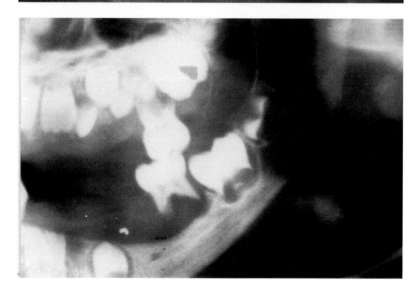

### Figs. 10.10 and 10.11

Leukemias are malignancies of the hematopoietic tissues. The disease is characterized by over-production of white blood cells with replacement of the normal bone marrow, circulation of abnormal cells in the blood, and infiltration of other tissues. The clinical features may be acute or chronic, and cells of either the lymphocytic or myeloid series are most commonly involved. Acute lymphocytic leukemia is one of the more common childhood malignancies; chronic lymphocytic leukemia, the most common form of leukemia, primarily affects older adults. Acute myeloid leukemia affects a broad age range that includes children and adults; chronic myeloid leukemia shows a peak incidence in the third and fourth decades of life.

Clinical manifestations of leukemia include fatigability, anemia, lymphadenopathy, hepatosplenomegaly, bone and abdominal pain, secondary infection, and hemorrhagic lesions secondary to thrombocytopenia. Oral lesions are more common in myelocytic/monocytic leukemias and may include gingival leukemic infiltrates, severe periodontal bone loss, oral ulcerations, and hemorrhagic lesions. Treatment and prognosis depend on the specific type of leukemia. Therapy primarily centers around chemotherapy and, in some cases, bone marrow transplantation. Children with acute lymphocytic leukemia now can expect a 50 to 70% 5-year survival rate, with 45% being long-term survivors. The myeloid leukemias have a more guarded prognosis. Although chronic myeloid leukemia may begin as a mild disease, the cells eventually undergo an acute blast transformation that can rapidly result in the patient's death. Acute myeloid leukemia has a 5-year survival rate of 10 to 30%. Although there is no cure for chronic lymphocytic leukemia, the disease is often slowly progressive; some patients have a life expectancy of greater than 10 years, depending on the stage of the disease.

### Fig. 10.12

Although complex classification systems have evolved to categorize lymphomas, they can be divided into two major categories: Hodgkin's disease and non-Hodgkin's lymphomas. Hodgkin's disease is seen most commonly in teenagers and young adults, with a second prevalence peak in middle-aged adults. Men are affected more frequently than women. Patients generally present with painless lymphadenopathy, usually involving the cervical, supraclavicular, and mediastinal lymph node chains. Intraoral involvement is exceedingly rare. Additional clinical symptoms noted in some patients include weight loss, fever, night sweats, and pruritus (itching). The treatment for Hodgkin's disease depends on the stage of involvement but typically involves radiation therapy, chemotherapy, or both. Patients with limited stage I or stage II disease are often managed with radiation therapy alone and have a nearly 90% 10-year survival rate. Patients with advanced stage III and stage IV disease require chemotherapy, possibly in conjunction with radiation therapy, and have a 50% or greater 10-year survival rate.

## Figure 10.10
### LEUKEMIA
Hemorrhagic gingival leukemic infiltrate. (Courtesy of Dr. M. Nazif.)

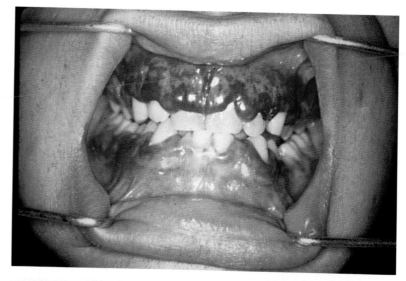

## Figure 10.11
### LEUKEMIA
Ulceration of the palate. (Courtesy of Dr. B. Roberts.)

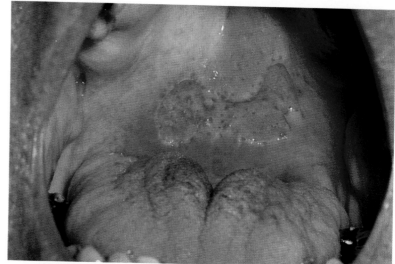

## Figure 10.12
### HODGKIN'S DISEASE
Cervical and supraclavicular lymphadenopathy.

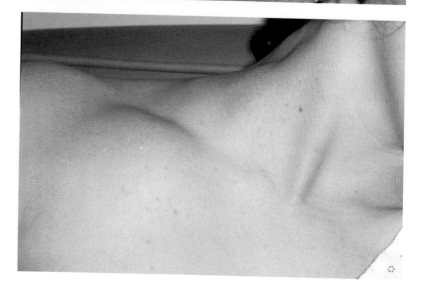

**Figs. 10.13, 10.14, and 10.15**

Non-Hodgkin's lymphomas are a heterogeneous group of lymphoid malignancies with clinical symptoms that are similar to Hodgkin's disease, although widespread systemic involvement is seen more frequently. They most frequently arise from cells of the B-lymphocyte series but also can arise from T-lymphocytes and rarely from histiocytes. Like Hodgkin's disease, non-Hodgkin's lymphomas are more common in men but with a peak prevalence in middle-aged and older adults. The condition usually begins as a slowly enlarging, nontender mass of one or more lymph nodes but sometimes occurs in extranodal locations. As the lymph nodes enlarge, they may become fixed to adjacent structures or matted together.

Oral involvement is most commonly seen in the lymphoid tissue of Waldeyer's ring, the hard palate, and buccal vestibule and gingiva. Oral lymphomas often present as a rapidly growing mass of short duration that may or may not be ulcerated. Primary bone involvement also may be seen. Concomitant systemic involvement may or may not already be present at the time of diagnosis.

Non-Hodgkin's lymphomas are usually treated with chemotherapy, radiation therapy, or both. The prognosis is highly variable, depending on the histopathologic subtype of lymphoma. Some low-grade tumors are slowly progressive, with many patients surviving for 10 years or more with limited therapy. The prognosis for high-grade tumors is more guarded, with a 60% mortality rate within 5 years of diagnosis.

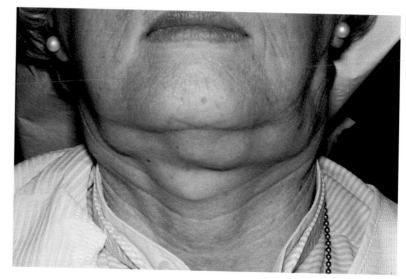

► **Figure 10.13**
**NON-HODGKIN'S LYMPHOMA**
Bilateral submandibular lymphadenopathy.

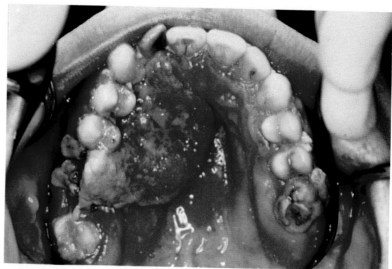

► **Figure 10.14**
**NON-HODGKIN'S LYMPHOMA**
Ulcerated mass of the hard palate.

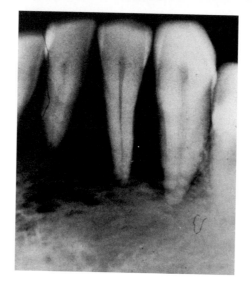

► **Figure 10.15**
**NON-HODGKIN'S LYMPHOMA**
Moth-eaten bone destruction in a primary bone lymphoma.

**Figs. 10.16 and 10.17**

Burkitt's lymphoma is a characteristic form of non-Hodgkin's lymphoma that was originally described in Central Africa and accounts for 50% of pediatric malignancies in that region. It has since been recognized throughout the world, including North America, although much less frequently. Burkitt's lymphoma is primarily a tumor of childhood, with occasional cases seen in young adults. The mean age of African cases is 7 years, compared with 11 years for American cases. The Epstein-Barr virus has been implicated in the etiology; evidence of Epstein-Barr virus DNA is found within the tumor cells in 95% of African cases, but virus can be demonstrated in only 15% of American cases. Approximately 60% of the African cases occur in the jaws; abdominal involvement is the most common presentation for American Burkitt's lymphoma, with only 15 to 18% of cases affecting the jaws. Jaw involvement is more frequent in younger patients.

Burkitt's lymphoma is more common in the maxilla than in the mandible, and it typically presents as a rapidly growing mass associated with bone destruction, loosening of teeth, and extension into adjacent soft tissues. Concomitant maxillary and mandibular involvement is not unusual. Loss of the lamina dura may be an early radiographic sign. Chemotherapy is the treatment of choice and usually results in disease remission, although recurrence is not uncommon. Prognosis depends on the clinical stage of the disease, with prolonged survival achieved in 50% of cases.

# MIDLINE LETHAL GRANULOMA (MIDLINE MALIGNANT RETICULOSIS, POLYMORPHIC RETICULOSIS, IDIOPATHIC MIDLINE DESTRUCTIVE DISEASE, ANGIOCENTRIC LYMPHOMA)

**Fig. 10.18**

Midline lethal granuloma is a progressive, destructive condition involving the nasal cavity, paranasal sinuses, palate, pharynx, and face. Clinically, it presents with ulceration of the palate or nasal septum, often in association with nasal stuffiness. This process gradually progresses, often resulting in total palatal destruction, bone sequestration, and destruction of facial tissues. Patients may become extremely debilitated, with death resulting from hemorrhage caused by large vessel erosion. Because of the variable histopathologic features of midline lethal granuloma, considerable confusion and controversy have arisen concerning the etiopathogenesis and classification of this condition. Most investigators currently believe that it represents a T-cell lymphoma with an affinity for involving blood vessels ("angiocentric"). Epstein-Barr virus has been implicated as a possible cause. Microscopically, some cases exhibit a benign-appearing inflammatory process ("idiopathic midline destructive disease"), whereas others show a proliferation of atypical mononuclear cells ("midline malignant reticulosis," "polymorphic reticulosis") or an obvious malignant lymphoma. Radiation therapy seems to be the most effective treatment, but chemotherapy is also sometimes used. Prolonged survival is achieved in 15 to 33% of cases.

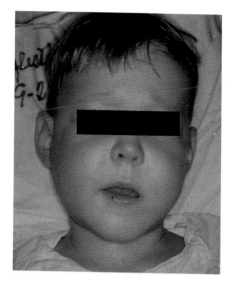

### ▶ Figure 10.16
### BURKITT'S LYMPHOMA
Right facial swelling. (Reprinted with permission from Budnick SD. Handbook of pediatric oral pathology. Chicago: Year Book, 1981.)

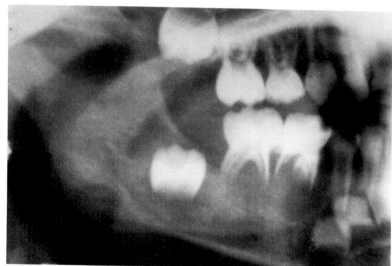

### ▶ Figure 10.17
### BURKITT'S LYMPHOMA
The tumor has destroyed the alveolar bone supporting the primary molar teeth. The teeth were mobile and painful. (Courtesy of Dr. Gregory Anderson.)

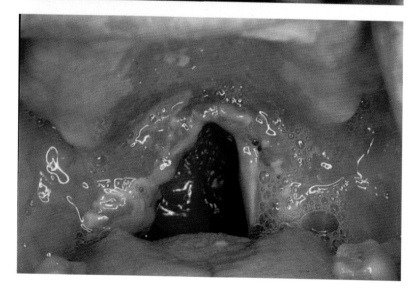

### ▶ Figure 10.18
### MIDLINE LETHAL GRANULOMA
Necrotic destruction of the soft palate.

## Figs. 10.19, 10.20, and 10.21

Mycosis fungoides is a T-cell lymphoma that preferentially involves the skin, tending to spare the lymph nodes and internal organs until late in the course of the disease. It occurs most commonly in middle-aged and older adults and affects men more often than women. Classic mycosis fungoides of the skin develops over many years, progressing through three stages: scaly patches, infiltrative plaques, and, finally, tumors. These stages often overlap, so that all three types of lesions may be present at the same time. Diagnosis in the early stages of the disease may prove difficult, with initial lesions being mistaken for psoriasis or eczema. In the fourth and final stage, tumor cells spread to lymph nodes and internal organs, causing death. Sézary syndrome is considered a leukemic variant of the disease in which patients exhibit circulating abnormal T-lymphocytes.

Oral involvement in mycosis fungoides is unusual and typically is discovered during the late stages of the disease. Oral lesions most commonly occur on the tongue and palate and usually are described as ulcerative or nodular in appearance. Treatment for mycosis fungoides depends on the stage of the disease and may include skin irradiation, topical chemotherapy, or systemic chemotherapy. The prognosis is variable, although some patients survive for 10 years or more before the disease disseminates and results in death. However, once oral involvement has been diagnosed, most patients die of disease complications within 3 years.

▶ **Figure 10.19**
**MYCOSIS FUNGOIDES**
Ulcerated plaque of the skin.

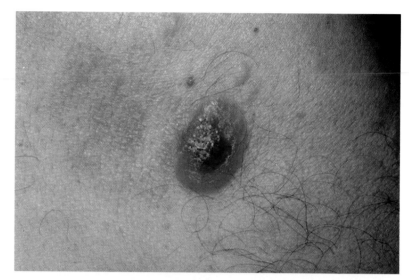

▶ **Figure 10.20**
**MYCOSIS FUNGOIDES**
Ulcerated tumor of the hard and soft palate. (Courtesy of Damm DD, White DK, Cibull ML, et al. Mycosis fungoides: initial diagnosis via palatal biopsy with discussion of diagnostic advantages of plastic embedding. Oral Surg Oral Med Oral Pathol 1984;58:413.)

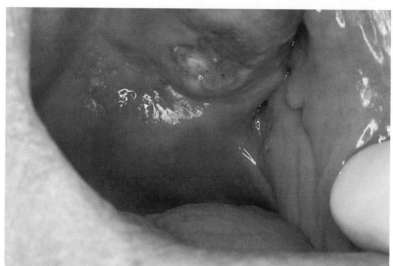

▶ **Figure 10.21**
**MYCOSIS FUNGOIDES**
Ulcerated lesions of the tongue.

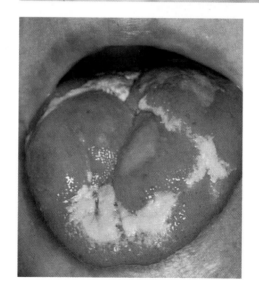

### Figs. 10.22 and 10.23

Multiple myeloma is a malignancy of plasma cells usually occurring in middle-aged and older adults. Men are more frequently affected than women. The disease is characterized by multiple destructive, "punched-out" bone lesions accompanied by pain and, sometimes, pathologic fracture. Typically, only one group of plasma cells becomes malignant, producing abnormal immunoglobulin proteins detectable on serum electrophoresis as a monoclonal gammopathy. In addition, excess immunoglobulin light chains may spill over into the urine as Bence Jones proteins. Other clinical features include anemia, thrombocytopenia, hypercalcemia, amyloidosis, and renal failure.

The spine, ribs, skull, and pelvis are common sites of involvement; the jaws are affected in 15 to 30% of cases. Jaw involvement may be characterized clinically by swelling, pain, paresthesia, tooth mobility, and root resorption. Treatment for multiple myeloma consists primarily of chemotherapy. Autologous stem cell transplantation and allogeneic bone marrow transplantation also have been used. Unfortunately, the prognosis is poor: the 5-year survival rate is about 25% and the median survival time is 3 years.

### Figure 10.22
**MULTIPLE MYELOMA**
Punched-out lesions of the skull. (Courtesy of Meyer I, Waldron C. Clinical pathologic conference. Oral Surg Oral Med Oral Pathol 1957;10:175.)

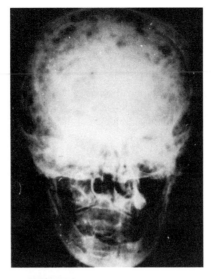

### Figure 10.23
**MULTIPLE MYELOMA**
Moth-eaten bone destruction and root resorption.

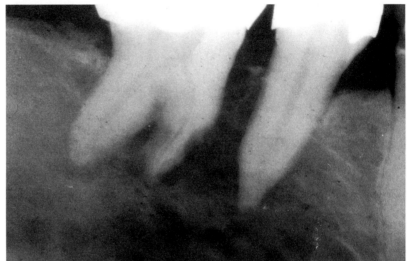

### Hemophilia

Djulbegovic B, Marasa M, Pesto A, et al. Safety and efficacy of purified factor IX concentrate and antifibrinolytic agents for dental extractions in hemophilia B. Am J Hematol 1996;51:168.

Kitchens CS. Approach to the bleeding patient. Hematol Oncol Clin North Am 1992;6:983.

Lusher JM, Arkin S, Abildgaard CF, et al. Recombinant factor VIII for the treatment of previously untreated patients with hemophilia A: safety, efficacy, and development of inhibitors: Kogenate Previously Untreated Patient Study Group. N Engl J Med 1993;328:453.

Lusher JM, Warrier I. Hemophilia A. Hematol Oncol Clin North Am 1992;6:1021.

Roberts HR, Eberst ME. Current management of hemophilia B. Hematol Oncol Clin North Am 1993;7:1269.

### Thrombocytopenia

Barrett AP, Tversky J, Griffiths CJ. Thrombocytopenia induced by quinine. Oral Surg Oral Med Oral Pathol 1983;55:351.

Goebel RA. Thrombocytopenia. Emerg Med Clin North Am 1993;11:445.

Karpatkin S. Autoimmune (idiopathic) thrombocytopenic purpura. Lancet 1997;349:1531.

Nishioka GJ, Chilcoat CC, Aufdemorte TB, et al. The gingival biopsy in the diagnosis of thrombotic thrombocytopenic purpura. Oral Surg Oral Med Oral Pathol 1988;65:580.

Souid A-K, Sadowitz PD. Acute childhood immune thrombocytopenic purpura. Clin Pediatrics 1995;34:487.

### Megaloblastic Anemia (Pernicious Anemia)

Colon-Otero G, Menke D, Hook CC. A practical approach to the differential diagnosis and evaluation of the adult patient with macrocytic anemia. Med Clin North Am 1992;76:581.

Drummond JF, White DK, Damm DD. Megaloblastic anemia with oral lesions: a consequence of gastric bypass surgery. Oral Surg Oral Med Oral Pathol 1985;59:149.

Field EA, Speechley JA, Rugman FR, et al. Oral signs and symptoms in patients with undiagnosed vitamin B12 deficiency. J Oral Pathol Med 1995;24:468.

Pruthi RK, Tefferi A. Pernicious anemia revisited. Mayo Clin Proc 1994;69:144.

### Plummer-Vinson Syndrome

Bredenkamp JK, Castro DJ, Mickel RA. Importance of iron repletion in the management of Plummer-Vinson syndrome. Ann Otol Rhinol Laryngol 1990;99:51.

Hoffman RM, Jaffe PE. Plummer-Vinson syndrome: a case report and literature review. Arch Intern Med 1995;155:2008.

Larsson L-G, Sandström A, Westling P. Relationship of Plummer-Vinson disease to cancer of the upper alimentary tract in Sweden. Cancer Res 1975;35:3308.

### Neutropenia

Kirstilä V, Sewón L, Laine J. Periodontal disease in three siblings with familial neutropenia. J Periodontol 1993;64:566.

Mishkin DJ, Akers JO, Darby CP. Congenital neutropenia: report of a case and a biorationale for dental management. Oral Surg Oral Med Oral Pathol 1976;42:738.

Spencer P, Fleming JE. Cyclic neutropenia: a literature review and report of case. J Dent Child 1985;52:108.

Yamalik N, Yavuzyilmaz E, Çaglayan F. Periodical gingival bleeding as a presenting symptom of periodontitis due to underlying cyclic neutropenia: case report. Aust Dent J 1993;38:272.

### Leukemia

Barrett AP. Gingival lesions in leukemia: a classification. J Periodontol 1984;55:585.

Dreizen S, McCredie KB, Keating MJ, et al. Malignant gingival and skin "infiltrates" in adult leukemia. Oral Surg Oral Med Oral Pathol 1983;55:572.

Hou G-L, Huang J-S, Tsai C-C. Analysis of oral manifestations of leukemia: a retrospective study. Oral Dis 1997;3:31.

Michaud M, Baehner RL, Bixler D, et al. Oral manifestations of acute leukemia in children. J Am Dent Assoc 1977;95:1145.

Pui C-H. Childhood leukemias. N Engl J Med 1995;332:1618.

Schaedel R, Goldberg MH. Chronic lymphocytic leukemia of B-cell origin: oral manifestations and dental treatment planning. J Am Dent Assoc 1997;128:206.

Weckx LLM, Hidal LBT, Marcucci G. Oral manifestations of leukemia. Ear Nose Throat J 1990;69:341.

## Hodgkin's Disease

Baden E, Al Saati T, Caverivière P, et al. Hodgkin's lymphoma of the oropharyngeal region: report of four cases and diagnostic value of monoclonal antibodies in detecting antigens associated with Reed-Sternberg cells. Oral Surg Oral Med Oral Pathol 1987;64:88.

Carbone A, Weiss LM, Gloghini A, et al. Hodgkin's disease: old and recent clinical concepts. Ann Otol Rhinol Laryngol 1996;105:751.

Urba WJ, Longo DL. Hodgkin's disease. N Engl J Med 1992;326:678.

Weinshel EL, Peterson BA. Hodgkin's disease. CA Cancer J Clin 1993;43:327.

## Non-Hodgkin's Lymphoma

Eisenbud L, Sciubba J, Mir R, et al. Oral presentations in non-Hodgkin's lymphoma: a review of thirty-one cases. Oral Surg Oral Med Oral Pathol 1983;56:151.

Howell RE, Handlers JP, Abrams AM, et al. Extranodal oral lymphoma, part II: relationships between clinical features and the Lukes-Collins classification of 34 cases. Oral Surg Oral Med Oral Pathol 1987;64:597.

Wallace C, Ramsey AD, Quiney RE. Non-Hodgkin's extranodal lymphoma: a clinico-pathological study of 24 cases involving head and neck sites. J Laryngol Otol 1988;102:914.

Wolvius EB, van der Valk P, van der Wal JE, et al. Primary non-Hodgkin's lymphoma of the salivary glands: an analysis of 22 cases. J Oral Pathol Med 1996;25:177.

Wright JM, Radman WP. Intrabony lymphoma simulating periradicular inflammatory disease. J Am Dent Assoc 1995;126:101.

## Burkitt's Lymphoma

Anavi Y, Kaplinsky C, Calderon S, et al. Head, neck, and maxillofacial childhood Burkitt's lymphoma: a retrospective analysis of 31 patients. J Oral Maxillofac Surg 1990;48:708.

Patton LL, McMillan CW, Webster WP. American Burkitt's lymphoma: a 10-year review and case study. Oral Surg Oral Med Oral Pathol 1990;69:307.

Svoboda WE, Aaron GR, Albano EA. North American Burkitt's lymphoma presenting with intraoral symptoms. Pediatr Dent 1991;13:52.

Wang MB, Strasnick B, Zimmerman MC. Extranodal American Burkitt's lymphoma of the head and neck. Arch Otolaryngol Head Neck Surg 1992;118:193.

## Midline Lethal Granuloma

Grange C, Cabane J, Dubois A, et al. Centrofacial malignant granulomas: clinicopathologic study of 40 cases and review of the literature. Medicine 1992;71:179.

Hartig G, Montone K, Wasik M, et al. Nasal T-cell lymphoma and the lethal midline granuloma syndrome. Otolaryngol Head Neck Surg 1996;114:653.

Mosqueda-Taylor A, Meneses-Garcia A, Zárate-Osorno A, et al. Angiocentric lymphomas of the palate: clinico-pathological considerations in 12 cases. J Oral Pathol Med 1997;26:93.

Nelson JF, Finkelstein MW, Acevedo A, et al. Midline "nonhealing" granuloma. Oral Surg Oral Med Oral Pathol 1984;58:554.

## Mycosis Fungoides

Brennan JA. The head and neck manifestations of mycosis fungoides. Laryngoscope 1995;105:478.

Damm DD, White DK, Cibull ML, et al. Mycosis fungoides: initial diagnosis via palatal biopsy with discussion of diagnostic advantages of plastic embedding. Oral Surg Oral Med Oral Pathol 1984;58:413.

Kasha EE Jr, Parker CM. Oral manifestations of cutaneous T-cell lymphoma. Int J Dermatol 1990;29:275.

Sirois DA, Miller AS, Harwick RD, et al. Oral manifestations of cutaneous T-cell lymphoma: a report of eight cases. Oral Surg Oral Med Oral Pathol 1993;75:700.

## Multiple Myeloma

Bataille R, Harousseau J-L. Multiple myeloma. N Engl J Med 1997;336:1657.

Epstein JB, Voss NJS, Stevenson-Moore P. Maxillofacial manifestations of multiple myeloma: an unusual case and review of the literature. Oral Surg Oral Med Oral Pathol 1984;57:267.

Joshua DE. Myeloma: new aspects of biology, prognosis and treatment. Pathology 1996;28:2.

Pisano JJ, Coupland R, Chen S-Y, et al. Plasmacytoma of the oral cavity and jaws: a clinicopathologic study of 13 cases. Oral Surg Oral Med Oral Pathol Oral Radiol Endod 1997;83:265.

Witt C, Borges AC, Klein K, et al. Radiographic manifestations of multiple myeloma in the mandible: a retrospective study of 77 patients. J Oral Maxillofac Surg 1997;55:450.

# chapter 11

# DISORDERS OF BONE

# OSTEOPETROSIS (MARBLE BONE DISEASE, ALBERS-SCHÖNBERG DISEASE)

## Figs. 11.1, 11.2, and 11.3

Osteopetrosis is a rare disorder characterized by a marked increase in bone density resulting from a defect in the bone-remodeling mechanism. Although the pattern of bone sclerosis is very distinctive, other diseases such as pyknodysostosis and dysosteosclerosis may produce similar changes and must be considered prior to definitive diagnosis. Several hereditary patterns of osteopetrosis are seen that are associated with variations in clinical severity.

The most severe form is autosomal recessive and noted at birth or early in life. Most of the skeleton shows extensive replacement of the bone marrow by dense bone, with resultant severe normocytic anemia, granulocytopenia, and significant hepatosplenomegaly caused by extramedullary hematopoiesis. Optic atrophy, loss of hearing, facial paralysis, and pathologic fractures are common complications; poor pneumatization of the paranasal sinuses usually is seen. Most patients with this form of the disease die before age 20 years as a result of anemia or infection caused by marrow replacement by sclerotic bone.

Clinically, the benign autosomal-dominant form is less severe and may not be detected until later in life. The extent of bone involvement and symptoms vary. Some cases are detected incidentally during a radiographic examination. These patients do not exhibit anemia or hepatosplenomegaly; blindness and deafness also usually are not present. Although variable, the life span usually is normal.

The jaws may be involved in both forms of the disease. Extensive osteosclerosis often obscures the outline of the roots of the teeth and blurs the separation between cortical and cancellous bone. Teeth abnormalities such as hypodontia, malformed crowns and roots, defective enamel, and extensive caries are common. Retardation of eruption caused by the densely sclerotic bone is common, particularly in the recessive form of the disease. In some cases, only a few teeth ever erupt. Osteomyelitis following extraction of teeth is a common complication. Excellent oral hygiene, use of topical fluorides, and regular professional care are important to decrease the necessity for tooth removal. When extraction of teeth is mandated, antibiotic coverage and primary closure of extraction sites have been recommended to decrease the prevalence of infection.

### Figure 11.1
### OSTEOPETROSIS

Photograph of the skin overlying the right mandible. Note numerous cutaneous fistulas that are draining purulent material from areas of necrosis within the underlying mandible.

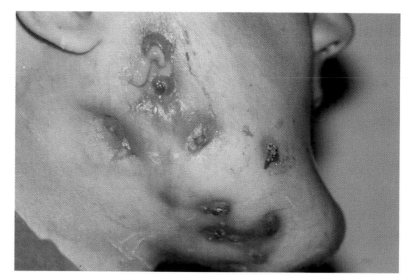

### Figure 11.2
### OSTEOPETROSIS

Intraoral photograph of an 8-year-old boy with severe recessive osteopetrosis. No permanent teeth have erupted.

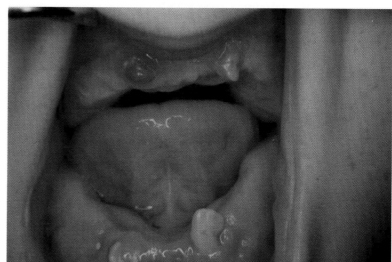

### Figure 11.3
### OSTEOPETROSIS

Radiograph of a mandible removed at autopsy from a 10-year-old girl who had severe childhood osteopetrosis showing the densely sclerotic bone and multiple malformed and unerupted teeth. (Courtesy of Younai F, Eisenbud L, Sciubba J. Osteopetrosis: a case report including gross and microscopic findings in the mandible at autopsy. Oral Surg Oral Med Oral Pathol 1988;65:214.)

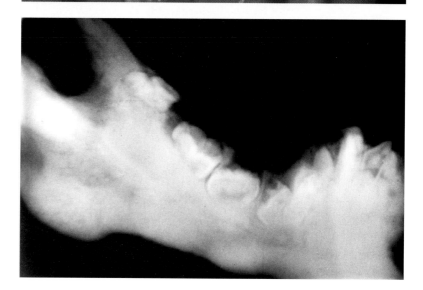

## Figs. 11.4, 11.5, and 11.6

Cleidocranial dysplasia is a skeletal disease often inherited as an autosomal-dominant trait. Up to 40% of the cases, however, seem to be spontaneous mutations. Although a variety of anomalies may be found in other bones, the defects chiefly involve membranous bones, with the skull and clavicles being the chief sites of the disorder. The patients tend to have short stature and a large head with frontal and parietal bossing and ocular hypertelorism. The sutures and fontanels show delayed closure or may remain open, and wormian bones commonly are observed on radiographic examination of the skull. Most patients also reveal hypoplasia or absence of nasal bones, diminished paranasal sinuses, and a broad base of the nose with a depressed nasal bridge. The midfacial skeleton may be hypoplastic, resulting in a relative mandibular prognathism.

The shoulder girdle defects vary from complete absence of the clavicles to a partial absence or marked thinning of one or both clavicles. The clavicular abnormalities result in a long-appearing neck, drooping shoulders, and an unusual mobility of the shoulders, with some patients being able to move their shoulders forward until they meet. Although the clavicular defects result in variations of the muscles related to the clavicles, function generally is not impaired.

Patients with cleidocranial dysplasia often show a narrow, high-arched palate and exhibit an increased prevalence of cleft palate. Multiple supernumerary teeth, prolonged retention of deciduous teeth and delay or failure of eruption of the permanent teeth are characteristic findings. Radiographic examination reveals multiple unerupted teeth, many of which show root dilaceration or root shortening.

No treatment is directed toward the skull and clavicular anomalies, but the dental problems represent a major source of morbidity. Without treatment, the retained deciduous dentition begins to rapidly deteriorate in late youth and early adulthood, leading to a premature aged facial appearance. In the past, total extraction of the dentition followed by full dentures was performed, but this has been abandoned. Removal of the deciduous and supernumerary teeth with overdentures placed on top of the impacted permanent teeth was associated with significant discomfort secondary to subsequent eruption of the remaining dentition and is in disfavor. In such cases, eruption has been noted as late as the sixth decade. Although no one method of approach is accepted universally, significant success has been obtained through removal of all deciduous and supernumerary teeth followed by surgical exposure and orthodontic or surgical repositioning of impacted permanent teeth. In many cases, the therapeutic protocol extends over many years and is timed to coincide with the developmental stages of the succedaneous dentition.

### Figure 11.4
### CLEIDOCRANIAL DYSPLASIA

This patient can approximate his shoulders. The enlarged skull with prominent frontal bossing is apparent. (Courtesy of Halstead CL, Blozis GG, Drinnan AJ, et al. Physical evaluation of the dental patient. St Louis: CV Mosby, 1982.)

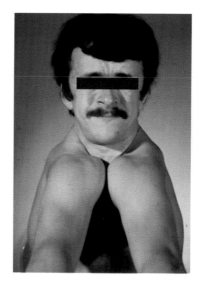

### Figure 11.5
### CLEIDOCRANIAL DYSPLASIA

Maxillary dentition of a young adult with cleidocranial dysplasia. Several deciduous teeth are still present, and several permanent teeth have not erupted. (Courtesy of Halstead CL, Blozis GG, Drinnan AJ, et al. Physical evaluation of the dental patient. St Louis: CV Mosby, 1982.)

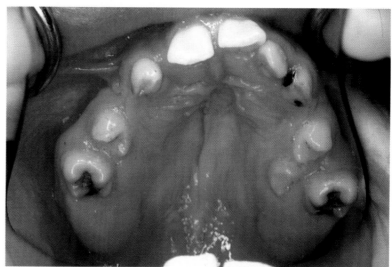

### Figure 11.6
### CLEIDOCRANIAL DYSPLASIA

Panographic radiograph of a 28-year-old male showing multiple impacted and supernumerary teeth and retention of deciduous teeth. (Courtesy of Dr. J. R. Cramer.)

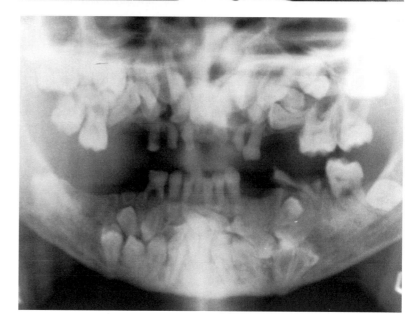

# FOCAL OSTEOPOROTIC MARROW DEFECT

## Fig. 11.7

An osteoporotic marrow defect is a normal anatomic variation that may be confused with a pathologic alteration. This nonneoplastic process presents as an asymptomatic radiolucent area that contains either hematopoietic or fibrofatty marrow. The lesion almost always is detected during a routine radiographic examination and is most commonly noted in mandibular edentulous areas of women. Many cases are noted in the site of a previous extraction, and rare patients report associated pain or swelling.

Radiographically, the radiolucency typically is ill-defined, seldom exceeds 1.0 cm in diameter, and usually reveals a central, faint trabecular pattern. In some cases, the fatty nature of the marrow defect can be predicted through the use of computed tomography and magnetic resonance imaging scans, possibly negating the necessity for biopsy. In many instances, the radiographic features are not diagnostic, simulate those of a number of different inflammatory or neoplastic lesions, and mandate biopsy. After the diagnosis is confirmed, no treatment is necessary. Although focal marrow defects have not been correlated to any systemic disease, the possibility of concurrent disorders associated with accelerated hematopoiesis, such as the hemolytic anemias, should be investigated in patients with widespread lucency associated with marrow enlargement.

# IDIOPATHIC OSTEOSCLEROSIS (DENSE BONE ISLAND, ENOSTOSIS)

## Figs. 11.8 and 11.9

Focal areas of increased radiodensity within the jaws unrelated to foci of infection are the most common causes of radiographic consultations received by oral and maxillofacial pathologists. These areas, which cannot be related to any inflammatory, dysplastic, or neoplastic process, are thought to occur in up to 10% of the population. Similar lesions have been seen in other bones.

Although idiopathic osteosclerosis occurs over a wide age range, most lesions are noted before 40 years of age, are asymptomatic, and occur in the premolar-molar areas of the mandible. Because the prevalence of the sclerotic zones does not seem to increase with age, these opacities most likely do not arise in later age or previous lesions are resorbed over time. The typical radiographic pattern is a well-defined or irregular area of radiopacity that does not demonstrate a radiolucent rim and that varies in size from 0.3 to 2.0 cm. Rare examples approach 7.0 cm in diameter. Although resorption and displacement of adjacent teeth are seen rarely, most cases do not reveal enlargement over time or buccolingual bony expansion. Bone adjacent to root apices is affected most frequently, but involvement of interradicular bone is not uncommon. Rarely, these islands of dense bone seem to surround the crown of impacted teeth in a distinctly pericoronal fashion. On occasion, the sclerotic area exhibits no relationship to a tooth.

Biopsy usually is not necessary because other radiographically similar processes such as superimposed soft-tissue calcifications, condensing osteitis, and overlying exostoses can be ruled out from clinical and radiographic features. No treatment is required because most demonstrate no tendency to enlarge or adversely affect adjacent structures.

### Figure 11.7
**FOCAL OSTEOPOROTIC MARROW DEFECT**

Irregular lytic area that was discovered during a routine radiographic examination of a female, age 49 years. Biopsy results revealed that the defect contained hematopoietic marrow. (Courtesy of Dr. Michael Sokolosky.)

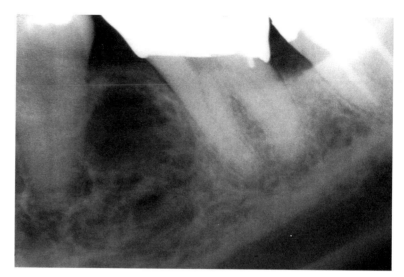

### Figure 11.8
**IDIOPATHIC OSTEOSCLEROSIS**

Localized zone of increased radiodensity between the maxillary premolars.

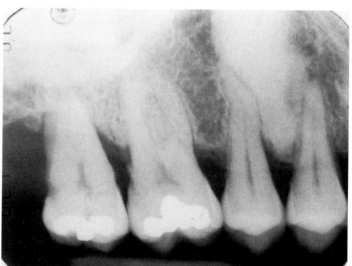

### Figure 11.9
**IDIOPATHIC OSTEOSCLEROSIS**

Localized zone of increased radiodensity associated with the distal root of the mandibular first molar. Note resorption of the distal root. (Courtesy of Dr. Lon Doles.)

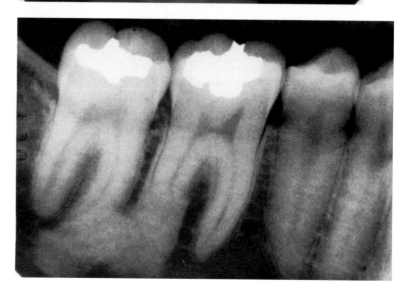

### Fig. 11.10

Skeletal osteomas are benign neoplasms of mature bone that essentially are restricted to the craniofacial skeleton. These lesions consist of mature compact or cancellous bone, and differentiation from exostoses or areas of idiopathic osteosclerosis often is difficult and arbitrary. Although most commonly found in the skull, osteomas do occur within the jaws, and they most frequently arise from the posterior lingual surface of the mandible in young adults. For a definitive diagnosis of osteoma, a history of sustained growth must be demonstrated. In many instances, the tumors seem to arise in close proximity to areas of muscle attachment; it has been suggested that these lesions represent nonneoplastic, but progressive, bony hyperplasia secondary to muscle traction in sites of previous trauma.

Osteomas of the jaws most frequently arise on the surface of the bone and present as slowly growing sessile or pedunculated masses. Endosteal osteomas generally produce no symptoms until they reach a large size and cause cortical expansion. Occasional osteomas arise in the paranasal sinuses and may be associated with symptoms such as sinusitis, headache, and ophthalmologic manifestations. Radiographically, most examples show a well-circumscribed lesion that is either densely sclerotic or has a trabecular pattern. Large osteomas associated with facial distortion or symptoms such as dysphagia or difficulties in mastication are treated by conservative surgical removal.

## GARDNER SYNDROME

### Figs. 11.11 and 11.12

Gardner syndrome is an autosomal-dominant condition characterized by the association of multiple osteomas, fibromatoses of the soft tissues and mesentery, epidermoid cysts of the skin, and adenomatous polyps of the gastrointestinal tract, usually in the colon. The intestinal polyps have a marked tendency to undergo rapid malignant transformation. Women with the syndrome also are predisposed dramatically to development of thyroid carcinoma and should be followed closely for this complication. Multiple osteomas, most frequently involving the mandible, maxilla, and frontal bone, appear during puberty, usually preceding the appearance of the gastrointestinal polyps. Supernumerary teeth, impacted teeth, and compound odontomas of the jaws also have been described in these patients, but the reported prevalence is variable.

Although some of the jaw osteomas may cause facial asymmetry, many merely represent areas of increased radiodensity similar to that seen in idiopathic osteosclerosis and often are discovered with panoramic radiographs or computed tomography. Some investigators have used panoramic radiographs as screening tools in first-degree relatives of affected individuals; those that demonstrate significant areas of osteosclerosis or clinically evident osteomas are evaluated further with fecal occult blood tests, flexible sigmoidoscopy, or colonoscopy. Because of the high prevalence of idiopathic osteosclerosis in the general population, its presence without a family history of Gardner syndrome is insufficient justification for further evaluation.

Therapy centers around prevention of carcinoma from the adenomatous polyps, with prophylactic colectomy performed soon after confirmation of the diagnosis. Without intervention, close to 50% of affected patients develop colorectal adenocarcinoma before age 30 years, with the frequency of carcinomatous transformation approaching 100% in older patients. The fibrous neoplasms are surgically removed as they are encountered, along with any jaw osteomas and epidermoid cysts that create aesthetic concerns.

## Figure 11.10
### OSTEOMA
A 16-year-old boy with a large, pedunculated osteoma arising from the mandibular cortex at the angle of the mandible.

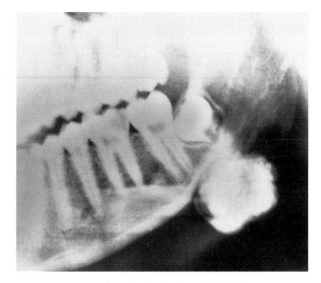

## Figure 11.11
### GARDNER SYNDROME
Clinical photograph of a 33-year-old male. The asymmetry beneath the mandible is caused by a large osteoma. (Courtesy of Dr. David Haddox.)

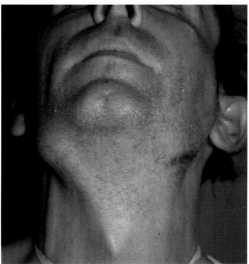

## Figure 11.12
### GARDNER SYNDROME
Panographic radiograph of the patient depicted in Figure 11.11 showing multiple osteomas of the mandible. (Courtesy of Dr. David Haddox.)

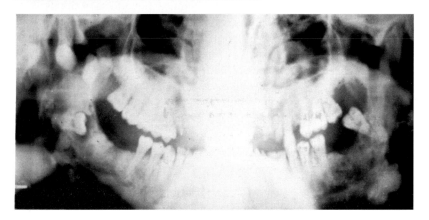

## Figs. 11.13, 11.14, and 11.15

Paget's disease is a chronic skeletal disorder characterized by abnormal resorption and deposition of bone that may be localized or widespread throughout the skeleton. Although most cases are polyostotic, involvement limited to a single bone may be seen. The jaws are affected in about 10 to 15% of the cases, with a significant maxillary predominance.

Affected bones become thickened, enlarged, and weakened. Severely involved weight-bearing long bones often develop a monkeylike bowing. Involvement of the skull with resultant narrowing of foramina occasionally results in neurologic complications such as deafness or visual disturbances. An increased hat size secondary to a progressive enlargement of head circumference is not rare.

The most common oral presentation is a progressive, symmetric maxillary enlargement that may reach massive proportions. Severe maxillary enlargement may result in a "lionlike" facies that has been termed "leontiasis ossea." With significant jaw enlargement, dentures often don't fit and remaining teeth become widely spaced or flared. Extensive root hypercementosis occasionally is detected.

Radiographically, Paget's disease demonstrates similarities to diffuse osseous dysplasia with early lucent alterations followed by the development of intermixed radiopacity. With maturation, the affected bone becomes predominantly radiopaque and exhibits the classic "cotton wool" appearance. Any patient demonstrating bony enlargements and multifocal mixed radiolucencies of the jaws should be evaluated further for the possibility of the disorder. In affected patients, serum alkaline phosphatase and urinary hydroxyproline levels usually are elevated, but blood calcium and phosphorus levels are normal.

In cases of Paget's disease with significant jaw enlargement, aesthetics and function may be improved by surgical reduction. Similar to end-stage osseous dysplasia, advanced osseous lesions of Paget's disease are sensitive to inflammation and develop osteomyelitis with little provocation. Elective surgery is not recommended in these patients, and all sources of bony inflammation must be kept to a minimum. When osteomyelitis develops, conservative surgical debridement of the affected area with appropriate antibiotic coverage is necessary.

Paget's disease rarely is a cause of death. Uncommonly, the hypervascularity of the pagetic bone acts as an arteriovenous shunt leading to high output heart failure or worsening of underlying cardiac disease. Parathyroid hormone antagonists such as calcitonin and biphosphonates have been used to minimize the effects of the disease by reducing bone turnover, especially early in the course of the disease. Two significant complications, giant cell tumor and sarcomatous transformation (usually osteosarcoma, malignant fibrous histiocytoma, or chondrosarcoma), demonstrate an increased prevalence in association with Paget's disease and must be considered in any patient who reveals accelerated growth of an affected bone. The most frequent associated malignancy, osteosarcoma, is aggressive and associated with a very poor prognosis, whereas most of the giant cell tumors respond to local surgical removal.

► **Figure 11.13**
**PAGET'S DISEASE OF BONE**
Marked symmetric maxillary enlargement
in a female, age 55. (Courtesy of Dr.
William McKenzie.)

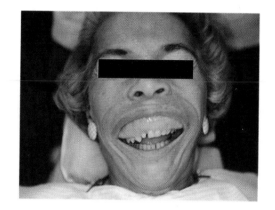

► **Figure 11.14**
**PAGET'S DISEASE OF BONE**
Periapical radiograph of a patient with
Paget's disease showing irregular
radiopaque foci ("cotton wool"
appearance). (Courtesy of Dr. Mona Ellis.)

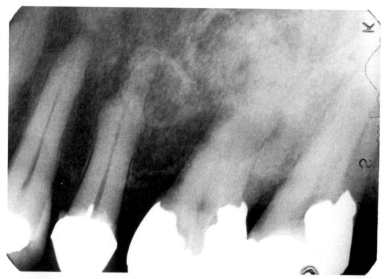

► **Figure 11.15**
**PAGET'S DISEASE OF BONE**
Skull film demonstrating multiple foci of
irregular increased radiodensity arranged
in the "cotton wool" pattern. (Courtesy of
Dr. Reg Munden.)

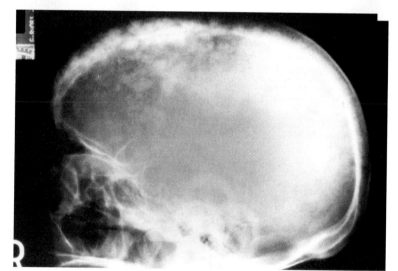

## MASSIVE OSTEOLYSIS (GORHAM-STOUT DISEASE)

### Figs. 11.16 and 11.17

Massive osteolysis is a rare chronic disease characterized by spontaneous and progressive destruction of one or more bones. Involvement of contiguous bones may occur. Although some investigators believe the process may represent an unusual intraosseous hemangiomatosis, the definitive cause is unknown and does not seem to be related to any known infectious, metabolic, endocrine, or neurologic disorder. Although most cases arise in children and young adults, examples have been reported in patients ranging from infancy to old age.

About one-fourth of cases have involved the craniofacial bones, with the jaws being two of the most commonly affected; occasional simultaneous involvement of both the maxilla and the mandible is reported. In the early stages, the disease is characterized by active bone lysis, often accompanied by mild to moderate pain. At this stage, radiographs show an ill-defined lysis of bone, with results of histopathologic examination demonstrating a vascular proliferation that closely resembles immature granulation tissue. With quiescence, the disease becomes painless and demonstrates no radiographic evidence of bone regeneration. Significant destruction of the jaws can lead to difficulty in mastication, swallowing, speaking, and respiratory function.

The progression of the destruction is variable, but in most cases, the process continues for months to a few years and leads to total loss of the affected bone. The diagnosis is made largely by exclusion of other diseases characterized by bone resorption and by failure to detect any biochemical abnormalities. Although there is no consistently satisfactory treatment for massive osteolysis, surgical excision of the affected area is the leading method of approach.

## LANGERHANS CELL HISTIOCYTOSIS (HISTIOCYTOSIS X)

### Fig. 11.18

Langerhans cell histiocytosis describes a group of uncommon diseases characterized by a proliferation of differentiated histiocyte-like cells often accompanied by a variable admixture of eosinophils, multinucleated giant cells, lymphocytes, and plasma cells. The distinctive histiocytic cells have been shown to represent Langerhans cells, and they possess unique ultrastructural and immunohistochemical features. Based on the type and extent of involvement, these histiocytoses can be divided into several major categories: (1) solitary or multiple involvement of bone without soft-tissue involvement, (2) chronic multifocal histiocytosis characterized by multiple bone involvement with skin and visceral involvement (see Figs. 11.19 to 11.21), and (3) acute disseminated disease. However, many patients show overlapping clinical features.

Solitary or multiple bone involvement without visceral involvement is termed "eosinophilic granuloma." The jaws are involved in 10 to 20% of cases and may be the only site of the disease. The most frequent gnathic site is the posterior mandible and typically is associated with mild, dull pain. In many instances, the disease mimics odontogenic infection and often is confused with periodontitis, apical inflammatory disease, and pericoronitis. Such similarities mandate histopathologic examination of supposedly inflammatory foci that do not respond to conventional therapy.

On discovery of isolated disease, thorough systemic evaluation for additional lesions is mandatory. In addition to evaluation of the soft tissues, a whole-body radiographic skeletal survey or bone scintigraphy is necessary. If no additional lesions are discovered, the focal site usually is treated surgically; intralesional injection with methylprednisolone also has been successful in a limited number of patients. Subsequent radiation therapy often is used in large or multifocal lesions.

### Figure 11.16
### MASSIVE OSTEOLYSIS

Ill-defined radiolucent area in the left mandibular premolar-molar area of a 22-year-old woman. This initially was considered to be related to pulp pathology; endodontic treatment was carried out. (Courtesy of Dr. J. R. Cramer.)

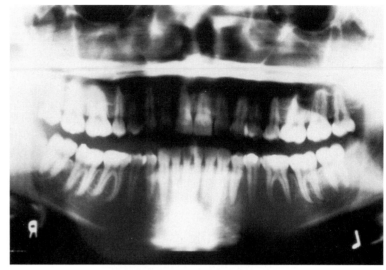

### Figure 11.17
### MASSIVE OSTEOLYSIS

Radiograph from the patient shown in Figure 11.16 taken 11 months later showing progressive destruction of the mandible, pathologic fracture, and loss of teeth. (Courtesy of Dr. J. R. Cramer.)

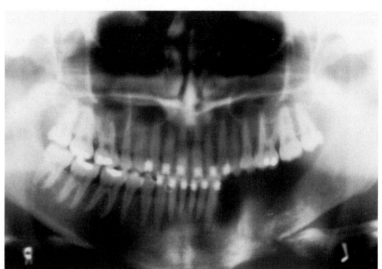

### Figure 11.18
### LANGERHANS CELL HISTIOCYTOSIS

Periapical radiograph demonstrating a lytic lesion enveloping the apices of the anterior incisors. After failure to respond to conventional endodontics, periapical surgery was performed. Results of histopathologic examination of the removed soft tissue revealed Langerhans cell histiocytosis. (Courtesy of Dr. James White.)

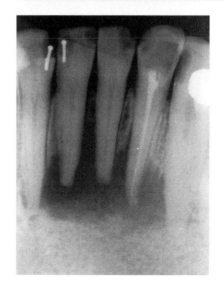

### Figs. 11.19, 11.20, and 11.21

The acute disseminated form of Langerhans cell histiocytosis is termed "Letterer-Siwe disease." Many authorities believe this form represents a separate, and most likely malignant, process whereas eosinophilic granuloma and chronic disseminated histiocytosis are variants of a single, less aggressive disease. The acute form primarily affects children before the age of 3 years and demonstrates rapid, widespread disease that exhibits both intraosseous and soft-tissue involvement. Commonly affected soft tissues include the skin, lung, liver, spleen, and lymph nodes. Although any bone may be involved, the skull, mandible, ribs, vertebrae, and femur are affected frequently. Treatment consists of multiagent chemotherapy with disappointing results and a poor prognosis.

The chronic disseminated form is nicknamed "Hand-Schüller-Christian disease" and demonstrates lesions in multiple bones with soft-tissue involvement. This pattern of histiocytosis may be encountered in patients over a wide age range, but most are children or young adults, with a definite male predilection. Bone lesions appear as sharply "punched-out" lytic defects, often with irregular margins. Infiltration of the alveolar bone often leads to severe horizontal bone loss and commonly exhibits involvement of the overlying soft tissues with ulcerative or proliferative gingival lesions. In advanced cases, the alveolar destruction gives a radiographic appearance of the teeth "floating in air." Proliferative periostitis in the absence of a focus of infection occasionally is a sign of underlying bone involvement. Accumulations of Langerhans cells may occur in any bone, with the skull, ribs, vertebrae, and jaws leading the list. Sites of soft-tissue infiltration commonly include the skin, mucosa, lymph nodes, and viscera.

In cases of chronic disseminated Langerhans cell histiocytosis, local symptomatic sites are treated surgically, with radiation used for those that are inaccessible surgically. The prognosis is variable, with occasional cases demonstrating spontaneous resolution, whereas others are resistant to therapy, disseminate, and require use of systemic chemotherapy. The prognosis in patients with localized lesions is good, but it becomes less favorable with widespread soft-tissue and organ involvement.

### Figure 11.19
### LANGERHANS CELL HISTIOCYTOSIS
Panoramic radiograph demonstrating multifocal areas of premature periodontal bone loss. Examination results of submitted soft tissue revealed Langerhans cell histiocytosis. (Courtesy of Dr. Robert Hobbs.)

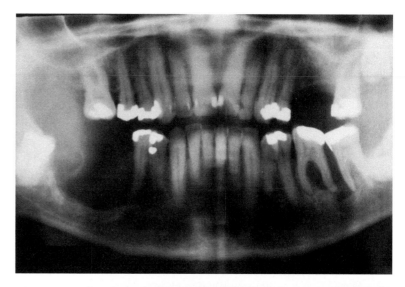

### Figure 11.20
### LANGERHANS CELL HISTIOCYTOSIS
Clinical photograph of a 16-year-old white male who presented with localized bone loss of the molar teeth in all four quadrants. This mirror view depicts the loss of attachment in the posterior maxilla on the right side.

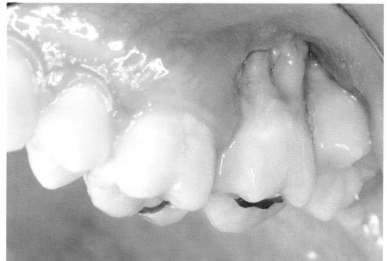

### Figure 11.21
### LANGERHANS CELL HISTIOCYTOSIS
Radiograph of the posterior maxillary dentition on the right side from the patient depicted in Figure 11.20. Note the significant loss of periodontal attachment of all three molar teeth.

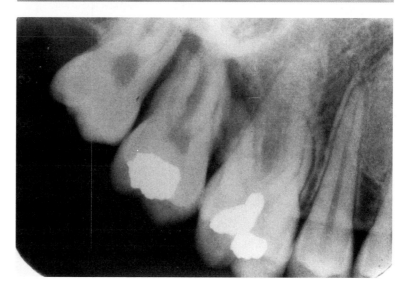

## Figs. 11.22, 11.23, and 11.24

The giant cell granuloma is a unique lesion of the oral cavity that occurs in gingival soft tissues or is located centrally within the jaws. Some lesions show both a soft-tissue and an intrabony component, and classification as to peripheral or central origin may be controversial. Most investigators believe that the giant cell granuloma is a nonneoplastic (reactive) lesion; however, some examples are similar histopathologically to the giant cell tumor of long bones and often behave like a true neoplasm. Whether or not true giant cell tumors occur in the jaws remains controversial, and some investigators believe giant cell granuloma and giant cell tumor represent two ends of a continuum of a single disease process. Many of the histopathologic features of giant cell granuloma suggest that the proliferation is an attempt at repair of an area of red blood cell extravasation and its contributing vessels.

Giant cell granulomas of the jaws occur in patients over a wide age range but are most common in the first three decades of life, with a slight female predilection. There is a 3:1 mandibular predominance with a predilection for occurrence in the anterior region, with occasional examples crossing the midline. Most cases involve the tooth-bearing areas, but examples may be found in the ascending ramus and tuberosity. Pain is not a common feature, and smaller lesions usually are discovered during a routine radiographic examination. Larger lesions tend to cause localized expansion of the affected bone, which is the most common presenting symptom. The radiologic findings are variable and may mimic those of several other odontogenic and nonodontogenic lesions.

Radiographically, giant cell granulomas produce a unilocular or multilocular radiolucency that may have sharp, well-defined or irregular, ragged margins. In a large radiographic review of giant cell granulomas, a direct correlation was seen between lesion size and the development of central loculations. The bone cortex may be thin and expanded or sometimes perforated by the lesion. Tooth displacement or resorption is not rare.

Most giant cell granulomas respond well to local curettage with few recurrences, and occasional reports have documented resolution following intralesional injection with corticosteroids. Some lesions, however, are locally aggressive and may require marginal resection for control. There is some degree of correlation between the clinical-radiologic-histopathologic features and behavior. Nonaggressive lesions generally show few or no symptoms, manifest slow growth, and do not demonstrate root resorption or cortical perforation. These lesions seldom recur after local curettage. The more aggressive forms of giant cell granuloma often are characterized by pain, rapid growth, root resorption, and cortical perforation. These lesions show a high prevalence of local recurrence after curettage and may require marginal resection to obtain a cure. In most instances, the histopathologic features of the giant cell granuloma are indistinguishable from those of cherubism and a brown tumor of hyperparathyroidism. Therefore, it is prudent to evaluate any patient with a central giant cell granuloma for these possibilities (see Figs. 11.25 and Figs 14.5 and 14.6).

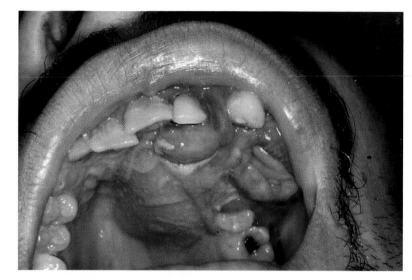

► **Figure 11.22**
**GIANT CELL GRANULOMA**
Expansile mass of the left anterior maxilla.

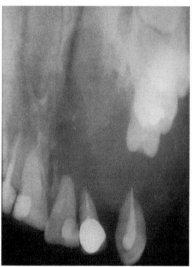

► **Figure 11.23**
**GIANT CELL GRANULOMA**
Occlusal radiograph of patient in Figure 11.22, showing a destructive radiolucent lesion.

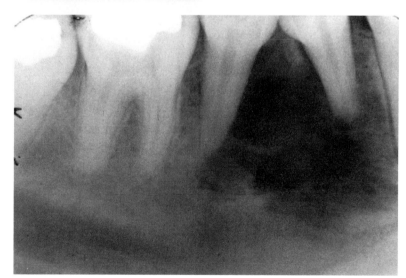

► **Figure 11.24**
**GIANT CELL GRANULOMA**
Multilocular radiolucent defect showing root resorption and tooth displacement in a 20-year-old female. (Courtesy of Dr. E. B. Bass.)

## Figs. 11.25, 11.26, and 11.27

Cherubism is an inherited disorder that is transmitted as an autosomal-dominant trait, but it often appears as a spontaneous mutation. The chief clinical feature is a bilateral, painless expansion of the mandible, especially over the angles. The initial presentation may be apparent as early as 1 year of age, although milder cases may not become apparent clinically until age 12 years. Less commonly, symmetric maxillary lesions also may be present, usually in the tuberosities. In severe cases, the entire mandible and maxilla are involved, resulting in marked facial deformity. The term "cherubism" arose from the common facial distortion that resembles plump-cheeked little angels (cherubs). Significant involvement of the maxilla can result in stretching of the skin of the upper face to expose the sclerae below the iris of the eye, resulting in an "eyes upturned to heaven" appearance.

Radiographically, the lesions present as unilocular or, more often, multilocular lytic defects that histopathologically closely resemble giant cell granuloma. Bilateral radiolucencies with significant cortical expansion are typical; and in some cases, the lesions extend continuously from the posterior region of one jaw to the posterior area of the contralateral quadrant. Involvement of the angle and ascending ramus is present in a large percentage of those affected. Displacement and delayed eruption of teeth are seen frequently. A similar radiographic pattern has been noted in patients who demonstrate numerous clinical features of Noonan syndrome. Although many similarities exist, this latter disorder seems to be separate from both cherubism and Noonan syndrome. As with any intraosseous lesion that resembles giant cell granuloma, further evaluation should be performed to rule out a brown tumor of hyperparathyroidism.

Treatment of cherubism is not standardized and is somewhat uncertain. Some cases have responded well to early curettage; others have shown increased growth after surgical intervention. In other cases, the lesions tend to stabilize or even partially regress with advancing age, but considerable functional or cosmetic deformity may persist. Overall, in patients with obvious cosmetic problems, surgical curettage appears to accelerate return to clinical and radiographic normalcy. Radiation therapy is contraindicated.

## Figure 11.25
### CHERUBISM

Characteristic facies of a young boy with cherubism. Extensive maxillary involvement has stretched the skin to expose the sclera, resulting in the "eyes upturned to heaven" appearance. (Courtesy of Dunlap C, Neville B, Vickers RA, et al. The Noonan syndrome/cherubism association. Oral Surg Oral Med Oral Pathol 1989;67:698.)

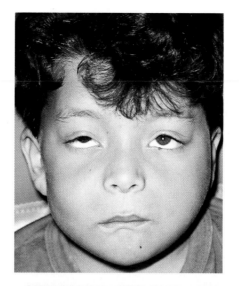

## Figure 11.26
### CHERUBISM

Intraoral view of the patient shown in Figure 11.25 showing marked enlargement of the right maxilla and multiple missing teeth.

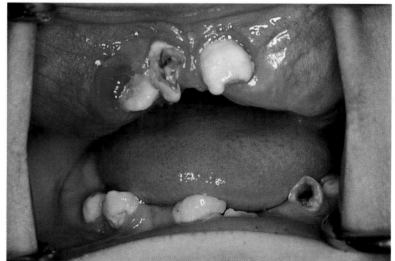

## Figure 11.27
### CHERUBISM

Panographic radiograph of the patient shown in Figure 11.25 showing extensive multilocular radiolucent lesions of the mandible and maxilla. (Courtesy of Dunlap C, Neville B, Vicker RA, et al. The Noonan syndrome/cherubism association. Oral Surg Oral Med Oral Pathol 1989;67:698.)

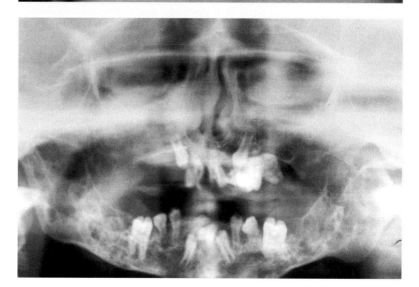

## SIMPLE BONE CYST (TRAUMATIC BONE CYST, HEMORRHAGIC BONE CYST)

### Figs. 11.28 and 11.29

Although the name implies an epithelium-lined cavity, the simple bone cyst consists of an idiopathic cavity within bone that may be empty or that may contain only a small amount of serous or serosanguineous fluid. Although controversial, many authorities believe the process is secondary to intraosseous hemorrhage in which the hematoma liquefies, resulting in a cavity within bone. The biochemical profile and protein electrophoresis of fluid removed from simple bone cysts demonstrate significant similarity with serum. When present within the jaws, most of these cavities occur in the mandible, with most cases presenting in patients younger than 20 years of age.

Although rare cases may produce clinically obvious swelling or pain, most examples are asymptomatic and are discovered during a routine radiographic examination as a well-defined radiolucent lesion. Large, simple bone cysts frequently show a scalloped or domelike superior margin extending between the roots of the teeth. Prompt resolution typically follows surgical exposure performed for diagnostic purposes. On occasion, the lumen of true cystic lesions may resemble closely a simple bone cyst on exploration. Therefore, scraping of the lesional walls and submission of any removed soft-tissue fragments are advantageous for diagnostic confirmation.

Occurrence in association with benign fibro-osseous lesions, such as osseous dysplasia or fibrous dysplasia, is not rare. Such lesions often are more difficult to resolve via surgical exploration, presumably because of the continued presence of the associated fibro-osseous process.

## ANEURYSMAL BONE CYST

### Fig. 11.30

Aneurysmal bone cyst is an intrabony accumulation of blood-filled spaces surrounded by reactive fibrous connective tissue that is not lined by either epithelium or endothelium. In many cases, the connective tissue wall contains numerous giant cells and may resemble closely a giant cell granuloma. Although the cause is idiopathic, many investigators believe the process may represent a secondary reaction to an intraosseous hematoma. Some aneurysmal bone cysts seem to arise de novo, whereas others are the result of the development of abnormal vascular communications within a preexisting bone lesion, such as fibrous dysplasia, osseous dysplasia, ossifying fibroma, and giant cell granuloma. Aneurysmal bone cyst, traumatic bone cyst, and giant cell granuloma share many similar features and may represent portions of a spectrum related to intraosseous vascular disturbances.

Although aneurysmal bone cysts are not rare in long bones, the process rarely occurs in the jaws. Most examples present in patients younger than age 20 years, and they are somewhat more common in the mandible. Clinically, there is a sudden increase in the size of the affected bone, often accompanied by pain. Radiographically, the lesion may present as a unilocular radiolucency or, more commonly, as a lytic expansion with thinning of the cortical plate and a honeycombed or soap-bubble appearance. The loculated radiographic appearance is not caused by true septa but rather is secondary to spurs and ridges on the inner surface of the expanded cortical plate.

On surgical exposure, the lesion usually resembles a blood-filled sponge from which slow hemorrhage may be evident. Although excessive hemorrhage during surgery has been seen in extragnathic lesions, extensive blood loss typically is not seen in aneurysmal bone cysts within the jaws. On curettage, hemorrhage may be abundant, but it is not difficult to control. Although venous-appearing blood may well up from the spongy tissue, removal of the bulk of the lesion usually controls the bleeding. Although surgical curettage is the treatment of choice, recurrence is not rare in those that are excised incompletely. In large or persistently recurrent lesions, surgical resection often combined with cryotherapy is necessary; radiation is contraindicated. Occasional successes have been obtained with preoperative angiography and embolization of the feeder vessels. Overall, the prognosis is good.

### Figure 11.28
### SIMPLE BONE CYST
Well-defined periapical radiolucency associated with the right mandibular cuspid. Pulp vitality was within normal limits. (Courtesy of Dr. C. W. Topp.)

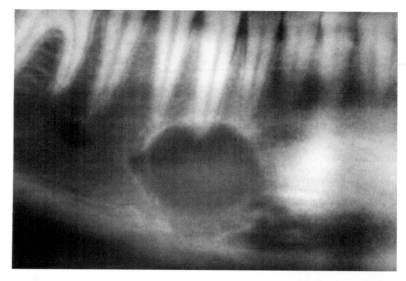

### Figure 11.29
### SIMPLE BONE CYST
Large radiolucency of the right body of the mandible that scallops in between teeth and thins the inferior border of the mandible. (Courtesy of Dr. Patrick Coleman.)

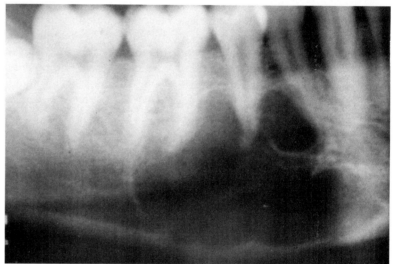

### Figure 11.30
### ANEURYSMAL BONE CYST
Large, multiloculated lesion of the posterior mandible in a 24-year-old woman. This was associated with buccal swelling.

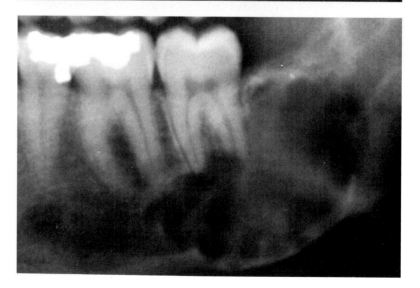

### Fig. 11.31

Intrabony hemangiomas are encountered most frequently in the craniofacial skeleton, and significant numbers of these vascular lesions involve the jaws, with the predominance occurring in the mandible. These lesions may be capillary or cavernous and represent hamartomas, reactive proliferations, or true neoplasms. Cases have been recorded in patients ranging from infancy to old age, with a peak prevalence in the third decade of life and a definite female predilection.

Although intraosseous hemangiomas often are asymptomatic, some may demonstrate signs or symptoms such as pain, paresthesia, swelling, mobile teeth, or localized gingival hemorrhage. Auscultation of a bruit is unusual without extension of the vascular lesion into the soft tissue overlying the affected bone. Although most lesions usually present as ill-defined and sometimes honeycombed lytic defects, the radiographic findings are variable and, unfortunately, nonspecific. Resorption or displacement of adjacent teeth and cortical expansion or sunburst trabeculation are not rare.

Failure to consider a central vascular lesion before intervention has resulted in severe bleeding and even exsanguination after incisional biopsy or extraction of teeth. Needle aspiration and angiography have been used as important diagnostic adjuncts before invasive procedures. Appropriate therapy is determined by the vascular supply, the age of the patient, and the size and location of the lesion. Although surgical removal is the leading therapeutic approach, cryotherapy, argon laser therapy, irradiation, and injection of sclerosing agents also have been used successfully in eradication of intraosseous hemangiomas. In significantly vascularized lesions, presurgical embolization has been used to reduce subsequent surgical hemorrhage.

## ARTERIOVENOUS MALFORMATION

### Figs. 11.32 and 11.33

An arteriovenous malformation represents an abnormal communication between the arterial and venous circulation, with the blood flow bypassing the capillary circulation. Arteriovenous malformations may be confused with hemangiomas and have been noted in both the oral soft tissues and the jawbones. In fact, some authorities believe hemangiomas of bone are rare, and most high-flow examples likely represent arteriovenous malformations. These anomalies may be congenital or acquired, most often as a result of trauma.

Clinically, intrabony arteriovenous malformations of the jaws typically are high-flow lesions and frequently demonstrate progressive pain, swelling of the bone, spontaneous gingival hemorrhage, tooth displacement or mobility, pulsation, and discoloration or hyperthermia of the overlying mucosa. Aspiration of intrabony lytic lesions always is a good practice; but if suspicion of a vascular malformation is high, arteriography without aspiration is most appropriate. Some lesions may exhibit no significant radiographic change; in other cases, a soap-bubble or honeycomb lucency may be seen.

Most cases are treated with surgical excision after preoperative embolization of the feeder vessels. Less frequently, permanent embolic obliteration has been performed by precise placement of an occlusive material within the central vasculature of the lesion. In surgically treated cases, extensive preoperative planning with use of quality angiography is mandatory. If blood flow is blocked in the proximal portion of a feeder vessel without simultaneously blocking the flow within the malformation, the residual feeder vessels compensate and maintain significant flow. In several reports, ligation of the external carotids without controlling flow through the malformation has been followed by extensive hemorrhage and fatal exsanguination on surgical exploration. Surgical removal of the lesion preferably is performed within 24 to 48 hours after completion of successful embolization. Although not ligated, the external carotid should be exposed at the time of surgery for ready access if uncontrollable hemorrhage is encountered during the procedure. Following successful resection, the defect usually is reconstructed immediately, occasionally by replantation of the resected segment after removal of the pathologic soft tissue. A postsurgical arteriogram should be performed after 1 year to detect any possible recurrence.

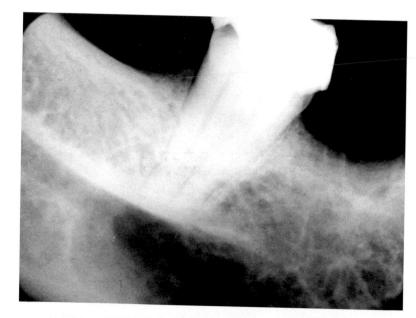

**Figure 11.31**
**HEMANGIOMA**
Irregular honeycombed radiolucent lesion in the mandible of a 65-year-old male. Biopsy of this lesion resulted in severe bleeding.

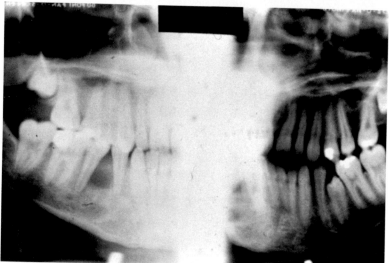

**Figure 11.32**
**ARTERIOVENOUS MALFORMATION**
Panographic radiograph showing a radiolucent lesion between the mandibular premolar teeth. This lesion was believed to be a lateral periodontal cyst, but pulsation was noted on clinical examination. (Courtesy of Dr. H. W. Allsup.)

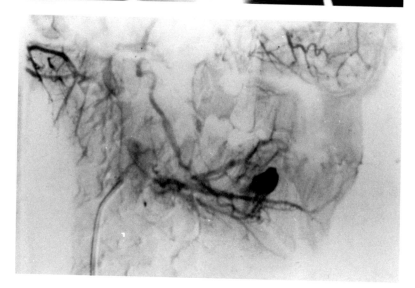

**Figure 11.33**
**ARTERIOVENOUS MALFORMATION**
Subtraction angiogram of the patient shown in Figure 11.32 showing the vascular defect in the premolar area. (Courtesy of Dr. H. W. Allsup.)

## DESMOPLASTIC FIBROMA (FIBROMATOSIS OF BONE)

**Fig. 11.34**

Desmoplastic fibroma is a neoplasm of fibroblastic cells that is histopathologically similar to the fibromatosis or desmoid tumor of soft tissues. Although most of these intraosseous fibrous neoplasms occur in various long bones, the jaws are not a rare site of involvement, with the mandible being one of the most commonly affected single bones. Although maxillary lesions may be seen, most of jaw examples present in the posterior mandible in patients with a mean age of less than 16 years.

The most common presentation is a painless swelling that may be associated with limited jaw opening. The proliferation creates a unilocular or multilocular lytic lesion that may be circumscribed or ill-defined. Cortical expansion and perforation with soft-tissue extension are not rare. On cortical perforation, a soft-tissue mass often is evident. Although metastasis is not seen, desmoplastic fibromas are locally aggressive neoplasms that tend to permeate bone and infiltrate soft tissue. Appropriate therapy is assured surgical removal.

## INTRAOSSEOUS NEUROFIBROMA

**Fig. 11.35**

Neurofibromas are slow-growing, benign neoplasms of nerve sheath origin. Intraosseous origin is uncommon; when noted, these tumors usually are solitary, without any signs of neurofibromatosis. When intraosseous examples are seen, the most commonly affected site in the entire skeleton is the mandible. Most of these tumors originate from the inferior mandibular nerve and present as a unilocular or multilocular radiolucency that rarely may demonstrate central radiopaque areas. These tumors demonstrate a female predominance and most frequently arise during young adulthood. The most common clinical presentation is swelling of the affected bone, often accompanied by pain or paresthesia.

Malignant transformation of neurofibromas is possible, but it most frequently is noted in association with neurofibromatosis. In addition, partial removal of solitary neurofibromas does not promote malignant change and may lead to regression. The recommended therapy is surgical excision of the tumor and its extension along the nerve.

## OSSEOUS DYSPLASIA (PERIAPICAL CEMENTO-OSSEOUS DYSPLASIA, CEMENTOMAS)

**Fig. 11.36**

Osseous dysplasia is a common, idiopathic, and nonneoplastic fibro-osseous replacement of bone that occurs only in the tooth-bearing areas of the jaws. Although its diverse clinical presentation has been known by a variety of names in the past, it finally is being clarified as a unified disease process under a single term. Currently, there are three recognized patterns of presentation: periapical, focal, and florid. However, these variants often demonstrate overlapping features. Osseous dysplasia has a predilection for black females between the ages of 30 and 50 years. Outside the United States, a significant number of cases also are noted in middle-aged Oriental females.

The most common form of osseous dysplasia is the periapical variant (periapical cemento-osseous dysplasia). The lesions usually are confined to bone surrounding the apices of the mandibular incisor teeth, but they also can involve other teeth. Typically, the condition is asymptomatic and is detected during a routine radiographic examination. Radiographically, the initial lesion appears as a circumscribed radiolucent defect about the apex of a tooth. The process may involve multiple apices that occasionally coalesce to form linear lytic areas enveloping multiple adjacent teeth. In the radiolucent stage, the alteration cannot be differentiated radiographically from chronic apical inflammatory disease, but the associated teeth are vital and seldom are restored. More advanced lesions show areas of mineralization within the radiolucent area; in the final stage, the lesion shows a dense central calcification often surrounded by a narrow radiolucent rim. Individual lesions seldom exceed 1.5 cm in diameter, with little tendency for progressive enlargement. Because the condition is benign and usually can be diagnosed on a clinical basis, biopsy is contraindicated and no treatment is necessary.

### Figure 11.34
### DESMOPLASTIC FIBROMA

Irregular radiolucency of the anterior maxilla in a 13-year-old female. (Courtesy of Dr. T. H. Daniel.)

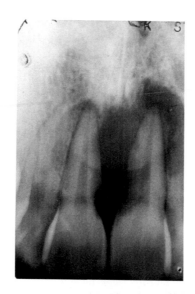

### Figure 11.35
### INTRAOSSEOUS NEUROFIBROMA

Large radiolucency of the right mandibular ramus. (Courtesy of Dr. Paul Allen.)

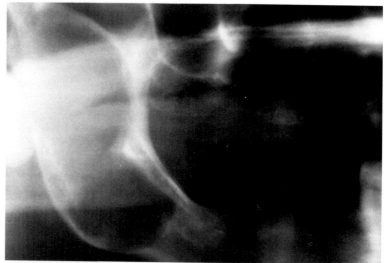

### Figure 11.36
### OSSEOUS DYSPLASIA

Periapical radiographs demonstrating multiple mixed radiolucencies of the anterior mandible. (Courtesy of Dr. Ken Peavy.)

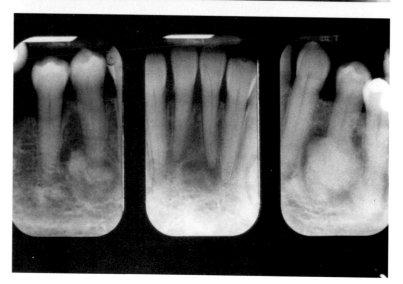

## FOCAL OSSEOUS DYSPLASIA (FOCAL CEMENTO-OSSEOUS DYSPLASIA)

**Fig. 11.37**

The second pattern of osseous dysplasia is known as the focal variant. About 80% occur in females in the fourth and fifth decades of life, and the condition has a relatively greater prevalence in blacks than whites. Of the three types of osseous dysplasia, the focal variant is the most common pattern discovered in Caucasians and often does not reveal future development of additional lesions. The affected areas are singular, generally asymptomatic, and often located in posterior regions of the tooth-bearing areas of the jaws. Frequently, the lesion develops at the site of a previous tooth extraction. Like the periapical variant, focal osseous dysplasia demonstrates several radiographic stages of development that reflect an increasing amount of mineralized product being formed within the lesion. It begins as a largely radiolucent defect, progressing to a mixed radiolucency, and finally becoming an almost totally radiopaque mass with a thin peripheral lucent border.

During its early radiolucent or mixed stage of maturation, focal osseous dysplasia may be confused easily with an ossifying fibroma because these processes demonstrate similar radiographic and histopathologic features. The most characteristic distinguishing feature is the appearance of these pathoses on surgical exploration. Focal osseous dysplasia exhibiting significant radiolucency is friable and difficult to remove intact, whereas ossifying fibroma is an adherent mass that separates cleanly from the surrounding bone. In addition, focal osseous dysplasia frequently is located in apical areas or in sites of previous extraction, whereas ossifying fibroma demonstrates no relationship to either.

The diagnosis of focal osseous dysplasia sometimes can be made on the basis of its clinical and radiographic features. Biopsy is necessary in other cases to rule out other more significant pathoses. Once the diagnosis has been made, only periodic observation is required because continued growth usually is not seen.

## FLORID OSSEOUS DYSPLASIA (DIFFUSE OSSEOUS DYSPLASIA, FLORID CEMENTO-OSSEOUS DYSPLASIA)

**Figs. 11.38 and 11.39**

Florid osseous dysplasia exhibits demographic and radiographic features that are similar to the periapical and focal forms of the condition. However, the florid form typically affects multiple sites in the posterior quadrants of either jaw, sometimes in association with identical periapical involvement of the anterior mandible. The process may be completely asymptomatic or may be associated with pain, an alveolar-mucosal fistula, and sequestration. The radiographic changes exhibit similarities with those seen in Paget's disease (see Figs. 11.13, 11.14, and 11.15), but patients with osseous dysplasia exhibit involvement of only the tooth-bearing areas of the jaws and usually do not reveal generalized expansion of the affected bone. Although cortical expansion typically is not seen, formation of simple bone cysts or aneurysmal bone cysts within the altered bone is not rare and may be associated with enlargement of the affected area. Generally, it is agreed that the clinical and radiographic features are sufficient for diagnosis; surgical intervention is not indicated and even may be contraindicated in the final radiopaque stage.

Once the lesions have matured into the predominantly radiopaque phase, the altered bone is extremely sensitive to inflammation. Inflammation introduced by periodontal disease, periapical pathosis, or overlying denture trauma can result in necrosis and sequestration of the sclerotic bone. Some patients have presented to their oral health care practitioner with several contiguous teeth embedded in necrotic, sclerotic bone that underwent sequestration and was removed by the affected individual.

Prophylactic removal of the altered bone would be problematic and without guarantee of redevelopment. The best therapy is maintenance of the dentition in an inflammatory-free state. Without introduction of inflammation, the altered bone remains asymptomatic. If all teeth are removed and replaced with complete dentures, normal ridge resorption often results in exposure and ultimate sequestration of the sclerotic masses. If infection does develop, saucerization of the dead bone may be required.

### Figure 11.37
### FOCAL OSSEOUS DYSPLASIA

A mixed radiolucent/radiopaque lesion in the edentulous second molar area of a 50-year-old female. (Courtesy of Waldron CA. Fibro-osseous lesions of the jaws. J Oral Maxillofac Surg 1985;43:249.)

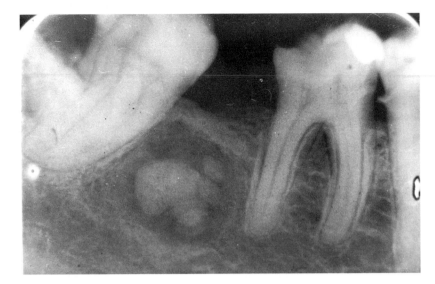

### Figure 11.38
### FLORID OSSEOUS DYSPLASIA

**(A)** Well-defined mixed radiolucency enveloping the apices of the mandibular first molar on the right side. **(B)** Contralateral side of the same patient exhibiting mixed radiolucency enveloping apices of the first molar and lytic lesion adjacent to the roots of the third molar.

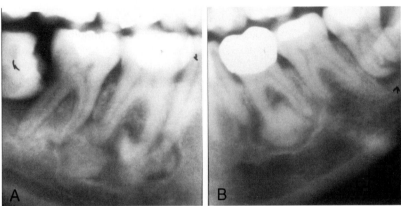

### Figure 11.39
### FLORID OSSEOUS DYSPLASIA

Extensive mandibular lesions in a 62-year-old black female. The lesions were asymptomatic and detected when radiographs were made before denture construction. (Courtesy of Waldron CA. Fibro-osseous lesions of the jaws. J Oral Maxillofac Surg 1985;43:249.)

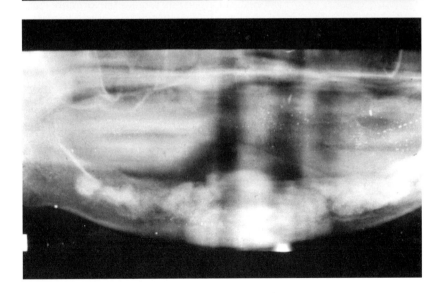

## Figs. 11.40, 11.41, 11.42, and 11.43

Fibrous dysplasia is considered a developmental, tumorlike (hamartomatous) lesion of bone. The disease may involve several or many bones (polyostotic fibrous dysplasia) or may be localized to a single bone (monostotic fibrous dysplasia). Polyostotic fibrous dysplasia is relatively rare and may, in some cases, involve more than 60% of the skeleton, with the mandible and craniofacial bones being some of the most commonly involved. Some affected individuals also show areas of skin pigmentation and a variety of endocrine abnormalities (McCune-Albright syndrome). Extensive polyostotic disease frequently results in pathologic fractures and severe bone deformity. Monostotic fibrous dysplasia is more commonly encountered. Maxillary fibrous dysplasia, although commonly included in this group, is not strictly monostotic because the process commonly involves a group of contiguous bones separated by sutures and is described more appropriately as craniofacial fibrous dysplasia.

A painless enlargement of the affected bone arising during childhood is the most common presenting symptom, and it may slowly increase to produce considerable deformity. Most examples are detected during the first two decades of life, although milder examples may not produce symptoms until later in life. When occurring in the jaws, there is a maxillary predominance. Radiographically, the characteristic finding is a "ground-glass" appearance best appreciated on periapical or occlusal views. Mandibular lesions may appear multilocular on lateral projections, but this is an optical illusion resulting from uneven endosteal erosion caused by the lesion, which contrasts with areas of preserved cortex. The area seldom is well-defined radiographically and tends to blend imperceptibly into adjacent normal bone. Complex maxillary lesions tend to cause obliteration of the maxillary sinus and involve the zygoma and orbit. Lateral skull films often demonstrate a characteristic thickening of the base of the skull involving the occipital, sphenoid, and frontal bones.

Most, but not all, examples of fibrous dysplasia of the jaws tend to stabilize and cease growing in adult life; accordingly, most therapeutic interventions are delayed until after the pubertal growth spurt and longer if possible. Milder forms of the disease may not require treatment, whereas other patients require one or more surgical reductions for correction of the cosmetic or functional deformity. The response to surgical contouring is variable, with some patients requiring multiple procedures before stabilization. Rare cases demonstrate accelerated growth and require resection for clinical improvement.

Although controversial, some surgeons recommend radical surgical excision and primary reconstruction of any cases of craniofacial fibrous dysplasia in which the surgery would not cause a greater functional or aesthetic disturbance. Such aggressive surgery is thought to prevent recurrence, stop further deformity, and avoid malignant transformation.

Radiation treatment is contraindicated and has been associated with development of postradiation bone sarcoma. Rare examples of "spontaneous" sarcomatous transformation also have been reported. The prevalence of malignant transformation is approximately 0.4%, 400 times the rate noted in normal individuals.

### Figure 11.40
### FIBROUS DYSPLASIA

Painless enlargement of the maxilla in a 32-year-old female. The enlargement was first detected when she was a teenager, and it has not grown appreciably in the past 6 years.

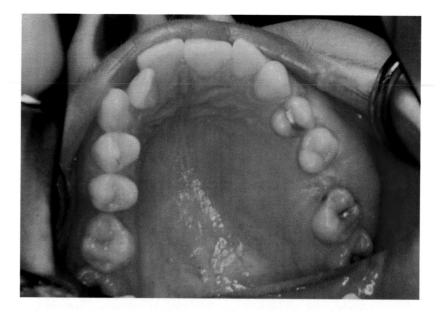

### Figure 11.41
### FIBROUS DYSPLASIA

Periapical radiographs of the patient shown in Figure 11.40 showing the characteristic "ground-glass" appearance of the lesional area with extension into the maxillary sinus. The altered bone pattern blends into a normal bone pattern in the incisor area. (Courtesy of Waldron CA. Fibro-osseous lesions of the jaws. J Oral Maxillofac Surg 1985;43:249.)

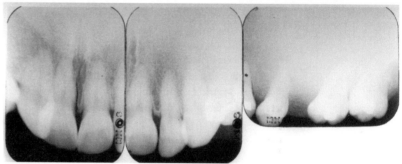

### Figure 11.42
### FIBROUS DYSPLASIA

Expansile lesion of the mandible in a 16-year-old boy.

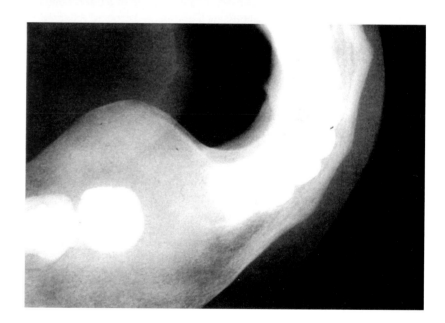

## SEGMENTAL ODONTOMAXILLARY DYSPLASIA (HEMIMAXILLOFACIAL DYSPLASIA)

### Figs. 11.44 and 11.45

Segmental odontomaxillary dysplasia is a unilateral developmental abnormality of the maxilla that was described initially under the term "hemimaxillofacial dysplasia" and often has been misdiagnosed as craniofacial fibrous dysplasia. Most affected patients present in the first two decades of life and demonstrate unilateral enlargement of the maxilla and the overlying gingival soft tissues. In a few patients, facial asymmetry and unilateral hypertrichosis are seen.

Radiographically, the involved quadrant exhibits an increased radiodensity with thickened bony trabeculae, decreased size of the adjacent maxillary sinus, one or more missing premolars, abnormal spacing of the erupted teeth, and delayed eruption of adjacent permanent teeth. Deciduous teeth within the zone of altered bone often demonstrate one or more developmental abnormalities, such as enlarged crowns, enlarged roots, splayed roots, or enlarged pulps.

Segmental odontomaxillary dysplasia seems to remain clinically and radiographically stable and does not require surgical intervention. Therapy is directed toward achieving adequate dental function and aesthetics in the involved quadrant.

### Figure 11.43
### FIBROUS DYSPLASIA

Computed tomography of a patient with unilateral craniofacial fibrous dysplasia of the maxilla that expands the alveolar ridge on the right side. (Courtesy of Dr. Craig Little.)

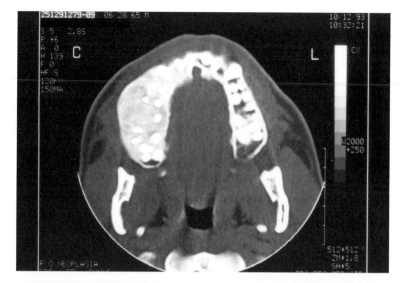

### Figure 11.44
### SEGMENTAL ODONTOMAXILLARY DYSPLASIA

Mirror view of maxillary arch. Note the unilateral enlargement of the alveolar ridge and the widely spaced dentition.

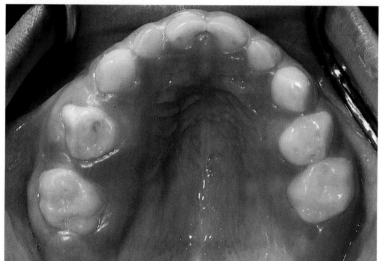

### Figure 11.45
### SEGMENTAL ODONTOMAXILLARY DYSPLASIA

Periapical radiograph of the left side of the maxilla from the patient depicted in Figure 11.44. Note the coarse trabecular pattern, the absence of the first premolar, and the widely spaced dentition.

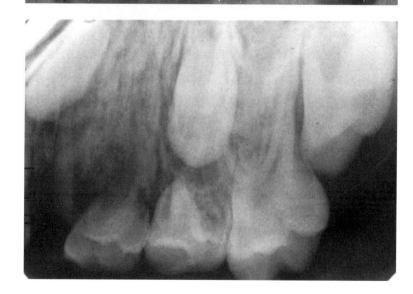

## Figs. 11.46, 11.47, and 11.48

Ossifying fibromas are true neoplasms of bone that demonstrate a mixture of cellular fibrous connective and cellular bone. On occasion, these tumors reveal psammomatoid differentiation in which acellular droplets of mineralized material are noted that previously have been termed "cementum." Because this pattern is present in ossifying fibromas outside of the jaws, it is recognized that this material is a variation of bone and not odontogenic. Therefore, the use of "cementifying fibroma" as a diagnostic term is being discontinued.

True ossifying fibromas are rare, and many jaw lesions that were previously assigned that diagnosis actually represent focal osseous dysplasia. Only through recent research have definitive criteria begun to emerge. As mentioned in the discussion of osseous dysplasia, ossifying fibroma is an adherent tumor that separates well from the surrounding bone, is not restricted to the tooth-bearing areas of the jaws, and does not occur predominantly in middle-aged black females.

Ossifying fibromas are somewhat more common in females, exhibit a mandibular predominance, and most frequently arise before 40 years of age. Smaller lesions are asymptomatic and usually are discovered during a radiographic examination, whereas larger ossifying fibromas produce a painless enlargement of the jaw. Some examples have reached a large size, resulting in considerable facial deformity.

The tumor is well-circumscribed, may be encapsulated, and typically is well-defined radiographically. Depending on the degree of mineralization in the tumor, the lesion may vary radiographically from completely radiolucent to a mixed radiolucent/radiopaque process. Teeth adjacent to the tumor may be displaced, but root resorption seldom is noted.

Ossifying fibromas show variable clinical behavior. Some have limited growth potential, and others may be aggressive clinically and show rapid or more extensive growth. These latter types sometimes are termed "juvenile," "active," or "aggressive" ossifying fibromas and most commonly are seen in patients younger than 15 years. Although the histopathologic criteria for juvenile ossifying fibromas are poorly defined and controversial, many exhibit significant psammomatoid differentiation. Most ossifying fibromas respond well to enucleation or curettage, and the prognosis is good. Larger and more clinically aggressive lesions may require marginal resection and bone grafting to eliminate the disease.

### Figure 11.46
### OSSIFYING FIBROMA
Circumscribed radiolucent defect in the mandibular molar area of a 28-year-old female. Localized expansion of the alveolus was present.

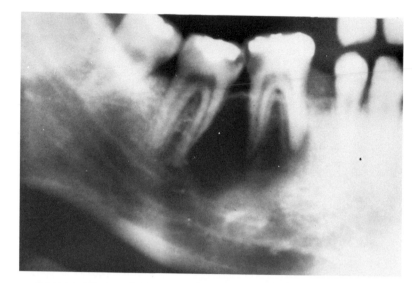

### Figure 11.47
### OSSIFYING FIBROMA
Surgical specimen from the lesion shown in Figure 11.46. The tumor was encapsulated and separated with ease from the bony defect.

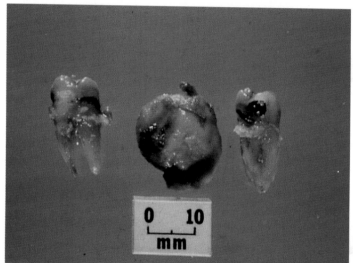

### Figure 11.48
### JUVENILE OSSIFYING FIBROMA
A magnetic resonance image of an enlargement of the maxilla on the left side in a 6-year-old black male. Note the tumor nearly filling the maxillary sinus.

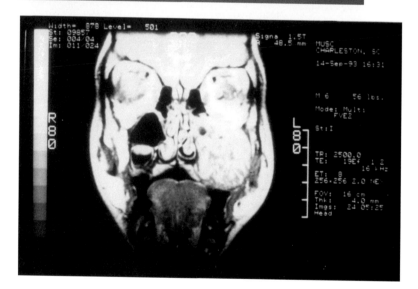

## OSTEOBLASTOMA

**Figs. 11.49**

Osteoblastoma is a true neoplasm of osteoblasts that typically exhibits plump, pleomorphic cells intermixed with irregular bone similar to that occasionally seen in osteosarcomas. This uncommon skeletal tumor rarely is seen in the jaws and demonstrates a mandibular predominance. Most osteoblastomas arise in patients between 10 and 20 years of age and are diagnosed more frequently in males (2:1). Pain is a fairly common symptom; in small lesions, the discomfort often is nocturnal and relieved by salicylate treatment. In addition, sensitivity to percussion may be seen and has been responsible for clinical misdiagnosis as periapical inflammatory disease. Radiographic findings are variable and consist of combinations of radiolucency and radiopacity. Some osteoblastomas present as circumscribed or ill-defined radiolucent areas that may contain focal areas of calcification, whereas others have shown a predominantly radiopaque mass surrounded by a thin radiolucent rim. Although some osteoblastomas may be aggressive locally, may recur, or may be associated with sarcomatous transformation, most tumors follow a benign course and respond to local curettage or en bloc resection.

## CEMENTOBLASTOMA

**Fig. 11.50**

Cementoblastoma is a true neoplasm of osteoblastlike cells thought to be derived from cells of the inner dental follicle that are termed "cementoblasts." Although many consider osteoblastoma and cementoblastoma to represent one pathologic process, others believe that cementoblastoma should remain as a separate entity because of its unique ability to fuse with dental hard tissue. From a practical standpoint, the diagnosis of cementoblastoma is made when the tumor is fused to the root surface of a tooth and demonstrates histopathologic features of an osteoblastoma.

Cementoblastomas most commonly arise in patients younger than age 30 years, with most cases affecting the mandibular first molars or premolars. These slow-growing tumors typically produce cortical expansion and often are associated with pain at night that can be relieved by aspirin. Although the lesion rarely may be radiolucent or mixed, most present as a radiopaque mass with a thin radiolucent border.

Typically, therapy involves surgical removal of the affected tooth along with the attached tumor. Incomplete removal usually results in recurrence. Occasionally, endodontic therapy followed by root resection coronal to the radicular tumor has been used successfully in examples that involved surgically accessible teeth.

## EWING'S SARCOMA

**Fig. 11.51**

Ewing's sarcoma is a malignancy of uncertain histogenesis that arises predominantly in bone and consists of a proliferation of undifferentiated small cells. Although these sarcomas account for 10 to 15% of all primary bone sarcomas, only about 2% occur in the jaws. When disseminated, tumor involvement of multiple bones is not rare. On discovery in the jaws, thorough evaluation should be performed to rule out a distant primary, but approximately 90% of reported cases in the jaws initially involved that location. Most of these cancers are seen in Caucasian children and adolescents, with less than 6% of cases noted in patients older than age 20 years.

The tumor often is associated with significant necrosis and may be confused with an inflammatory process. Pain and swelling often are early complaints. Radiographically, the tumor shows an irregular osteolytic lesion with or without cortical expansion. Although not commonly detected in the jaws, Ewing's sarcoma frequently produces laminated periosteal hyperplasia (onion-skinning) of the cortical bone overlying the tumor bed. When present in the jaws, widening of the periodontal ligament space; destruction of unerupted tooth follicles; and tooth displacement, mobility, and resorption may be seen; swelling and erythema of the overlying soft tissues are not rare. The prognosis of Ewing's sarcoma has shown a dramatic improvement in recent years. Radiation therapy and multiple drug chemotherapy have resulted in 90% local control and 40% long-term survival rates. When compared with mandibular lesions, primary maxillary tumors have been associated with faster growth and a greater resistance to therapy.

### ▶ Figure 11.49
### OSTEOBLASTOMA
Computed tomography of an ill-defined mixed radiolucency of the anterior mandible in a 3-year-old Caucasian male. (Courtesy of Dr. Ed Marshall.)

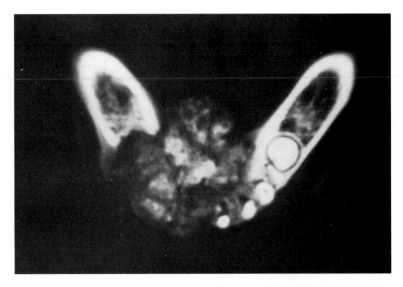

### ▶ Figure 11.50
### CEMENTOBLASTOMA
Panoramic radiograph exhibiting a radiopaque mass attached to the distal root of the left mandibular first molar. (Courtesy of Dr. John Wright.)

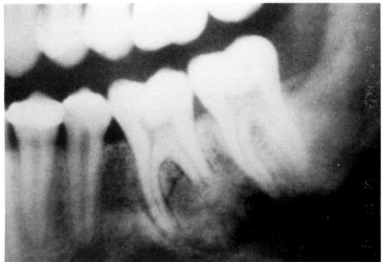

### ▶ Figure 11.51
### EWING'S SARCOMA
A 15-year-old girl with an ill-defined radiolucent lesion of the tuberosity causing extrusion of the maxillary second molar. She presented with facial swelling that was believed to be caused by periapical inflammatory disease. (Courtesy of Damm DD, White DK, Drummond JF, et al. Ewing's tumor of the jaws. Pediatr Dent 1985;7:57.)

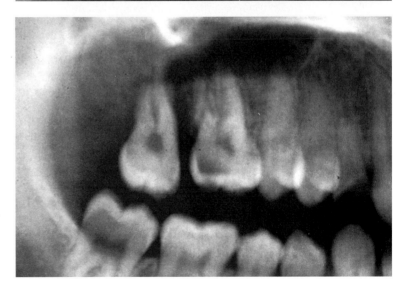

## Figs. 11.52 to 11.57

Osteosarcoma is a primary malignancy of bone-forming cells and is the most frequent type of primary cancer of bone, but it still represents an uncommon tumor. About 7% of all osteosarcomas occur in the jaws, and they tend to occur in older patients more often than do osteosarcomas of the extragnathic skeleton. The mean age (36 years) for patients with osteosarcoma of the jaws is about a decade and a half greater than that recorded for osteosarcomas of the long bones. The disease is somewhat more common in males than in females, with the mandible and maxilla being about equally involved.

Swelling and pain are the most common initial complaints, followed by loosening of teeth, paresthesia, and nasal obstruction in the case of maxillary tumors. Some patients report symptoms for relatively long periods, suggesting slow growth of the tumor. Depending on the degree of mineralization of the neoplastic osteoid produced by the tumor, the radiographic findings may reveal a densely sclerotic process, a mixed radiolucency, or a completely radiolucent process. The margins of the lesion are ill-defined. Penetration of the cortex with growth of the tumor outside the cortex results in the radiographic appearance of trabeculae of new bone radiating out from the bone surface, the so-called "sunburst" appearance. This radiographic feature is observed in about 25% of jaw osteosarcomas and is best appreciated on an occlusal view of a mandibular lesion. Teeth involved in the area frequently show irregular ("spiking") root resorption.

In their early stages, jaw osteosarcomas may present only subtle radiographic changes, consisting only of a slight variation in the trabecular pattern. An important radiographic change consisting of a symmetric widening of the periodontal ligament space around one or several teeth may be noted in some cases but is not specific for osteosarcoma. This has been shown to be the result of tumor infiltration in the periodontal ligament. This radiographic change, when accompanied by pain, discomfort, or minor changes in the trabecular pattern, may be of great importance in early diagnosis of osteosarcoma of the jaws.

Radical surgery is the usual treatment, with radiation and chemotherapy sometimes used adjunctively. The tumor tends to extend through intramedullary spaces beyond the apparent clinical or radiographic margins, and local recurrence after surgical removal is a major problem. Osteosarcomas are prone to develop hematogenous metastases, chiefly to the lungs. Jaw osteosarcomas do not metastasize as readily as those arising in long bones; local recurrence after inadequate initial surgery is the chief problem.

The overall survival rate for patients with osteosarcoma of the jaws is about 40%, which is considerably better than that for patients with osteosarcomas of the long bones. Recently, large and multicenter studies of patients with osteosarcoma have demonstrated improved survival through use of specific presurgical chemotherapeutic regimens. This initial therapy is followed by radical surgical removal, with thorough review of the histopathologic specimen to evaluate the response to the initial chemotherapy. In those patients with significant local residual tumor, further chemotherapy or radiation often is used. Overall, the prognosis of osteosarcoma of the jaws seems to be related to prompt diagnosis, tumor grade and size, aggressive chemotherapy, and definitive surgical resection. Because secondary malignancies are not rare in patients treated for osteosarcoma, lifelong follow-up is mandatory.

Juxtacortical osteosarcoma is an uncommon variety that occasionally involves the jaws, originates close to the surface of the bone, and presents in two different patterns. In the parosteal variant, the tumor is ill-defined and often involves the cortex and medullary bone. Histopathologically, the tumor exhibits a high degree of structural differentiation, with its bland features making separation from a benign neoplasm difficult. Although these tumors initially demonstrate a good prognosis and minimal metastatic potential, recurrence is likely after less than radical initial excision, and the lesion often then develops into a typical higher grade osteosarcoma. In the periosteal variant, the tumor grows outward from an intact periosteum and exhibits features of malignancy that are obvious histopathologically. Although the process exhibits a better prognosis than typical osteosarcoma, local recurrence and distant metastasis is possible if the tumor is not promptly and adequately treated by wide surgical resection. Adjunctive radiation therapy or chemotherapy typically is not used.

Osteosarcoma also is a well-known late sequela of radiation therapy given for other purposes. Jaw osteosarcomas have developed 10 to 15 years after radiation therapy was administered to benign (or occasionally malignant) lesions of the jaws or overlying soft tissues. Finally, an increased prevalence of osteosarcoma is noted in patients with Paget's disease of bone.

### Figure 11.52
### OSTEOSARCOMA

**(A)** Painful expansion of the posterior mandible in a 44-year-old female. Two molar teeth had been extracted several weeks previously, and the patient had been treated with antibiotics for a presumed infection. **(B)** Occlusal radiograph of same patient showing destruction of the buccal cortex with "sunburst" production of tumor bone.

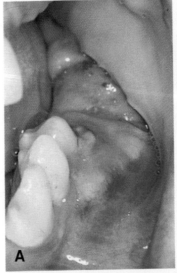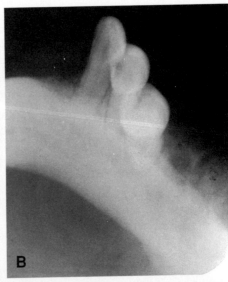

### Figure 11.53
### OSTEOSARCOMA

Periapical radiograph of the patient depicted in Figure 11.52 showing symmetric widening of the periodontal ligament space of the premolar teeth.

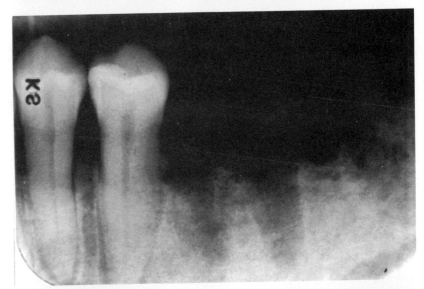

### Figure 11.54
### OSTEOSARCOMA

Occlusal radiograph of a 40-year-old female who presented with a firm lobular mass on the buccal aspect of the mandible. This demonstrates the "sunburst" tumor bone formation with cortical bone destruction.

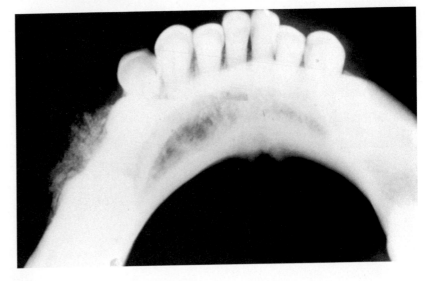

**Figure 11.55**
**OSTEOSARCOMA**
Periapical radiographs of a 32-year-old female who had a painful swelling over the second molar. Note the ill-defined radiolucent lesion in the furcation area. (Courtesy of Dr. E. B. Bass.)

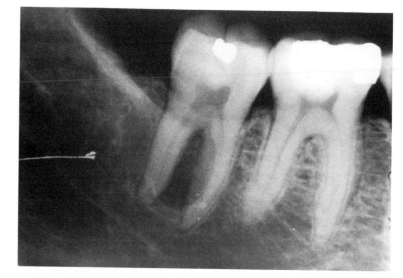

**Figure 11.56**
**OSTEOSARCOMA**
Same patient depicted in Figure 11.55. Endodontic treatment was performed, and the filling material was extruded into the furcation area. Biopsy specimen revealed an osteosarcoma. (Courtesy of Dr. E. B. Bass.)

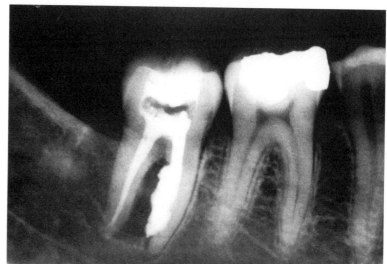

**Figure 11.57**
**JUXTACORTICAL OSTEOSARCOMA, PAROSTEAL VARIANT**
Periapical radiograph showing a low-grade osteosarcoma arising on the alveolar bone surface between the mandibular canine and lateral incisor teeth.

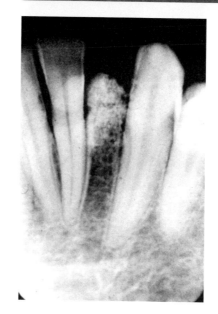

## Figs. 11.58, 11.59, and 11.60

Chondrosarcoma is the primary malignancy of cartilage-forming cells within bone. This cancer is uncommon in the jaws and exhibits a lower prevalence than osteosarcoma. Although examples have been recorded in patients over a wide age range, the peak prevalence for jaw tumors is in the third and fourth decades of life. Chondrosarcoma occurs with equal frequency in both jaws. The most common initial complaint is a swelling or mass, although a few patients complain initially of pain. Dental complaints, such as localized periodontal bone loss and loosening or migration of teeth, are not uncommon. Maxillary tumors may cause initial symptoms of nasal obstruction.

Radiographically, chondrosarcomas characteristically show a destructive radiolucent lesion with ill-defined margins. The radiolucent area frequently contains scattered radiopaque foci resulting from calcification of the neoplastic cartilage. Symmetric widening of the periodontal ligament space and irregular root resorption may be noted in teeth involved by the tumor. The radiographic features usually suggest a malignant tumor but cannot be differentiated from osteosarcoma.

Because chondrosarcomas are not radiosensitive and are less responsive to chemotherapy than are osteosarcomas, treatment typically consists of radical surgical resection, with adjuvant therapies often reserved for patients with postsurgical residual disease. Overall, metastasis of chondrosarcomas of the jaws is uncommon, and most treatment failures are caused by uncontrollable local disease secondary to inadequate removal during the initial therapy. Because recurrence may develop as late as 20 years after initial therapy, follow-up must be lifelong.

One exception to the typical pattern is mesenchymal chondrosarcoma, a variant that is not rare within the jaws. Although the aggressiveness of the tumor is variable, this pattern on occasion may be highly malignant, and it demonstrates significant recurrence along with lymphatic and hematogenous metastasis. Radical surgery, often combined with chemotherapy and radiation therapy, is the treatment of choice; overall, the prognosis is poor, with approximately 70% of those affected succumbing to their tumor.

### Figure 11.58
### CHONDROSARCOMA

Clinical photograph of a 50-year-old woman showing a massive tumor projecting lingually in the posterior molar area. She stated that the tumor had been present for many years with slow growth.

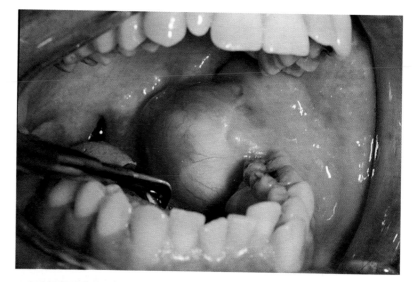

### Figure 11.59
### CHONDROSARCOMA

Panographic radiograph from the patient depicted in Figure 11.58 showing a destructive radiolucent lesion containing numerous radiopaque foci.

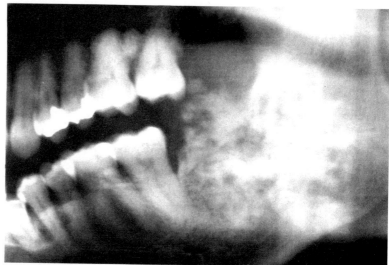

### Figure 11.60
### CHONDROSARCOMA

Same patient depicted in Figures 11.58 and 11.59. Computed tomography exhibiting a large lesion projecting lingually from the mandible.

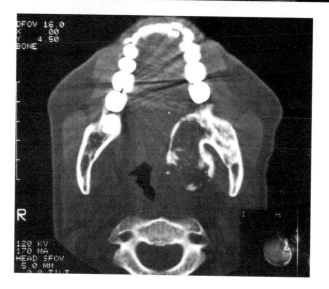

### Osteopetrosis

Dyson DP. Osteomyelitis of the jaws in Albers-Schönberg disease. Br J Oral Surg 1970;7:178.

Elster AD, Theros EG, Key LL, et al. Cranial imaging in autosomal recessive osteopetrosis, part I: facial bones and calvarium. Radiology 1992;183:129.

Mintz SM, Martone CH, Anavi Y. Avoiding problems in patients with craniotubular disorders. J Am Dent Assoc 1993;124:116.

Steiner M, Gould AR, Means WR. Osteomyelitis of the mandible associated with osteopetrosis. J Oral Maxillofac Surg 1983;41:395.

Younai F, Eisenbud L, Sciubba JJ. Osteopetrosis: a case report including gross and microscopic findings in the mandible at autopsy. Oral Surg Oral Med Oral Pathol 1988;65:214.

### Cleidocranial Dysplasia

Becker A, Lustmann J, Shteyer A. Cleidocranial dysplasia, part 1: general principles of the orthodontic and surgical treatment modality. Am J Orthod Dentofacial Orthop 1997;111:28.

Becker A, Shteyer A, Bimstein E, et al. Cleidocranial dysplasia, part 2 B: treatment protocol for the orthodontic and surgical modality. Am J Orthod Dentofacial Orthop 1997;111:173.

Farrar EL, Van Sickels JE. Early surgical management of cleidocranial dysplasia: a preliminary report. J Oral Maxillofac Surg 1983;41:527.

Jensen BL, Kreiborg S. Development of the dentition in cleidocranial dysplasia. J Oral Pathol Med 1990;19:89.

Jensen BL, Kreiborg S. Dental treatment strategies in cleidocranial dysplasia. Br Dent J 1992;172:243.

Jensen BL, Kreiborg S. Craniofacial abnormalities in 52 school-age and adult patients with cleidocranial dysplasia. J Craniofac Genet Dev Biol 1993;13:98.

Richardson A, Deussen FF. Facial and dental anomalies in cleidocranial dysplasia: a study of 17 cases. Int J Paediatr Dent 1994;4:225.

Trimble LD, West RA, McNeill RW. Cleidocranial dysplasia: comprehensive treatment of the dentofacial abnormalities. J Am Dent Assoc 1982;105:661.

### Focal Osteoporotic Marrow Defect

Barker BF, Jensen JL, Howell FV. Focal osteoporotic marrow defects of the jaws. Oral Surg Oral Med Oral Pathol 1974;38:404.

Crawford BE, Weathers DR. Osteoporotic marrow defects of the jaws. J Oral Surg 1970;28:600.

Gordy FM, Crews KM, O'Carroll MK. Focal osteoporotic bone marrow defect in the anterior maxilla. Oral Surg Oral Med Oral Pathol 1993;76:537.

Sa'do B, Ozeki S, Higuchi Y, et al. Osteoporotic bone marrow defect of the mandible: report of a case diagnosed by computed tomography scanning. J Oral Maxillofac Surg 1992;50:80.

Schneider LC, Mesa ML, Fraenkel D. Osteoporotic bone marrow defect: radiographic features and pathogenic factors. Oral Surg Oral Med Oral Pathol 1988;65:127.

Standish SM, Shafer WG. Focal osteoporotic bone marrow defects of the jaws. J Oral Surg 1962;20:123.

### Idiopathic Osteosclerosis

Geist JR, Katz JO. The frequency and distribution of idiopathic osteosclerosis. Oral Surg Oral Med Oral Pathol 1990;69:388.

Kawai T, Hirakuma H, Murakami S, et al. Radiographic investigation of idiopathic osteosclerosis of the jaws in Japanese dental outpatients. Oral Surg Oral Med Oral Pathol 1992;74:237.

Kawai T, Murakami S, Kishino M, et al. Gigantic dense bone island of the jaw. Oral Surg Oral Med Oral Pathol Oral Radiol Endod 1996;82:108.

McDonnell D. Dense bone island: a review of 107 patients. Oral Surg Oral Med Oral Pathol 1993;76:124.

### Osteoma

Cutilli BJ, Quinn PD. Traumatically induced peripheral osteoma: report of a case. Oral Surg Oral Med Oral Pathol 1992;73:667.

Kaplan I, Calderon S, Buchner A. Peripheral osteoma of the mandible: a study of 10 new cases and analysis of the literature. J Oral Maxillofac Surg 1994;52:467.

Richards HE, Strider JW Jr, Short SG, et al. Large peripheral osteoma arising from the genital tubercle area. Oral Surg Oral Med Oral Pathol 1986;61:268.

Schneider LC, Dolinski HB, Grodjesk JE. Solitary peripheral osteoma of the jaws: report of a case and review of the literature. Oral Surg Oral Med Oral Pathol 1980;38:452.

Swanson KS, Guttu RL, Miller ME. Gigantic osteoma of the mandible: report of a case. J Oral Maxillofac Surg 1992;50:635.

## Gardner Syndrome

Haggitt RC, Reid BJ. Hereditary gastrointestinal polyposis syndromes. Am J Surg Pathol 1986;10:871.

Ida M, Nakamura T, Utsunomiya J. Osteomatous changes and tooth abnormalities found in the jaws of patients with adenomatosis coli. Oral Surg Oral Med Oral Pathol 1981;52:2.

Kaffe I, Rozen P, Horowitz I. The significance of idiopathic osteosclerosis found in panoramic radiographs of sporadic colorectal neoplasia patients and their relatives. Oral Surg Oral Med Oral Pathol 1992;74:366.

Sondergaard J, Bulow S, Jarvinen H, et al. Dental anomalies in familial adenomatous polyposis. Acta Odontol Scand 1987;45:61.

Wesley RK, Cullen CL, Bloom WS. Gardner's syndrome with bilateral osteomas of the coronoid process resulting in limited opening. Pediatr Dent 1987;9:53.

Williams SC, Peller PJ. Gardner's syndrome: case report and discussion of the manifestations of the disorder. Clin Nucl Med 1994;19:668.

Yuasa K, Yonetsu K, Kanda S, et al. Computed tomography of the jaws in familial adenomatosis coli. Oral Surg Oral Med Oral Pathol 1993;76:251.

## Paget's Disease

Bhambhani M, Lamberty BGH, Clements MR, et al. Giant cell tumours in mandible and spine: a rare complication of Paget's disease of bone. Ann Rheum Dis 1992;51:1335.

Carrillo R, Morales A, Rodriguez-Peralto JL, et al. Benign fibro-osseous lesions in Paget's disease of the jaws. Oral Surg Oral Med Oral Pathol 1991;71:588.

Ellis GL, Connole PW. Diffuse mandibular enlargement caused by osteitis deformans. Ear Nose Throat 1985;64:466.

Fisher EW. Rhinological manifestations of Paget's disease of bone (osteitis deformans). J Craniomaxillofac Surg 1990;18:169.

Gleich LL, Eberle RC, Shanha AR, et al. Paget's sarcoma of the mandible. Head Neck 1995;17:425.

Hoffman CD, Huntley TA, Wiesenfeld D, et al. Maxillary giant cell tumour associated with Paget's disease of bone. Int J Oral Maxillofac Surg 1994;23:161.

Smith BJ, Eveson JW. Paget's disease of bone with particular reference to dentistry. J Oral Pathol 1981;10:233.

Tillman H. Paget's disease of bone: a clinical, radiographic and histopathologic study of 24 cases involving the jaws. Oral Surg Oral Med Oral Pathol 1962;15:1225.

## Massive Osteolysis

Frederikson NL, Wesley RK, Sciubba JJ, et al. Massive osteolysis of the maxillofacial skeleton: a clinical, radiographic, histologic and ultrastructural study. Oral Surg Oral Med Oral Pathol 1983;55:470.

Gorham LW, Stout AP. Hemangiomatosis and its relationship to massive osteolysis. Trans Assoc Am Phys 1954;67:302.

Heffez L, Doku HC, Carter BL, et al. Perspectives on massive osteolysis: report of case and review of the literature. Oral Surg Oral Med Oral Pathol 1983;55:331.

Ohnishi T, Yano Y, Nakazawa M, et al. Massive osteolysis of the mandible: a case report. J Oral Maxillofac Surg 1993;51:932.

Ohya T, Shibata S, Takeda Y. Massive osteolysis of the maxillofacial bones: report of two cases. Oral Surg Oral Med Oral Pathol 1990;70:698.

Yayada Y, Yoshiga K, Takada K, et al. Massive osteolysis of the mandible with subsequent obstructive sleep apnea syndrome: a case report. J Oral Maxillofac Surg 1995;53:1463.

## Langerhans Cell Histiocytosis

Dagenais M, Pharoah MJ, Sikorski PA. The radiographic characteristics of histiocytosis X: a study of 29 cases that involve the jaws. Oral Surg Oral Med Oral Pathol 1992;74:230.

Hartman KH. A review of 114 cases of histiocytosis X. Oral Surg Oral Med Oral Pathol 1980;49:38.

Howarth DM, Mullan BP, Wiseman GA, et al. Bone scintigraphy evaluated in diagnosing and staging Langerhans' cell histiocytosis and related disorders. J Nucl Med 1996;37:1456.

Piattelli A, Paolantonio M. Eosinophilic granuloma of the mandible involving the periodontal tissues: a case report. J Periodontol 1995;66:731.

Pringle GA, Daley TD, Veinot LA, et al. Langerhans' cell histiocytosis in association with periapical granulomas and cysts. Oral Surg Oral Med Oral Pathol 1992;74:186.

Stewart JCB, Regezi JA, Lloyd RV. Immunohistochemical study of idiopathic histiocytosis of the mandible and maxilla. Oral Surg Oral Med Oral Pathol 1986;61:48.

Yu Q, Wang P-Z, Shi H-M, et al. Radiographic findings in Langerhans' cell disease affecting the mandible. Oral Surg Oral Med Oral Pathol Oral Radiol Endod 1995;79:251.

## Giant Cell Granuloma

Auclair PL, Kratochvil FJ, Slater LJ, et al. A clinical and histomorphologic comparison of the central giant cell granuloma and the giant cell tumor. Oral Surg Oral Med Oral Pathol 1988;66:197.

Eisenbud L, Stern M, Rothberg M, et al. Central giant cell granuloma of the jaws: experience in management of thirty-seven cases. J Oral Maxillofac Surg 1988;46:376.

El-Labban NG. Intravascular fibrin thrombi and endothelial cell damage in central giant cell granuloma. J Oral Pathol Med 1997;26:1.

Ficarra G, Kaban LB, Hansen LS. Central giant cell lesions of the mandible and maxilla: a clinicopathologic and cytometric study. Oral Surg Oral Med Oral Pathol 1987;64:44.

Kaffe I, Ardekian L, Taicher S, et al. Radiologic features of central giant cell granuloma of the jaws. Oral Surg Oral Med Oral Pathol Oral Radiol Endod 1996;81:720.

Kermer C, Millesi W, Watzke IM. Local injection of corticosteroids for central giant cell granuloma: a case report. Int J Oral Maxillofac Surg 1994;23:366.

Minic A, Stajcic Z. Prognostic significance of cortical perforation in the recurrence of central giant cell granulomas of the jaws. J Craniomaxillofac Surg 1996;24:104.

Stolovitzky JP, Waldron CA, McConnel FMS. Giant cell lesions of the maxilla and paranasal sinuses. Head Neck 1994;16:143.

Tallan EM, Olsen KD, McCaffrey TV, et al. Advanced giant cell granuloma: a twenty-year study. Otolaryngol Head Neck Surg 1994;110:413.

Whitaker SB, Waldron CA. Central giant cell lesions of the jaws: a clinical, radiologic and histopathologic study. Oral Surg Oral Med Oral Pathol 1993;75:199.

## Cherubism

Betts NJ, Stewart JCB, Fonseca RJ, et al. Multiple central giant cell lesions with a Noonan-like phenotype. Oral Surg Oral Med Oral Pathol 1993;76:601.

Cohen MM Jr, Gorlin RJ. Noonan-like/multiple giant cell lesion syndrome. Am J Med Genet 1991;40:159.

Dunlap C, Neville B, Vickers RA, et al. The Noonan syndrome/cherubism association. Oral Surg Oral Med Oral Pathol 1989;67:698.

Hamner JE, Ketcham AS. Cherubism: an analysis of treatment. Cancer 1963;23:1133.

Hitomi G, Nishide N, Mitsui K. Cherubism. Diagnostic imaging and review of the literature in Japan. Oral Surg Oral Med Oral Pathol Oral Radiol Endod 1996;81:623.

Kaugers GE, Niamtu J III, Svirsky JA. Cherubism: diagnosis, treatment, and comparison with central giant cell granulomas and giant cell tumors. Oral Surg Oral Med Oral Pathol 1992;73:369.

Koury ME, Stella JP, Epker BN. Vascular transformation in cherubism. Oral Surg Oral Med Oral Pathol 1993;76:20.

Peters WJN. Cherubism: a study of 20 cases from one family. Oral Surg Oral Med Oral Pathol 1979;47:307.

## Simple Bone Cyst

Donkor P, Punnia-Moorthy A. Biochemical analysis of simple bone cyst fluid: report of a case. Int J Oral Maxillofac Surg 1994;23:296.

Fielding CG. The traumatic bone cyst: review of literature and report of two cases. Mil Med 1992;157:676.

Hara H, Ohishi M, Higuchi Y. Fibrous dysplasia of the mandible associated with large solitary bone cyst. J Oral Maxillofac Surg 1990;48:88.

Heubner GR, Turlington EG. So-called traumatic (hemorrhagic) bone cysts of the jaws. Oral Surg Oral Med Oral Pathol 1971;33:334.

Horner K, Forman GH, Smith NJD. Atypical simple bone cysts of the jaws, I: recurrent lesions. Clin Radiol 1988;39:53.

Howe GL. Haemorrhagic cysts of the mandible. Br J Oral Surg 1965;3:55.

Kaugars GE, Cale AE. Traumatic bone cyst. Oral Surg Oral Med Oral Pathol 1987;63:318.

Kuroi M. Simple bone cyst of the jaw: review of the literature and report of a case. J Oral Surg 1980;38:456.

Saito Y, Hoshina Y, Nagamine T, et al. Simple bone cyst: a clinical and histopathologic study of fifteen cases. Oral Surg Oral Med Oral Pathol 1992;74:487.

## Aneurysmal Bone Cyst

Bataineh AB. Aneurysmal bone cysts of the maxilla: a clinicopathologic review. J Oral Maxillofac Surg 1997;55:1212.

Matt BH. Aneurysmal bone cyst of the maxilla: case report and review of the literature. Int J Pediatr Otorhinolaryngol 1993;25:217.

Struthers PJ, Shear M. Aneurysmal bone cysts of the jaws, I. Int J Oral Surg 1984;13:85.

Struthers PJ, Shear M. Aneurysmal bone cysts of the jaws, II: pathogenesis. Int J Oral Surg 1984;13:92.

Toljanic JR, Lechewski E, Huvos AG, et al. Aneurysmal bone cysts of the jaws: a case study and review of the literature. Oral Surg Oral Med Oral Pathol 1987;64:72.

Trent C, Byl FM. Aneurysmal bone cyst of the mandible. Ann Otol Rhinol Laryngol 1993;102:917.

Wiatrak BJ, Myer CM III, Andrews TM. Alternatives in the management of aneurysmal bone cysts of the mandible. Int J Pediatr Otorhinolaryngol 1995;31:247.

## Hemangioma

Beziat J-L, Marcelino J-P, Bascoulergue Y, et al. Central vascular malformation of the mandible: a case report. J Oral Maxillofac Surg 1997;55:415.

Bunel K, Sindet-Pedersen S. Central hemangioma of the mandible. Oral Surg Oral Med Oral Pathol 1993;75:565.

Greene LA, Freedman PD, Freidman JM, et al. Capillary hemangioma of the maxilla: a report of two cases in which angiography and embolization were used. Oral Surg Oral Med Oral Pathol 1990;70:268.

Hayward JR. Central cavernous hemangioma of the mandible: report of 4 cases. J Oral Surg 1981;39:526.

Lamberg MA, Tasanen A, Jääskelainen J. Fatality from central hemangioma of the mandible. J Oral Surg 1979;37:578.

Yeoman CM. Management of hemangioma involving facial, mandibular and pharyngeal structures. Br J Oral Maxillofac Surg 1987;25:195.

## Arteriovenous Malformation

Behnia H, Motamedi MHK. Treatment of central arteriovenous malformation of the mandible via resection and immediate replantation of the segment: a case report. J Oral Maxillofac Surg 1997;55:79.

Darlow LD, Murphy JB, Berrios RJ, et al. Arteriovenous malformation of the sinus: an unusual clinical presentation. Oral Surg Oral Med Oral Pathol 1988;66:21.

Flandroy P, Pruvo J-P. Treatment of mandibular arteriovenous malformations by direct transosseous puncture: report of two cases. Cardiovasc Intervent Radiol 1994;17:222.

Kelley D, Terry B, Small E. Arteriovenous malformation of the mandible: report of case. J Oral Maxillofac Surg 1977;35:387.

Kula K, Blakey G, Wright JT, et al. High-flow vascular malformations: literature review and case report. Pediatr Dent 1996;18:322.

Larsen PE, Peterson LJ. A systematic approach to management of high-flow vascular malformations of the mandible. J Oral Maxillofac Surg 1993;51:62.

Mohammadi H, Said-Al-Naief NAH, Heffez LB. Arteriovenous malformation of the mandible: report of a case with a note on the differential diagnosis. Oral Surg Oral Med Oral Pathol Oral Radiol Endod 1997;84:286.

Resnick SA, Russell EJ, Hanson DH, et al. Embolization of a life-threatening mandibular vascular malformation by direct percutaneous transmandibular puncture. Head Neck 1992;14:372.

## Desmoplastic Fibroma

Freedman PD, Cardo VA, Kerpel SM, et al. Desmoplastic fibroma (fibromatosis) of the jawbones. Oral Surg Oral Med Oral Pathol 1978;46:386.

Hopkins KM, Huttula CS, Kahn MA, et al. Desmoplastic fibroma of the mandible: review and report of two cases. J Oral Maxillofac Surg 1996;54:1249.

Inwards CY, Unni KK, Beabout JW, et al. Desmoplastic fibroma of bone. Cancer 1991;68:1978.

Kwon PHJ, Horswell BB, Gatto DJ. Desmoplastic fibroma of the jaws. Head Neck 1989;11:67.

Makek M, Lello GE. Desmoplastic fibroma of the mandible: literature review and report of three cases. J Oral Maxillofac Surg 1986;44:385.

Templeton K, Glass N, Young SK. Desmoplastic fibroma of the mandible in a child: report of a case. Oral Surg Oral Med Oral Pathol Oral Radiol Endod 1997;84:620.

## Intraosseous Neurofibroma

Ellis GL, Abrams AM, Melrose RJ. Intraosseous benign neural sheath neoplasms of the jaws: report of seven new cases and review of the literature. Oral Surg Oral Med Oral Pathol 1977;44:731.

Papadopoulos H, Zachariades N, Angelopoulos AP. Neurofibroma of the mandible: review of the literature and report of a case. Int J Oral Maxillofac Surg 1981;10:293.

Papageorge MB, Doku HC, Lis R. Solitary neurofibroma of the mandible and infratemporal fossa in a young child: report of a case. Oral Surg Oral Med Oral Pathol 1992;73:407.

Polak M, Polak A, Brocheriou C, et al. Solitary neurofibroma of the mandible: case report and review of the literature. J Oral Maxillofac Surg 1989;47:65.

## Osseous Dysplasia

Groot RH, van Merkesteyn JPR, Bras J. Diffuse sclerosing osteomyelitis and florid osseous dysplasia. Oral Surg Oral Med Oral Pathol Oral Radiol Endod 1996;81:333.

Higuchi Y, Nakamura N, Tashiro H. Clinicopathologic study of cemento-osseous dysplasia producing cysts of the mandible. Oral Surg Oral Med Oral Pathol 1988;65:339.

MacDonald-Jankowski DS. Florid osseous dysplasia in Hong Kong Chinese. Dentomaxillofac Radiol 1996;25:39.

Melrose RJ, Abrams AA, Mills BC. Florid osseous dysplasia. Oral Surg Oral Med Oral Pathol 1976;41:62.

Robinson HBG. Osseous dysplasia: reaction of bone to injury. J Oral Surg 1956;14:3.

Schneider LC, Mesa ML. Differences between florid osseous dysplasia and diffuse sclerosing osteomyelitis. Oral Surg Oral Med Oral Pathol 1990;70:308.

Su L, Weathers DR, Waldron CA. Distinguishing features of focal cemento-osseous dysplasia and cemento-ossifying fibromas, I: a pathologic spectrum of 316 cases. Oral Surg Oral Med Oral Pathol Oral Radiol Endod 1997;84:301.

Su L, Weathers DR, Waldron CA. Distinguishing features of focal cemento-osseous dysplasia and cemento-ossifying fibromas, II: a clinical and radiologic spectrum of 316 cases. Oral Surg Oral Med Oral Pathol Oral Radiol Endod 1997;84:540.

Summerlin D-J, Tomich CE. Focal cemento-osseous dysplasia: a clinicopathologic study of 221 cases. Oral Surg Oral Med Oral Pathol 1994;78:611.

Waldron CA. Fibro-osseous lesions of the jaws. J Oral Maxillofac Surg 1993;51:828.

## Fibrous Dysplasia

Chen Y-R, Noordhoff MS. Treatment of craniomaxillofacial fibrous dysplasia: how early and how extensive. Plast Reconstr Surg 1991;87:799.

Harris WH, Dudley HR Jr, Barry RJ. The natural history of fibrous dysplasia. J Bone Joint Surg 1962;44A:207.

Pfeffer S, Molina E, Feuillan P, et al. McCune-Albright syndrome: the patterns of scintigraphic abnormalities. J Nucl Med 1990;31:1474.

Schwartz DT, Alpert M. The malignant transformation of fibrous dysplasia. Am J Med Sci 1964;247:1.

Waldron CA. Fibro-osseous lesions of the jaws. J Oral Maxillofac Surg 1993;51:828.

Waldron CA, Giansanti JS. Benign fibro-osseous lesions of the jaws: a clinical-radiologic-histologic review of sixty-five cases. Oral Surg Oral Med Oral Pathol 1973;35:190.

## Segmental Odontomaxillary Dysplasia

Danforth RA, Melrose RJ, Abrams AM, et al. Segmental odontomaxillary dysplasia: report of eight cases and comparison with hemimaxillofacial dysplasia. Oral Surg Oral Med Oral Pathol 1990;70:81.

DeSalvo MS, Copete MA, Riesenberger RE, et al. Segmental odontomaxillary dysplasia (hemimaxillofacial dysplasia): case report. Pediatr Dent 1996;18:154.

Miles DA, Lovas JL, Cohen MM Jr. Hemimaxillofacial dysplasia: a newly recognized disorder of facial asymmetry, hypertrichosis of the facial skin, unilateral enlargement of the maxilla, and hypoplastic teeth in two patients. Oral Surg Oral Med Oral Pathol 1987;64:445.

Packota GV, Pharoah MJ, Petrikowski CG. Radiographic features of segmental odontomaxillary dysplasia: a study of 12 cases. Oral Surg Oral Med Oral Pathol Oral Radiol Endod 1996;82:577.

## Ossifying Fibroma

Eversole LR, Leider AS, Nelson K. Ossifying fibroma: a clinicopathologic study of 64 cases. Oral Surg Oral Med Oral Pathol 1985;60:505.

Johnson LC, Yousefi M, Vinh T, et al. Juvenile active ossifying fibroma: its nature, dynamics and origin. Acta Otolaryngol (Stockh) Suppl 1991;488:1.

Makek MS. So-called "fibro-osseous lesions" of tumorous origin: biology confronts terminology. J Cranio-maxillofac Surg 1987;15:154.

Margo C, Ragsdale B, Perman K, et al. Psammomatoid (juvenile) ossifying fibroma of the orbit. Ophthalmology 1985;92:150.

Su L, Weathers DR, Waldron CA. Distinguishing features of focal cemento-osseous dysplasia and cemento-ossifying fibromas, I: a pathologic spectrum of 316 cases. Oral Surg Oral Med Oral Pathol Oral Radiol Endod 1997;84:301.

Su L, Weathers DR, Waldron CA. Distinguishing features of focal cemento-osseous dysplasia and cemento-ossifying fibromas, II: a clinical and radiologic spectrum of 316 cases. Oral Surg Oral Med Oral Pathol Oral Radiol Endod 1997;84:540.

Summerlin D-J, Tomich CE. Focal cemento-osseous dysplasia: a clinicopathologic study of 221 cases. Oral Surg Oral Med Oral Pathol 1994;78:611.

Waldron CA. Fibro-osseous lesions of the jaws. J Oral Maxillofac Surg 1993;51:828.

## Osteoblastoma

Ataoglu O, Oygur T, Yamalik K, et al. Recurrent osteoblastoma of the mandible: a case report. J Oral Maxillofac Surg 1994;52:86.

Eisenbud L, Kahn L, Friedman E. Benign osteoblastoma of the mandible: fifteen year follow-up showing spontaneous regression after a biopsy. J Oral Maxillofac Surg 1987;45:53.

El-Mofty S, Refai H. Benign osteoblastoma of the maxilla. J Oral Maxillofac Surg 1987;47:60.

Peters TED, Oliver DR, McDonald JS. Benign osteoblastoma of the mandible: report of a case. J Oral Maxillofac Surg 1995;53:1347.

Ribera MJ. Osteoblastoma in the anterior maxilla mimicking periapical pathosis of odontogenic origin. J Endod 1996;22:142.

Smith RA, Hansen LS, Resnik D, et al. Comparison of osteoblastoma in gnathic and extra-gnathic sites. Oral Surg Oral Med Oral Pathol 1982;54:285.

Strand-Pettinen I, Lukinmaa PL, Holstrom T, et al. Benign osteoblastoma of the mandible. Br J Oral Maxillofac Surg 1990;28:311.

## Cementoblastoma

Biggs JT, Benenati FW. Surgically treating a benign cementoblastoma while retaining the involved tooth. J Am Dent Assoc 1995;126:1288.

Jelic JS, Loftus MJ, Miller AS, et al. Benign cementoblastoma: report of an unusual case and analysis of 14 additional cases. J Oral Maxillofac Surg 1993;51:1033.

Keyes G, Hildebrand K. Successful surgical endodontics for benign cementoblastoma. J Endod 1987;13:566.

Makek M, Lello G. Benign cementoblastoma: case report and literature review. J Oral Maxillofac Surg 1982;10:182.

Monks FT, Bradley JC, Turner EP. Central osteoblastoma or cementoblastoma: a case report and 12 year review. Br J Oral Surg 1981;19:29.

Slootweg PJ. Cementoblastoma and osteoblastoma: a comparison of histologic features. J Oral Pathol Med 1992;21:385.

Ulmansky M, Hjørting-Hansen E, Praetorius F, et al. Benign cementoblastoma: a review and five new cases. Oral Surg Oral Med Oral Pathol 1994;77:48.

## Ewing's Sarcoma

Arafat A, Ellis GL, Adrian JC. Ewing's sarcoma of the jaws. Oral Surg Oral Med Oral Pathol 1983;55:589.

Berk R, Heller A, Heller D, et al. Ewing's sarcoma of the mandible: a case report. Oral Surg Oral Med Oral Pathol Oral Radiol Endod 1995;79:159.

Damm DD, White DK, Drummond JF, et al. Ewing's tumor of the jaws. Pediatr Dent 1985;7:57.

Fiorillo A, Tranfa F, Canale G, et al. Primary Ewing's sarcoma of the maxilla, a rare and curable localization: report of two new cases, successfully treated by radiotherapy and systemic chemotherapy. Cancer Lett 1996;103:177.

Kissane JM, Askin FB, Foulkes M, et al. Ewing's sarcoma of bone: clinicopathologic aspects of 303 cases from the Intergroup Ewing's Sarcoma Study. Hum Pathol 1983;14:773.

Mamede RM, Mello FV, Barbieri J. Prognosis of Ewing's sarcoma of the head and neck. Otolaryngol Head Neck Surg 1990;102:650.

Wang C-L, Yacobi R, Pharoah M, et al. Ewing's sarcoma: metastatic tumor to the jaw. Oral Surg Oral Med Oral Pathol 1991;71:597.

Wood RE, Nortjé CL, Hesseling P, et al. Ewing's tumor of the jaw. Oral Surg Oral Med Oral Pathol 1990;69:120.

## Osteosarcoma

August M, Magennis P, Dewitt D. Osteogenic sarcoma of the jaws: factors influencing prognosis. Int J Oral Maxillofac Surg 1997;26:198.

Bras JM, Donner R, van der Kwast WAM. Juxtacortical osteogenic sarcoma. Oral Surg Oral Med Oral Pathol 1980;50:535.

Clark JL, Unni KK, Dahlin DC, et al. Osteosarcoma of the jaws. Cancer 1983;51:2311.

Garrington GE, Scofield HH, Cornyn J, et al. Osteosarcoma of the jaws. Cancer 1967;20:377.

Lewis M, Perl A, Som PM, et al. Osteogenic sarcoma of the jaw: a clinicopathologic review of 12 patients. Arch Otolaryngol Head Neck Surg 1997;123:169.

Patterson A, Greer RO, Howard D. Periosteal osteosarcoma of the maxilla: a case report and review of the literature. J Oral Maxillofac Surg 1990;48:522.

Slootweg PJ, Müller H. Osteosarcoma of the jawbones. J Oral Maxillofac Surg 1985;13:158.

Tanzawa H, Uchiyama S, Sato K. Statistical observation of osteosarcoma of the maxillofacial region in Japan: analysis of 114 Japanese cases reported between 1930 and 1989. Oral Surg Oral Med Oral Pathol 1991;72:444.

van Es RJJ, Keus RB, van der Waal I, et al. Osteosarcoma of the jaw bones: long-term follow up of 48 cases. Int J Oral Maxillofac Surg 1997;26:191.

Zarbo RJ, Regezi JA, Baker SR. Periosteal osteogenic sarcoma of the mandible. Oral Surg Oral Med Oral Pathol 1984;57:643.

## Chondrosarcoma

Finn DG, Goepfert H, Batsakis JG. Chondrosarcoma of the head and neck. Laryngoscope 1984;94:1539.

Garrington GE, Collett WK. Chondrosarcoma, I: a selected literature review. J Oral Pathol 1988;17:1.

Garrington GE, Collett WK. Chondrosarcoma, II: chondrosarcoma of the jaws: analysis of 37 cases. J Oral Pathol 1988;17:12.

Hackney FL, Aragon SB, Aufdemorte TB, et al. Chondrosarcoma of the jaws: clinical findings, histopathology, and treatment. Oral Surg Oral Med Oral Pathol 1991;71:139.

Ormiston IW, Piette E, Tideman H, et al. Chondrosarcoma of the mandible presenting as periodontal lesions: report of 2 cases. J Craniomaxillofac Surg 1994;22:231.

Ruark DS, Schlehaider UK, Shah JP. Chondrosarcomas of the head and neck. World J Surg 1992;16:1010.

Saito K, Unni KK, Wollan PC, et al. Chondrosarcoma of the jaw and facial bones. Cancer 1995;76:1550.

Zakkak TB, Flynn TR, Boguslaw B, et al. Mesenchymal chondrosarcoma of the mandible: case report and review of the literature. J Oral Maxillofac Surg 1998;56:84.

# chapter 12
## ODONTOGENIC CYSTS AND TUMORS

## Figs. 12.1, 12.2, and 12.3

The dentigerous cyst is the most common of the developmental odontogenic cysts of the jaws and accounts for approximately 20 to 24% of all epithelial-lined jaw cysts. It develops when fluid or a space occurs between follicular tissue lined by reduced enamel epithelium and the crown of an unerupted tooth. It is attached to the tooth at the cervix. The pathogenesis of this process is unknown, but its growth may involve not only osmotic pressure but independent growth of the lining epithelium. It also has been suggested that periapical inflammation from a deciduous tooth may stimulate the follicular tissue of the corresponding, unerupted permanent tooth to detach and undergo cystic change.

Third molars are the most commonly involved teeth, and the maxillary permanent canines are the second most common site. Dentigerous cysts, in rare instances, develop in association with unerupted deciduous teeth. A dentigerous cyst may also involve unerupted supernumerary teeth and odontomas. A patient may have more than one dentigerous cyst. It is most often initially detected in teenagers and young adults.

Radiographically, the dentigerous cyst presents as a well-defined, unilocular radiolucency surrounding the crown of an unerupted tooth. It often has a sclerotic border. Depending on the position of the unerupted tooth, the cyst may appear to involve the lateral surface of the tooth root, or it may appear to completely engulf it. It must be emphasized that the radiographic appearance is not diagnostic, though, as odontogenic keratocysts, unilocular ameloblastomas, and a number of other lesions may show a similar radiographic appearance. Radiographic distinction between a follicle and a small dentigerous cyst is not clear-cut. However, a radiolucency of 3 to 4 mm or larger is suggestive of cyst formation. Dentigerous cysts may display considerable growth potential, resulting in destruction of medullary bone and expansion of the jaw. The involved tooth may be displaced for a considerable distance from its original location, and the cyst may cause root resorption of adjacent erupted teeth.

An ameloblastoma may arise from neoplastic alteration of the epithelial lining of a dentigerous cyst, but this tumor also may arise de novo from dental lamina of follicular tissue. The epithelial lining of a dentigerous cyst also may undergo carcinomatous transformation in rare instances. The lining of the dentigerous cyst also is believed to be responsible for the rare development of intraosseous mucoepidermoid carcinoma of the jaws (Fig. 10.21). The treatment of the dentigerous cyst is enucleation and removal of the associated tooth.

### Figure 12.1
### DENTIGEROUS CYST
A small dentigerous cyst involving an unerupted lower third molar. (Courtesy of Dr. C. W. Topp.)

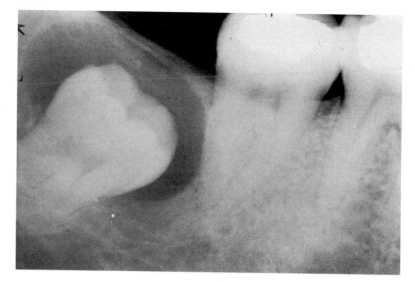

### Figure 12.2
### DENTIGEROUS CYST
A large dentigerous cyst involving a mandibular first premolar. The developing premolar has been displaced toward the lower border of the mandible. (Courtesy of Dr. Pat Coleman.)

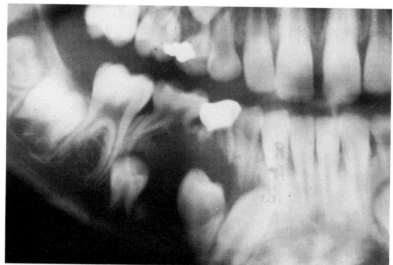

### Figure 12.3
### DENTIGEROUS CYST
Gross specimen of a dentigerous cyst surrounding the crown of the tooth and attached at the cervix.

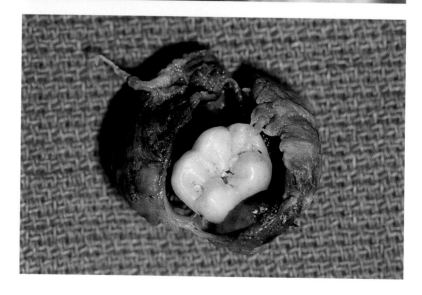

# ERUPTION CYST (ERUPTION HEMATOMA)

## Figs. 12.4 and 12.5

The eruption cyst is a variation of the dentigerous cyst in which an epithelial-lined cavity is associated with the crown of an erupting deciduous or permanent tooth. Most occur in the first decade of life and involve the maxilla. The cyst forms in the gingival mucosa above the crown of the erupting tooth from accumulation of fluid or blood in the dilated follicle. Clinically, the lesion presents as a soft, often translucent gingival swelling. If the cystic cavity contains considerable blood, the swelling may have a blue or purplish color. Such lesions are sometimes referred to as "eruption hematomas." Treatment may not be required because the cyst often ruptures spontaneously, permitting the tooth to erupt. In other instances, eruption is impeded and simple excision of the roof of the cyst is needed to facilitate eruption.

# GINGIVAL CYST OF THE NEWBORN

## Fig. 12.6

These are small, superficial cysts filled with keratin that occur on the alveolar mucosa of newborns. The cysts are derived from remnants of the dental lamina. Clinically, they present as small, usually multiple, whitish papules on the alveolar ridge. They are a common finding and more often seen on the maxilla. Gingival cysts of the newborn are asymptomatic lesions that do not require treatment. Typically, they rupture spontaneously and healing occurs.

## Figure 12.4
### ERUPTION CYST
Clinical photograph of an eruption cyst involving the mandibular second premolar in a 13-year-old girl.

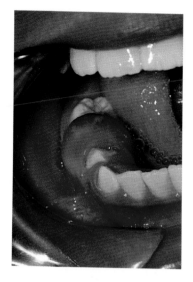

## Figure 12.5
### ERUPTION CYST
Radiograph of the same patient depicted in Figure 12.4 showing a pericoronal radiolucency and the overlying soft-tissue shadow representing the soft-tissue portion of the cyst.

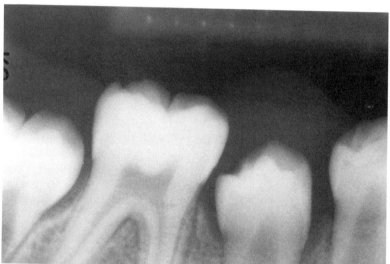

## Figure 12.6
### GINGIVAL CYST OF THE NEWBORN
Multiple whitish papules on the maxillary alveolar ridge.

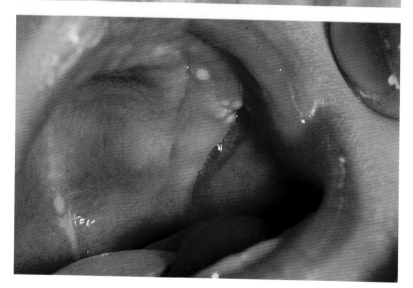

## GINGIVAL CYST OF THE ADULT

**Fig. 12.7**

The gingival cyst of the adult is a rare lesion that is widely considered to be the soft-tissue counterpart of the lateral periodontal cyst and most likely is derived from dental lamina rests in the gingiva (rests of Serres). Surface or crevicular epithelium may be the source in some instances. These cysts are typically located on the facial gingiva or alveolar mucosa in the mandibular premolar-canine area and are usually seen in middle-aged or older adults. Clinically, they present as painless swellings seldom exceeding 1.0 cm in diameter. Larger gingival cysts may cause a superficial "cupping-out" of the underlying cortical bone, but this is seldom apparent on a radiograph. They may exhibit a blue, translucent hue. Gingival cysts are treated by simple surgical excision.

## LATERAL PERIODONTAL CYST

**Figs. 12.8 and 12.9**

The lateral periodontal cyst is an uncommon developmental odontogenic cyst that seems to be derived from remnants of dental lamina within interdental bone. It is thought to be the intraosseous counterpart of the gingival cyst of the adult. Its histopathologic picture is specific, and the name should be used only with those characteristic microscopic features. Other specific odontogenic cysts, such as a lateral radicular cyst, odontogenic keratocyst, or calcifying odontogenic cyst, can appear radiographically identical to the lateral periodontal cyst.

The lateral periodontal cyst is usually asymptomatic and is discovered on a routine radiographic examination. It typically presents as a well-circumscribed, unilocular radiolucent lesion located between the roots of vital, erupted teeth in middle-aged and older adults. There is a significant predilection for the mandibular premolar-canine area. In the maxilla, it is most often observed in the canine-lateral incisor area. Most examples are less than 1.0 cm in diameter. Those lateral periodontal cysts that exhibit a loculated radiographic appearance and/or a polycystic lesion on gross or microscopic examination have been termed "botryoid odontogenic cysts."

The lateral periodontal cyst is treated by conservative surgical enucleation. Recurrence is uncommon. However, there seems to be an increased possibility of recurrence in the polycystic variant.

### Figure 12.7
**GINGIVAL CYST OF THE ADULT**
Cystic lesion of gingiva adjacent to a mandibular canine.

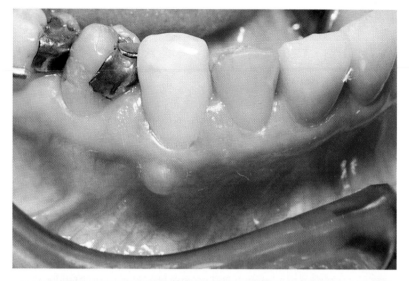

### Figure 12.8
**LATERAL PERIODONTAL CYST**
Typical location between the roots of vital mandibular premolars.

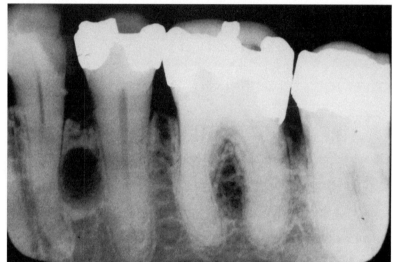

### Figure 12.9
**INFLAMMATORY CYST SIMULATING A LATERAL PERIODONTAL CYST**
This lesion cannot be radiographically differentiated from a lateral periodontal cyst. This lesion proved to be an inflammatory cyst related to a necrotic pulp in the second premolar. (Courtesy of Dr. Richard Ziegler.)

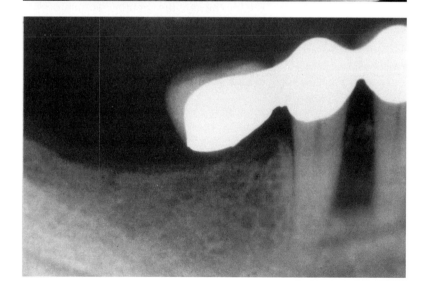

## Figs. 12.10 to 12.14

The odontogenic keratocyst is a developmental odontogenic cyst that deserves special consideration because of its clinical behavior. It seems to arise from remnants of dental lamina and represents 3 to 12% of all odontogenic cysts. The chief concerns with this lesion are its potentially aggressive growth and a recurrence rate that is higher than that of other odontogenic cysts. The odontogenic keratocyst also is the jaw cyst found in the nevoid basal cell carcinoma syndrome. It is encountered over a wide age range, but the peak prevalence is seen in patients in the second and third decades of life. In contrast, those that develop in the anterior midline of the maxilla have a mean age of nearly 70 years.

The odontogenic keratocyst can occur within any region of the jaws, but approximately 65 to 75% of them are located in the mandible, usually in the posterior body and ascending ramus. The cyst characteristically grows within the medullary spaces of the bone in an anteroposterior direction and may reach a large size without causing clinically obvious expansion of the jaw. Radiographically, the odontogenic keratocyst shows a well-circumscribed radiolucent area with a smooth and often sclerotic margin. Smaller lesions are unilocular, whereas larger cysts may present a multilocular radiolucent appearance.

It must be emphasized that the diagnosis of odontogenic keratocyst is made histopathologically; the radiographic appearance may resemble that of many other odontogenic cysts and neoplasms. In 25 to 40% of cases, an odontogenic keratocyst is associated with the crown of an unerupted tooth, suggesting a radiologic diagnosis of dentigerous cyst. A keratocyst located in an edentulous area cannot be differentiated radiographically from residual periapical inflammatory disease. In addition, the odontogenic keratocyst may develop between teeth, giving the radiographic appearance of a lateral periodontal cyst, or in the midline of the maxilla, mimicking a nasopalatine duct cyst. In some instances, the cyst develops in place of a tooth, usually the mandibular third molar. The earlier classifications of odontogenic cysts include the term "primordial cyst" for this situation. However, primordial cysts invariably exhibit the characteristic histopathology of the odontogenic keratocyst, and this term has been dropped from the current classification. Multiple odontogenic keratocysts strongly suggest the possibility of the nevoid basal cell carcinoma syndrome, but multiple cysts also have been described in patients who have no other signs of this condition. In rare instances, the cyst develops in the gingiva from remnants of dental lamina and clinically resembles the gingival cyst of the adult.

The treatment of the odontogenic keratocyst is variable, and no single method can be universally applied to all patients. All treatment modalities should include complete removal of the cyst and treatment of the bony cavity. The chief long-term complication of the cyst is recurrence, which has been estimated to be between 25 and 30%. Recurrence may appear more than 10 years after initial therapy, and an extended follow-up period is necessary. Squamous cell carcinoma is an extremely rare complication of the odontogenic keratocyst.

### Figure 12.10
### ODONTOGENIC KERATOCYST

This large keratocyst is associated with the crown of an unerupted mandibular third molar. (Courtesy of Dr. S. C. Roddy.)

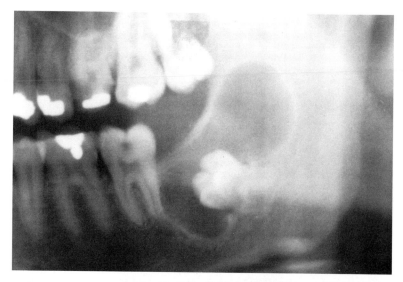

### Figure 12.11
### ODONTOGENIC KERATOCYST

A small odontogenic keratocyst located between the roots of vital second premolar and first molar teeth. Radiographically, the lesion suggests a lateral periodontal cyst.

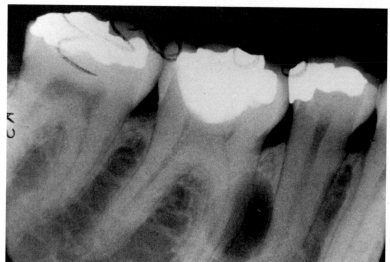

### Figure 12.12
### ODONTOGENIC KERATOCYST

An asymptomatic odontogenic keratocyst that has developed in place of the third molar. The patient denied a history of previous third molar removal.

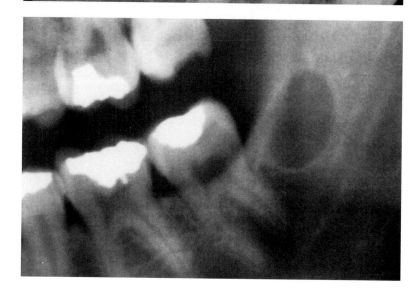

ODONTOGENIC CYSTS AND TUMORS

## ORTHOKERATINIZED ODONTOGENIC CYST

**Fig. 12.15**

The orthokeratinized odontogenic cyst is a developmental odontogenic cyst that forms a distinctive layer of luminal orthokeratin but is *not* considered to be an odontogenic keratocyst because of other histopathologic and clinical features. Misdiagnosis may result in overtreatment. The cyst usually occurs in the posterior mandible, and up to 75% are associated with an unerupted third molar, appearing like a dentigerous cyst. It is most often seen in the second and third decades of life, and there is a male predilection. Treatment is conservative surgical removal. The recurrence rate has been reported to be approximately 2%, in contrast to 25 to 30% for the odontogenic keratocyst. This cyst is not associated with the nevoid basal cell carcinoma syndrome.

### Figure 12.13
**ODONTOGENIC KERATOCYST**
Large multilocular lesion involving the posterior mandible and ascending ramus. (Courtesy of Dr. Jerry Merrell.)

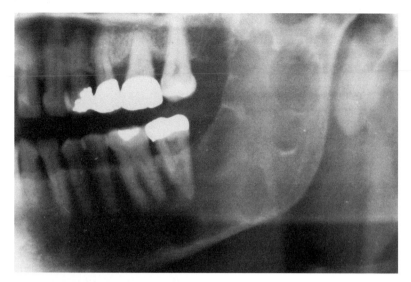

### Figure 12.14
**ODONTOGENIC KERATOCYST**
An odontogenic keratocyst positioned between vital maxillary incisors. The radiographic appearance is identical to a lateral periodontal cyst or a small nasopalatine duct cyst (Fig. 1.28).

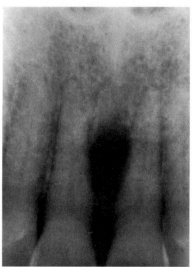

### Figure 12.15
**ORTHOKERATINIZED ODONTOGENIC CYST**
Unilocular radiolucency associated with crown of impacted third molar. Radiograph also could represent a dentigerous cyst, odontogenic keratocyst, or ameloblastoma.

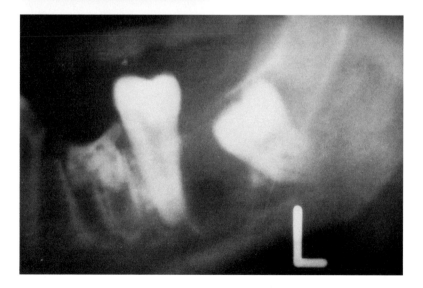

## Figs. 12.16, 12.17, and 12.18

The nevoid basal cell carcinoma syndrome is inherited as an autosomal-dominant trait with high penetrance and variable expressivity. It seems to be related to a mutation in a tumor suppressor gene on chromosome 9. The chief components are multiple basal cell carcinomas of the skin, jaw cysts, rib and vertebral anomalies, palmar and plantar pits, epidermal cysts, and intracranial calcifications (also see Figs. 12.19, 12.20, and 12.21). A host of other anomalies also have been reported in these patients, including ovarian fibromas and rare but nonrandom cases of cleft lip/palate and medulloblastoma. There is great variability in the expressivity of the various components, and no single component is present in all patients. Affected patients often present a characteristic facies with frontal and temporoparietal bossing, resulting in an increased cranial circumference. The eyes may appear widely separated, and about 40% of patients have true ocular hypertelorism. Mild mandibular prognathism is also a common finding.

Basal cell carcinomas of the skin are the most significant clinical finding. Approximately 80% of whites and 40% of African-Americans exhibited basal cell carcinomas in a large series of patients reported from the National Institute of Arthritis and Musculoskeletal and Skin Disease. The carcinomas are usually multiple; some patients have had more than 1000 separate tumors. The tumors usually develop after puberty or in the second and third decades of life but can first appear in young children. They usually involve the face, neck, back, and thorax, often in non–sun-exposed areas. Nevoid basal cell carcinomas cannot be microscopically differentiated from the ordinary type of basal cell carcinoma, and they demonstrate all of the histologic variants of that tumor. Clinically, the skin tumors may vary from small, flesh-colored papules to plaque-like or ulcerated lesions. Palmar and plantar pits are present in most patients.

### Figure 12.16
### NEVOID BASAL CELL CARCINOMA SYNDROME

This patient shows the characteristic frontal bossing. The right mandibular asymmetry is caused by a large keratocyst of the right mandible. The flame nevus of the left face is an incidental finding not related to the syndrome.

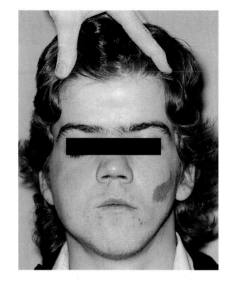

### Figure 12.17
### NEVOID BASAL CELL CARCINOMA SYNDROME

This 49-year-old man has had several hundred basal cell carcinomas removed from his face over a 20-year period. Several ulcerating basal cell carcinomas are present. The patient had multiple jaw cysts as a young man, and his son is also affected.

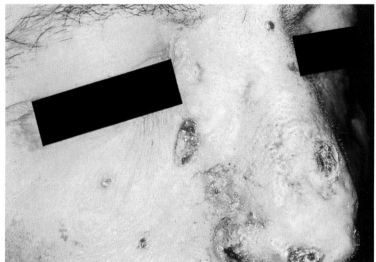

### Figure 12.18
### NEVOID BASAL CELL CARCINOMA SYNDROME

Plantar pits in a patient with this syndrome.

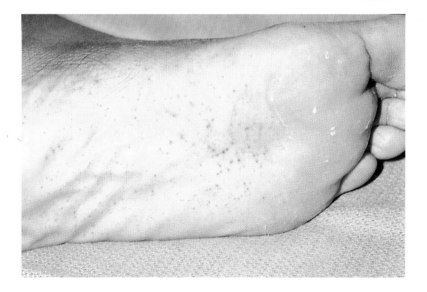

## Figs. 12.19, 12.20, and 12.21

Jaw cysts are one of the more constant features of the nevoid basal cell carcinoma syndrome and are present in three-fourths of affected persons. The cysts are more common in the mandible than in the maxilla and particularly involve the lower third molar and canine areas. The cysts commonly appear during the first decade of life and are a common initial manifestation of the syndrome because of swelling, pain, or intraoral drainage from a cyst. The cysts are usually multiple; some patients may have as many as 10 separate cysts. These cysts are invariably odontogenic keratocysts, although histopathologically they may show more florid epithelial proliferation and a greater tendency to form daughter cysts. Recurrence after enucleation is common. The multiple cysts frequently cause displacement of adjacent teeth or dilaceration of developing roots. The cysts in this syndrome are frequently associated with the crowns of developing teeth and radiographically resemble a dentigerous cyst. Patients with multiple jaw cysts should be evaluated for other manifestations of this syndrome.

Skeletal anomalies are present in about three-fourths of all patients. The most common anomaly is a bifid or splayed rib. This may involve several ribs and may be bilateral. Other skeletal anomalies include kyphoscoliosis, hemivertebrae, and fusion of vertebral bodies. A distinctive lamellar calcification of the falx cerebri, which can be noted on an anteroposterior skull film, is a highly consistent finding and is present in most patients with this syndrome. Most of the anomalies present in this syndrome are not life threatening. The prognosis largely depends on the behavior of the skin basal cell carcinomas.

**Figure 12.19**
**NEVOID BASAL CELL CARCINOMA SYNDROME**
Radiograph of a 26-year-old male showing multiple impacted teeth with pericoronal radiolucencies. (Courtesy of Dr. T. R. Kerley.)

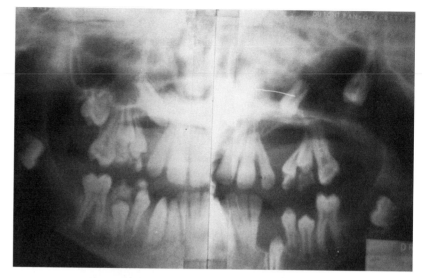

**Figure 12.20**
**NEVOID BASAL CELL CARCINOMA SYNDROME**
Chest radiograph showing several bifid ribs.

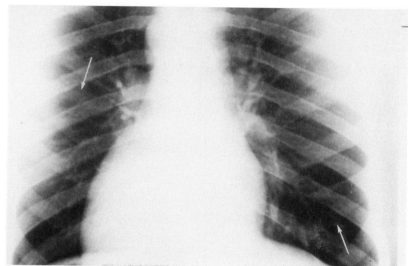

**Figure 12.21**
**NEVOID BASAL CELL CARCINOMA SYNDROME**
Skull radiograph of the patient depicted in Figure 12.16 showing calcification of the falx cerebri.

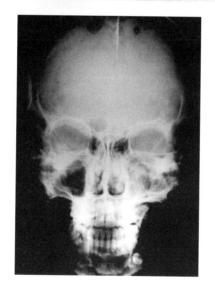

## CALCIFYING ODONTOGENIC CYST (GORLIN CYST)

### Figs. 12.22 and 12.23

The calcifying odontogenic cyst is an uncommon lesion that appears to arise from remnants of odontogenic epithelium either within bone or in the gingival soft tissues. Up to 30% of cases present as firm, localized gingival lesions without primary underlying bone involvement. About 85% of the cases represent cystic lesions, but the remaining grow in a solid fashion and are considered neoplasms. The term "dentinogenic ghost cell tumor" has been used to designate the solid form.

There is an equal distribution between the maxilla and the mandible, and the calcifying odontogenic cyst may occur at any age, with the peak occurrence in the second and third decades of life. Most cases are found in the incisor/canine region. Radiographically, the lesions usually exhibit a well-delineated, unilocular radiolucency, but they can be multilocular. The radiolucency may contain scattered radiopacities in up to half of the cases. About one-third of the lesions are associated with an impacted tooth; another common location is between the roots of teeth. They also frequently develop in association with odontomas. Most lesions are less than 3.0 cm in diameter, but examples up to 12.0 cm in diameter have been reported. Treatment is conservative surgical removal. Recurrences are uncommon and malignant transformation is rare.

## GLANDULAR ODONTOGENIC CYST

### Fig. 12.24

The glandular odontogenic cyst is a recently described developmental odontogenic cyst that has an epithelial lining exhibiting glandular differentiation. It occurs over a wide age range, with most persons being middle aged or older. Most cases develop in the anterior mandible, but they also occur in the anterior maxilla. Radiographically, the lesions present as well-defined unilocular or multilocular radiolucencies. An occasional lesion may develop in association with an impacted tooth. The glandular odontogenic cyst may exhibit aggressive growth, and a recurrence rate of 25% has been reported. Most cases have been treated by enucleation or curettage, but some authors have recommended en bloc resection for some lesions.

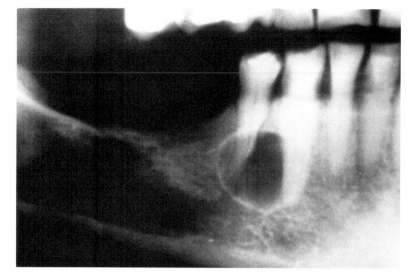

▶ **Figure 12.22**
**CALCIFYING ODONTOGENIC CYST**
Unilocular radiolucent lesion in the premolar-canine area. (Courtesy of Dr. S. R. Tucker.)

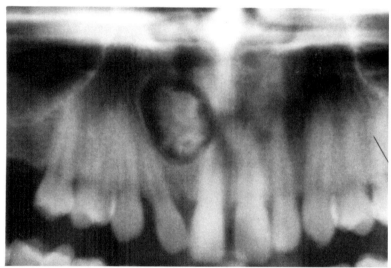

▶ **Figure 12.23**
**CALCIFYING ODONTOGENIC CYST**
Well-defined, unilocular lesion of the anterior maxilla with central odontoma. (Courtesy of Dr. Pinckney Harper.)

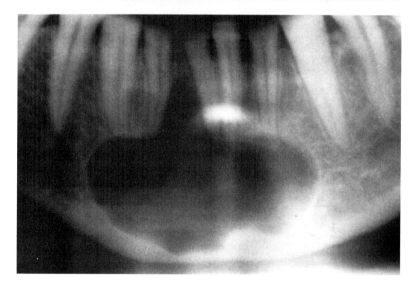

▶ **Figure 12.24**
**GLANDULAR ODONTOGENIC CYST**
Well-defined radiolucency of the anterior mandible with extension between roots of vital incisors. (Courtesy of Dr. Carroll Gallagher.)

## Figs. 12.25, 12.26, and 12.27

Squamous cell carcinoma arising from the epithelial lining of an odontogenic cyst is rare but may be somewhat more common than is generally appreciated. Carcinomatous change has been observed in the lining of dentigerous cysts, periapical cysts, residual cysts, odontogenic keratocysts, and orthokeratinized odontogenic cysts. About 40% have been associated with "residual cysts," and about 20% have been related to dentigerous cysts. Most develop in middle-aged or older persons, and there is a marked male predilection. Nearly 80% occur in the mandible. The radiographs frequently do not suggest a malignant lesion, and the diagnosis is made only after microscopic examination of the presumed cyst. Some patients complain of pain in the involved area. The prognosis is variable, but about half the patients survive for 5 years.

▶ **Figure 12.25**
**CARCINOMA ARISING IN ODONTOGENIC CYST**
Radiolucent lesion surrounding the crown of an unerupted mandibular third molar in a 58-year-old man. The operative diagnosis was dentigerous cyst, but microscopic examination revealed a squamous cell carcinoma arising in the cyst lining.

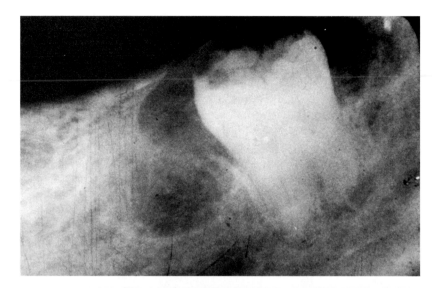

▶ **Figure 12.26**
**CARCINOMA ARISING IN ODONTOGENIC CYST**
Massive tumor involving face of a patient who was treated for an odontogenic keratocyst 19 years previously. Review of the original biopsy sample showed severe epithelial dysplasia in the cyst lining. She had multiple recurrences and received radiation therapy 7 years earlier.

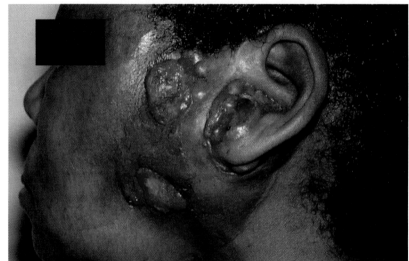

▶ **Figure 12.27**
**CARCINOMA ARISING IN ODONTOGENIC CYST**
Nuclear magnetic resonance image from the patient shown in Figure 12.26 showing an extensive tumor of the jaws and face.

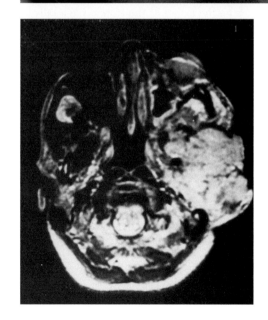

## Figs. 12.28 to 12.33

The ameloblastoma is a locally aggressive odontogenic neoplasm in which ameloblastic differentiation is present. It is the most common true odontogenic tumor, excluding the relatively common odontoma, which in most cases represents a hamartoma of odontogenic tissue rather than a neoplasm. Its prevalence exceeds that of all other odontogenic tumors combined. The ameloblastoma is derived from remnants of dental lamina, and it can arise from the lining of dentigerous cysts. Peripheral ameloblastomas also may develop from surface epithelium of the gingiva. It is capable of causing significant oral and facial deformity and has a high recurrence rate if inadequately treated. Based on the clinical and radiographic findings and histopathologic appearance, three categories of ameloblastoma have been designated to help manage patients because the individual categories exhibit differences in behavior and recurrence rates and do not require the same extent of surgical management. The three categories or types are conventional, unicystic, and peripheral (extraosseous).

The conventional type of ameloblastoma is the most common type and consists of a solid, infiltrating component, but areas of cyst formation may be present. It may arise de novo or from a preexisting unicystic type. The conventional ameloblastoma is more common in adults, with the average age of the patient at the time of diagnosis being approximately 36 years. Eighty-five percent of cases occur in the mandible, with 60% developing in the molar region and ramus. It usually presents as a multilocular radiolucency. It often is described as having a "soap bubble" appearance when the loculations are large or as "honeycombed" when small loculations are present. The margins are usually well defined, but there may be areas that are less well demarcated. Conventional ameloblastomas also may be unilocular, and they often are associated with an unerupted tooth. Root resorption of teeth adjacent to the tumor is frequently noted. One histopathologic form of the conventional type, the desmoplastic variant, induces new bone formation in the supporting connective tissue, and the radiographic picture may appear as a mixed radiolucent-radiopaque lesion that may be interpreted as a fibro-osseous lesion. In contrast to the other histopathologic forms of the conventional ameloblastoma, this variant is most common in the maxilla and anterior regions of the jaws.

As a rule, conventional ameloblastomas are painless, slow-growing tumors that remain asymptomatic until they reach a large size. A painless swelling of the bone is the most common presenting symptom, and buccal and lingual cortical expansion is frequently present. Treatment depends on the extent of the tumor. Generally, these tumors are treated by en bloc removal because this type of ameloblastoma tends to infiltrate between trabeculae of intact bone before resorption is evident. Therefore, the margins of the tumor often extend beyond the apparent clinical or radiographic margins. Removal of the tumor by curettage will likely leave small islands of tumor within the bone, which will later manifest as a recurrence. Involvement of cortical bone and/or overlying soft tissue usually requires more extensive surgery. The overall recurrence rate of conventional ameloblastoma is approximately 23%. However, it is nearly 35% for cases treated by conservative therapy. Ameloblastomas of the posterior maxilla are particularly dangerous because of their anatomic location and difficulty in establishing an adequate surgical margin. Death has resulted from direct extension into the base of the skull.

The unicystic variant of ameloblastoma is a relatively new category that has been created because of the differences between it and the conventional type. It represents approximately 6% of reported cases of ameloblastoma, but this figure probably is too low in light of current cases of ameloblastoma being reported. This type most often is discovered in the second and third decades of life, and the peak prevalence is about one and a half decades earlier than that of the conventional type. The average age at time of diagnosis is approximately 22 years. Its typical radiographic presentation is that of a well-defined, unilocular radiolucency associated with the crown of an unerupted tooth, usually a mandibular third molar, that cannot be differentiated from a dentigerous cyst or an odontogenic keratocyst. It also may appear as a unilocular radiolucency that is nonspecific. The definitive diagnosis of the unicystic ameloblastoma requires correlation of the clinical finding of a cyst at the time of surgery and the histopathologic findings of a unicystic structure lined by ameloblastic epithelium. They probably arise from neoplastic alteration of a preexisting cyst or develop de novo as a unicystic neoplasm from remnants of primitive dental lamina. Conservative surgical management such as curettage has been used for the unicystic ameloblastoma when the neoplastic epithelium is confined to the lumen of the cyst. If the ameloblastic epithelium has penetrated into the adjacent connective tissue stroma, more aggressive treatment of the surrounding bone usually is required. The recurrence rate for true unicystic ameloblastoma is approximately 14%. Long-term follow-up is required for both this type of ameloblastoma and the conventional type.

**AMELOBLASTOMA**
Large multilocular ("soap bubble") lesion of
the mandible. An impacted premolar is
displaced to the lower border of the
mandible. (Courtesy of Dr. Tony
Traynham.)

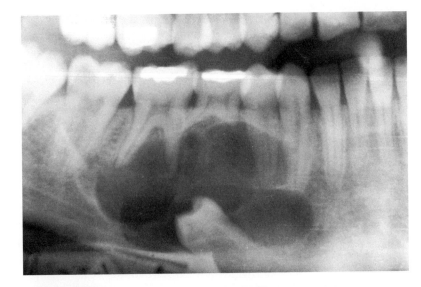

▶ **Figure 12.29**
**AMELOBLASTOMA**
Large multilocular lesion of the mandible.
An impacted third molar is located near
the angle of the mandible.

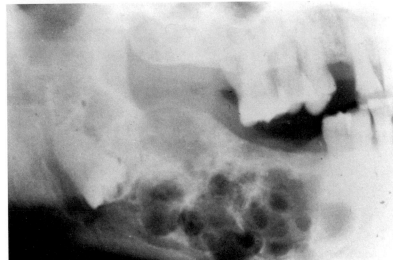

▶ **Figure 12.30**
**AMELOBLASTOMA**
Unicystic ameloblastoma associated with
the crown of an unerupted lower third
molar. Radiographically, the lesion
resembles a typical dentigerous cyst.

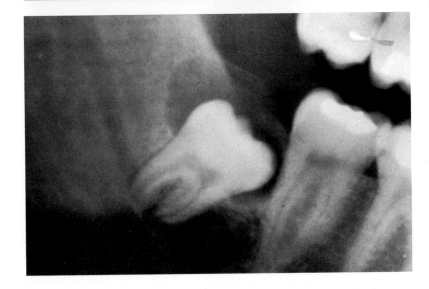

Large unicystic ameloblastoma of the left
mandible associated with impacted third
molar and causing significant destruction
of ramus.

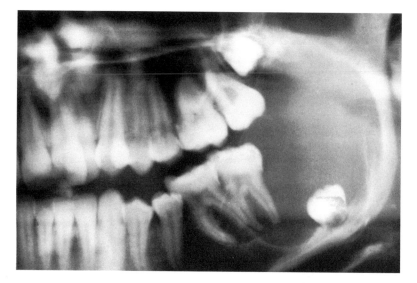

▶ **Figure 12.32**
**AMELOBLASTOMA**

A 15-year-old female with expansion of
palate from maxillary ameloblastoma.

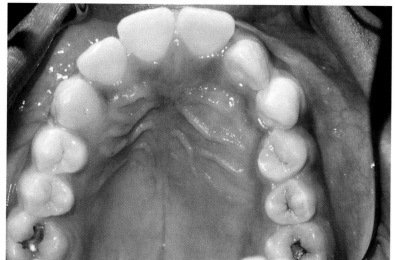

▶ **Figure 12.33**
**AMELOBLASTOMA**

Computed tomographic scan of the same
patient depicted in Figure 12.32 showing
an ameloblastoma that has almost filled
the sinus and has encroached on nasal
cavity. Buccal and palatal cortical plates
are expanded, and there is perforation of
the buccal plate in one area. The tumor
was primarily cystic in nature but showed
areas of mural invasion.

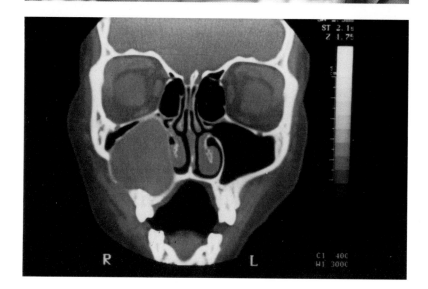

## PERIPHERAL (EXTRAOSSEOUS) AMELOBLASTOMA

### Fig. 12.34

Peripheral (extraosseous) ameloblastomas are rare lesions that present as pedunculated or sessile gingival masses seldom exceeding 2 cm in diameter. They usually are mucosal colored. They originate from rests of dental lamina in gingival connective tissue or from overlying surface epithelium. Other odontogenic neoplasms also develop in soft tissue, but the ameloblastoma accounts for approximately 50% of all peripheral odontogenic tumors. The average age at diagnosis is 51 years, and 65% of the tumors arise in the anterior regions of the jaws. There is a mandibular predilection of 5:1. Multicentric cases have been reported, and rare cases of malignant peripheral ameloblastomas have been described. The tumor originates in soft tissue, although superficial erosion of the underlying bone is occasionally present. The peripheral ameloblastoma seems to be less aggressive than its intraosseous counterpart, and the prognosis after local excision is excellent. A recurrence rate of 8% has been reported.

## MALIGNANT AMELOBLASTOMA AND AMELOBLASTIC CARCINOMA

### Figs. 12.35 and 12.36

In rare instances, an ameloblastoma may exhibit the true features of malignancy. In some situations, a cytologically benign ameloblastoma has metastasized and the cytologic features of the metastatic focus appear like the primary jaw lesion without dysplastic cellular alterations. This type of ameloblastoma has been designated as "malignant ameloblastoma." The term "ameloblastic carcinoma" is used to designate an ameloblastoma that exhibits cytologic features of malignancy in the primary tumor or in any metastasis.

In both situations there is a significant mandibular predilection. In cases of malignant ameloblastoma, the clinical history often includes extensive local disease and a long history of duration of the tumor, with recurrences and several surgical procedures. Most metastases are solitary, and the most common site is the lung. Other sites of metastasis have included the lymph nodes, spine, liver, and brain. In ameloblastic carcinoma, the disease often exhibits aggressive local behavior with rapid growth and pain. The radiographs may show a poorly defined destructive lesion, and there may be perforation of cortical bone and extension into surrounding soft tissue. The lungs are the most common site for metastasis.

Treatment of the primary tumor is surgical resection. In both situations the prognosis is poor, with death usually occurring 1 to 2 years after metastasis has been detected. Metastasis and carcinomatous transformation of peripheral ameloblastomas also have been described.

### Figure 12.34
### PERIPHERAL AMELOBLASTOMA
This lobulated soft-tissue ameloblastoma cannot be distinguished clinically from a number of gingival tumors. There was no involvement of the underlying bone. (Courtesy of Dr. S. R. Tucker.)

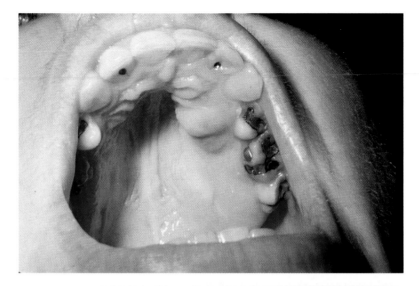

### Figure 12.35
### AMELOBLASTIC CARCINOMA
This 64-year-old woman has noted mandibular swelling for 3 months. It recently has become painful.

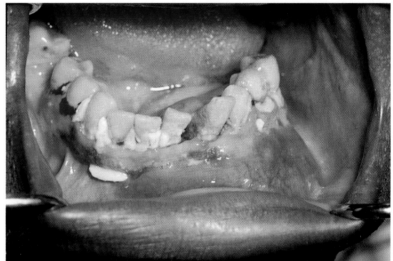

### Figure 12.36
### AMELOBLASTIC CARCINOMA
Panoramic radiograph of the same patient depicted in Figure 12.35 showing extensive destruction of the mandible with loss of the lower border.

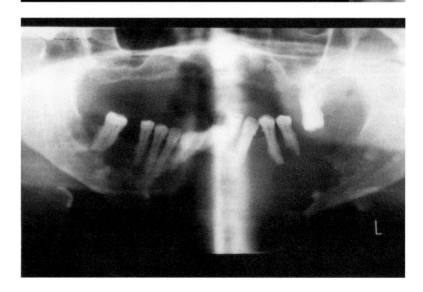

## Figs. 12.37, 12.38, and 12.39

The adenomatoid odontogenic tumor represents 3 to 7% of all odontogenic tumors and is chiefly found in patients younger than age 20 years. There is a female predilection, and 75% of cases are located in the anterior regions of the jaws. About 65% of cases are found in the maxilla. The tumor is asymptomatic, and small lesions are discovered on routine radiographic examination or when failure of tooth eruption is investigated. Larger tumors cause a painless swelling of the affected bone. Radiographically, the lesion presents as a well-demarcated radiolucent area that, in about 75% of patients, surrounds or is adjacent to the crown of an unerupted tooth, usually the cuspid. This radiographic appearance is often indistinguishable from that of a dentigerous cyst. The other cases usually occur between the roots of teeth and cause separation of the involved tooth roots and displacement of teeth. Histopathologically, many adenomatoid odontogenic tumors demonstrate small calcifications associated with the proliferating epithelial elements. These may appear on the radiograph as small "snowflake" calcifications interspersed within the radiolucent area. Most adenomatoid odontogenic tumors are less than 3 cm in diameter, although a few examples of large tumors have been reported. The adenomatoid odontogenic tumor is an encapsulated lesion that tends to enucleate with relative ease. The prognosis is excellent, and only one reported case of recurrence has been identified. Extraosseous adenomatoid odontogenic tumors are rare and present as small swellings on the anterior facial gingiva.

► **Figure 12.37**
**ADENOMATOID ODONTOGENIC TUMOR**
Painless enlargement of the maxillary
lateral incisor-canine area. (Courtesy of Dr.
Louis Belinfante.)

► **Figure 12.37**
**ADENOMATOID ODONTOGENIC TUMOR**
Painless enlargement of the maxillary
lateral incisor-canine area. (Courtesy of Dr.
Louis Belinfante.)

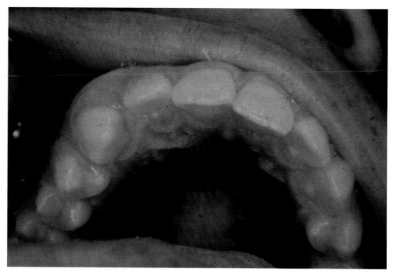

► **Figure 12.38**
**ADENOMATOID ODONTOGENIC TUMOR**
Periapical radiograph of the same patient
depicted in Figure 12.37 showing a
circumscribed radiolucent lesion containing
small focal calcifications. (Courtesy of
Louis Belinfante.)

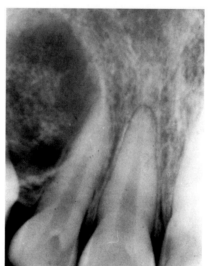

► **Figure 12.39**
**ADENOMATOID ODONTOGENIC TUMOR**
Large radiolucent lesion in the anterior
mandible associated with an unerupted
canine tooth.

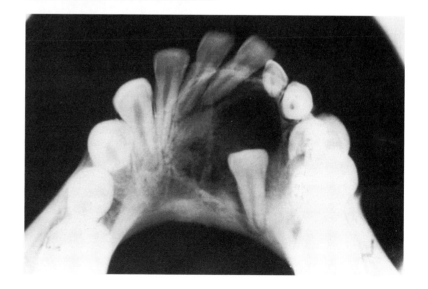

## Figs. 12.40 and 12.41

The calcifying epithelial odontogenic tumor is a rare odontogenic neoplasm that accounts for about 1% of all odontogenic tumors. There is a wide age range, but most patients are in the third to sixth decades of life. About 5% of the tumors are extraosseous and occur on the anterior gingiva. Approximately two-thirds of the intrabony lesions are located in the mandible, usually the premolar-molar region. Most present as a slowly growing, painless swelling. The radiographic findings are variable. Most are associated with an impacted tooth and are radiolucent. Smaller tumors tend to be unilocular; larger lesions often assume a multilocular, honeycombed appearance. It may be well defined or more poorly delineated. The neoplasm also may have a radiopaque component. Calcifications of varying size may be diffusely distributed within the radiolucency or concentrated near the crown of the associated, unerupted tooth. The calcifying epithelial odontogenic tumor seems to be less aggressive than the ameloblastoma, and treatment consists of conservative surgical removal. Recent studies have indicated a recurrence rate of approximately 15%. However, one histopathologic variant, the clear cell type, may be more aggressive and has a higher recurrence rate. Rare carcinomatous transformation has been documented.

# SQUAMOUS ODONTOGENIC TUMOR

## Fig. 12.42

The squamous odontogenic tumor is a rare, benign odontogenic neoplasm that may arise from the epithelial rests of Malassez. There is a wide age range, but the prevalence peaks in the third decade of life. There is almost an equal distribution between the mandible and maxilla. The most commonly affected area of the mandible is the premolar-molar region; in the maxilla, the most common site is the anterior region. The lesion usually presents as a radiolucency within alveolar bone between erupted teeth. Some cases have been well-defined masses, but others have resembled periodontal disease. In addition, cases have developed in association with unerupted teeth, simulating a dentigerous cyst. About 30% of the patients have had multiple lesions, including multiple members of one family. An extraosseous case also has been documented. Local surgical excision of the lesion seems to be effective therapy. Recurrence is rare.

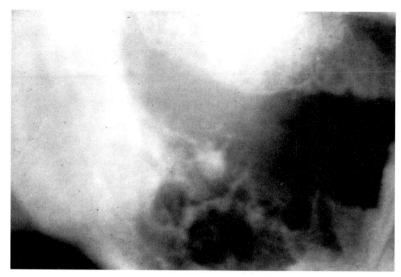

### ▶ Figure 12.40
### CALCIFYING EPITHELIAL ODONTOGENIC TUMOR

Irregular radiolucent lesion in the mandible of a 58-year-old female. Calcified foci of various size are present within the lesion.

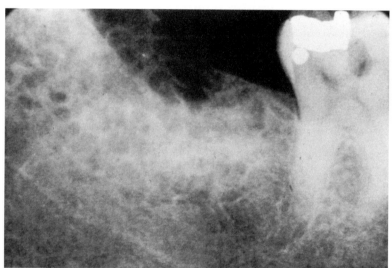

### ▶ Figure 12.41
### CALCIFYING EPITHELIAL ODONTOGENIC TUMOR

This posterior mandibular tumor shows a fine honeycombed multilocular radiolucent appearance.

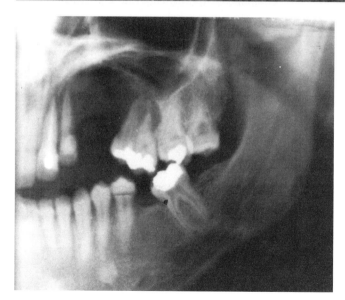

### ▶ Figure 12.42
### SQUAMOUS ODONTOGENIC TUMOR

Marginal alveolar bone defect in the maxillary premolar area, suggesting vertical periodontal bone loss. (Courtesy of Dr. Ed McGaha.)

## AMELOBLASTIC FIBROMA

### Fig. 12.43

The ameloblastic fibroma is characterized by neoplastic proliferation of both odontogenic epithelium and odontogenic ectomesenchyme and represents about 2% of all odontogenic tumors. The epithelial component can mimic that of the ameloblastoma, but this tumor is much less aggressive. Most cases occur in the first two decades of life, with peak prevalence in the second decade. The ameloblastic fibroma is found in the posterior mandible about 80% of the time. The tumor is generally asymptomatic, although large lesions may result in bone expansion. Radiographically, the lesion presents as a unilocular or occasionally multilocular radiolucency often associated with an unerupted tooth. The margins usually are well outlined with a sclerotic border. A cumulative recurrence rate of 18% has been reported after conservative excision. Malignant transformation to ameloblastic fibrosarcoma is rare but has been documented.

## AMELOBLASTIC FIBRO-ODONTOMA

### Figs. 12.44 and 12.45

The ameloblastic fibro-odontoma is one of the more common odontogenic neoplasms and represents a combination of an ameloblastic fibroma and developing complex odontoma. It is seen almost exclusively in the first two decades of life, with the average age of the patient being 9 years. The mandible and maxilla are involved with about equal frequency, and most occur in the posterior regions of the jaws. Smaller lesions are generally discovered when radiographs are taken to determine the reason for failure of a tooth to erupt. However, some ameloblastic fibro-odontomas have grown to a large size, causing bony expansion. Radiographically, the lesion presents as a sharply circumscribed, unilocular or multilocular radiolucency that contains variable amounts of calcified material with the radiodensity of enamel and dentin. If the tumor contains only a small amount of uncalcified or slightly calcified enamel and dentinal matrix, it appears completely radiolucent and cannot be radiographically differentiated from a number of other odontogenic and nonodontogenic lesions. Some lesions, however, exhibit a significant radiopaque component. Approximately 80% are associated with an unerupted tooth. The ameloblastic fibro-odontoma enucleates with relative ease from the bony defect, and recurrence is essentially nonexistent.

**AMELOBLASTIC FIBROMA**
Unilocular radiolucent lesion involving the posterior body and ascending ramus of the mandible in a young male. The developing second molar has been displaced to the lower border of the mandible.

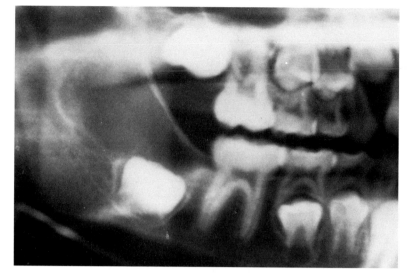

► **Figure 12.44**
**AMELOBLASTIC FIBRO-ODONTOMA**
Large tumor with prominent central calcified component in an 8-year-old girl.

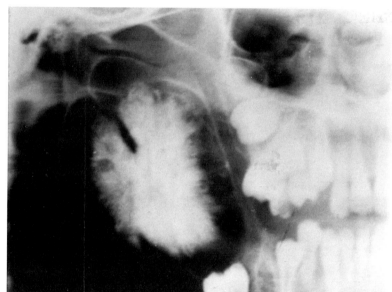

► **Figure 12.45**
**AMELOBLASTIC FIBRO-ODONTOMA**
Large, well-defined radiolucency of the posterior mandible associated with an impacted tooth. Small flecks of calcification are concentrated in the superior portion of the lesion. The inferior border has been expanded.

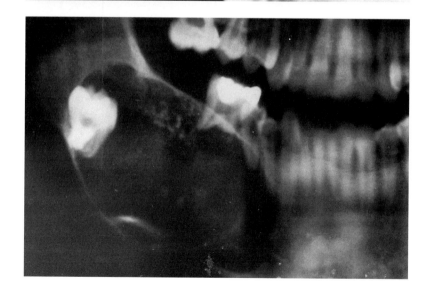

**Fig. 12.46 and 12.47**

The ameloblastic fibrosarcoma is a rare odontogenic cancer that consists of ameloblastic fibroma elements but with a malignant stroma. About half of the reported cases seem to have evolved from recurrent ameloblastic fibromas. The average age of 27.5 years is about a decade older than that for the typical ameloblastic fibroma. Approximately 80% occur in the mandible, and radiographically they present as radiolucencies with poorly defined margins. Treatment consists of radical surgical removal. Several patients have died of extension of local disease or as the result of metastasis.

## CLEAR CELL ODONTOGENIC CARCINOMA

**Fig. 12.48**

The clear cell odontogenic carcinoma is a rare odontogenic neoplasm that has the capacity for locally aggressive behavior, recurrence, and metastasis. It primarily occurs in middle-aged and older adults, with a peak prevalence in the seventh decade of life. There is a marked female predominance, and the mandible is affected in about 75% of the cases. Most develop in the anterior regions of the jaws. Radiographically, the tumor usually presents as a nonspecific, ill-defined radiolucency. Jaw expansion is usually present, and pain is not uncommon. Regional lymph node and disseminated metastasis has occurred in affected patients. Treatment of the primary tumor is surgical resection. As of this writing, 4 of 19 reported patients have died of their disease.

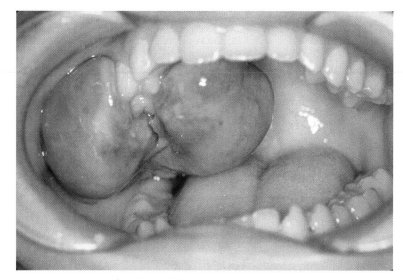

### Figure 12.46
**AMELOBLASTIC FIBROSARCOMA**

Extensive swelling of the posterior maxilla. (Courtesy of Tajima Y, Utsumi N, Suzuki S, et al. Ameloblastic fibrosarcoma arising de novo in the maxilla. Pathol Int 1997;47:564.)

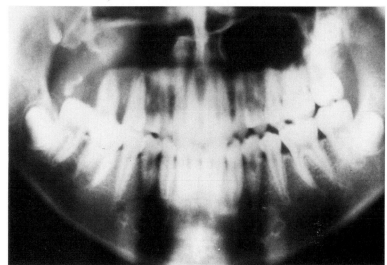

### Figure 12.47
**AMELOBLASTIC FIBROSARCOMA**

Ill-defined, destructive radiolucency of the posterior maxilla in the same patient depicted in Figure 12.46. (Courtesy of Dr. Yoshifumi Tajima.)

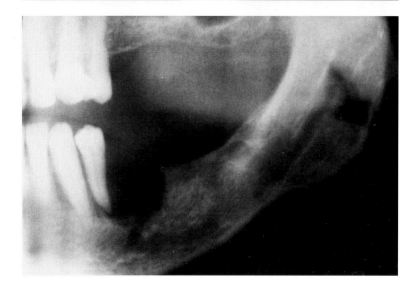

### Figure 12.48
**CLEAR CELL ODONTOGENIC CARCINOMA**

Unilocular radiolucency of the mid-body of the mandible in a middle-aged adult. The patient has a history of previous extraction of loose teeth. The lesion is not well-delineated.

## Figs. 12.49, 12.50, and 12.51

Odontomas are benign hamartomatous proliferations composed of enamel, dentin, cementum, and pulp in varying amounts. They are relatively common and are subclassified into compound and complex types. Compound odontomas are composed of multiple (occasionally 100 or more) toothlike structures. Complex odontomas consist of a mass of enamel, dentin, and cementum arranged in a haphazard fashion. The compound and complex types occur with about equal frequency and are seen somewhat more often in the maxilla than in the mandible. Compound odontomas are noted more commonly in the anterior parts of the jaws, whereas the greatest number of complex odontomas occur in the molar regions.

Most odontomas are detected in the first three decades of life and are usually found on a routine radiographic examination or when films are taken to determine the cause for failure of tooth eruption. Most odontomas are relatively small, seldom exceeding the size of a tooth in the anatomic site where they are found. Some odontomas, however, have grown to a significant size and caused bone expansion. Most are associated with the crowns of unerupted teeth, but they also occur between the roots of erupted teeth. The radiographic appearance is usually diagnostic, with a small radiolucent rim separating the proliferation from surrounding normal bone. However, some complex odontomas may mimic a fibro-osseous lesion such as focal osseous dysplasia (Fig. 11.37). Odontomas also have developed in association with other odontogenic cysts and neoplasms, and this possibility should be considered if significant areas of radiolucency are present. Rare extraosseous odontomas have occurred in the gingiva. The treatment for odontomas is enucleation. True recurrence has not been reported.

▶ **Figure 12.49**
**COMPOUND ODONTOMA**
This lesion in the anterior maxilla of a 10-year-old girl contains several dozen rudimentary teeth. (Courtesy of Dr. Roland Lafond.)

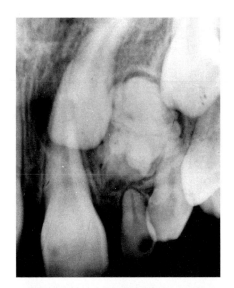

▶ **Figure 12.50**
**COMPOUND ODONTOMA**
Three miniature, toothlike structures surrounded by a thin rim of radiolucency between mandibular first and second molars.

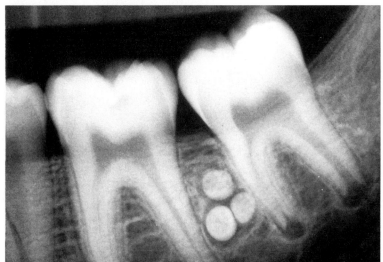

▶ **Figure 12.51**
**COMPLEX ODONTOMA**
Radiograph of a large, complex odontoma associated with an impacted second molar in a 13-year-old girl. (Courtesy of Dr. D. C. Wetmore.)

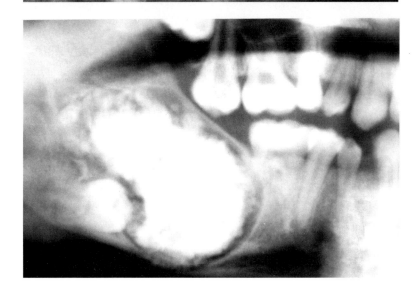

## Fig. 12.52

The odontogenic fibroma is a rare odontogenic neoplasm whose exact definition is still not clearly delineated. Two histopathologic patterns exist that have been accepted within the framework of this term. The neoplasm has been seen over a wide age range, with the mean age being approximately 40 years. There is a significant female predilection and a slight mandibular predominance. Most cases in the maxilla have occurred in the anterior region, and in the mandible it is usually seen the posterior areas. Radiographically, the lesion presents as a unilocular or occasionally multilocular radiolucency with well-defined margins. It usually arises between the roots of teeth, but nearly one-third of the reported cases have been associated with the crown of an unerupted tooth. Most cases have been treated by curettage; recurrence is uncommon. A peripheral form of the odontogenic fibroma involves the gingiva and clinically cannot be differentiated from the more common peripheral ossifying fibroma or other peripheral odontogenic tumors.

## ODONTOGENIC MYXOMA

## Figs. 12.53 and 12.54

The odontogenic myxoma is believed to arise from primitive odontogenic ectomesenchyme and bears a close histologic resemblance to the mesodermal portion of the developing tooth (dental papilla). Myxomas of the jaws have been reported in patients over a wide age range, with a peak prevalence in the second and third decades of life. The mandible is somewhat more often involved than the maxilla. The tumor may grow to a large size, causing swelling and distortion of the affected bone. A painless, localized swelling is the most common initial complaint. Radiographically, the tumor presents as a radiolucency, often with irregular or scalloped margins. The radiolucent area frequently contains fine residual trabeculae, often arranged at acute angles to one another. Large myxomas often show a multilocular appearance closely simulating that of an ameloblastoma.

Myxomas tend to infiltrate adjacent bone and to recur after enucleation and curettage. Large tumors may require en bloc resection. Recurrence rates have varied considerably in series of reported cases. However, the prognosis is good after surgical removal. An exceedingly rare cytologically atypical and clinically aggressive form has been designated as "odontogenic myxosarcoma."

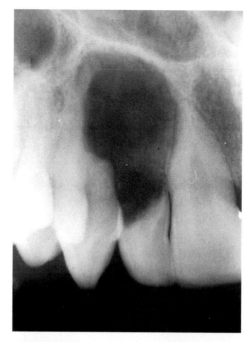

▶ **Figure 12.52**
**ODONTOGENIC FIBROMA**
Radiolucent lesion in the anterior maxilla of a 37-year-old female. The tumor has caused resorption of the roots of the lateral incisor and canine teeth. (Courtesy of Dr. Mark Bowden.)

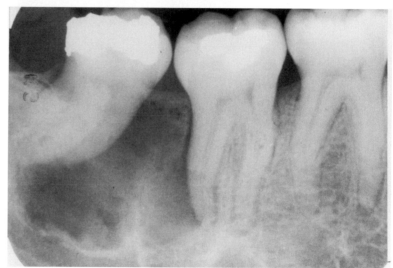

▶ **Figure 12.53**
**ODONTOGENIC MYXOMA**
This mandibular lesion in a 43-year-old female was asymptomatic and was detected during a routine radiographic examination.

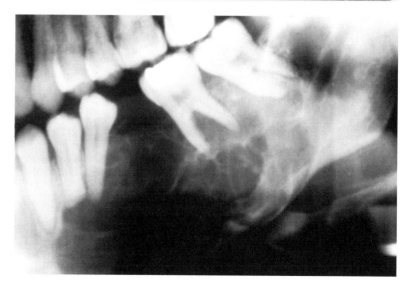

▶ **Figure 12.54**
**ODONTOGENIC MYXOMA**
Large multilocular lesion of the mandible in a 28-year-old woman. Root resorption is present on several teeth. (Courtesy of Dr. T. R. Kerley.)

ODONTOGENIC CYSTS AND TUMORS

# SUGGESTED READINGS

## Odontogenic Cysts—General Considerations

Daley TED, Wysocki GP. New developments in selected cysts of the jaws. J Can Dent Assoc 1997;63:526.

Daley TD, Wysocki GP, Pringle GA. Relative incidence of odontogenic tumors and oral and jaw cysts in a Canadian population. Oral Surg Oral Med Oral Pathol 1994;77:276.

Kramer IRH, Pindborg JJ, Shear M. Histological typing of odontogenic tumors. 2nd ed. Berlin: Springer-Verlag, 1992.

Kreidler JF, Raubenheimer EJ, van Heerden WF. A retrospective analysis of 367 cystic lesions of the jaw: the Ulm experience. J Craniomaxillofac Surg 1993;21:339.

Li T, Browne RM, Matthews JB. Immunocytochemical expression of growth factors by odontogenic jaw cysts. Mol Pathol 1997;50:21.

Shear M. Developmental odontogenic cysts: an update. J Oral Pathol Med 1994;23:1.

## Dentigerous Cyst/Eruption Cyst

Anderson RA. Eruption cysts: a retrograde study. J Dent Child 1990;57:124.

Been A, Altini M. Dentigerous cysts of inflammatory origin: a clinicopathologic study. Oral Surg Oral Med Oral Pathol Oral Radiol Endod 1996;81:203.

Boyczuk MP, Berger JR, Lazow SK. Identifying a deciduous dentigerous cyst. J Am Dent Assoc 1995; 126:643.

Brookstone MS, Huvos AG. Central salivary gland tumors of the maxilla and mandible: a clinicopathologic study of 11 cases with an analysis of the literature. J Oral Maxillofac Surg 1992;50:229.

Carr MM, Anderson RD, Clarke KD. Multiple dentigerous cysts in childhood. J Otolaryngol 1996;25:267.

Daley TD, Wysocki GP. The small dentigerous cyst: a diagnostic dilemma. Oral Surg Oral Med Oral Pathol Oral Radiol Endod 1995;79:77.

Gardner DG. Plexiform unicystic ameloblastoma: a diagnostic problem in dentigerous cysts. Cancer 1981;47:1358.

Leider AS, Eversole LR, Barkin ME. Cystic ameloblastoma. Oral Surg Oral Med Oral Pathol 1985;60:624.

Manganaro AM, Cross SE, Startzell JM. Carcinoma arising in a dentigerous cyst with neck metastasis. Head Neck 1997;19:436.

Seward MH. Eruption cyst: an analysis of its clinical features. J Oral Surg 1973;31:31.

Som PM, Shangold LM, Biller HF. A palatal dentigerous cyst arising from a mesiodente. Am J Neuroradiol 1992;13:212.

## Gingival Cyst of the Newborn/Adult

Bell RC, Chauvin PJ, Tyler MT. Gingival cyst of the adult: a review and a report of eight cases. J Can Dent Assoc 1997;63:533.

Buchner A, Hansen LS. Histomorphologic spectrum of the gingival cyst in the adult. Oral Surg Oral Med Oral Pathol 1979;48:532.

Cataldo E, Berkman MD. Cysts of the oral mucosa in newborns. Am J Dis Child 19687;116:44.

Fromm A. Epstein's pearls, Bohn's nodules and inclusion cysts of the oral cavity. J Dent Child 1967;34:275.

Jorgenson RJ, Shapiro SD, Salinas CF, et al. Intraoral findings and anomalies in neonates. Pediatrics 1982;69:577.

Nxumalo TN, Shear M. Gingival cysts of the adult. J Oral Pathol Med 1992;21:309.

## Lateral Periodontal Cyst

Altini M, Shear M. The lateral periodontal cyst: an update. J Oral Pathol Med 1992;21:245.

Carter LC, Carney YL, Perez-Pudlewski D: Lateral periodontal cyst: multifactorial analysis of a previously unreported series. Oral Surg Oral Med Oral Pathol Oral Radiol Endod 1996;81:210.

Gurol M, Burkes EJ Jr, Jacoway J. Botryoid odontogenic cyst: analysis of 33 cases. J Periodontol 1995;66:1069.

Rasmusson LG, Magnusson BC, Borrman H. The lateral periodontal cyst: a histopathological and radiographic study of 32 cases. Br J Oral Maxillofac Surg 1991;29:54.

Wysocki GP, Brannon RB, Gardner DG, et al. Histogenesis of the lateral periodontal cyst and gingival cysts of the adult. Oral Surg Oral Med Oral Pathol 1980;50:327.

## Odontogenic Keratocyst

Ahlfors E, Larsson A, Sjögren S. The odontogenic keratocyst: a benign cystic neoplasm? J Oral Maxillofac Surg 1984;42:10.

Anand VK, Arrowood JP, Krolls SO. Odontogenic keratocyst: a study of 50 patients. Laryngoscope 1995; 105:14.

Brannon RB. The odontogenic keratocyst: a clinicopathologic study of 312 cases, part I: clinical features. Oral Surg Oral Med Oral Pathol 1976;42:54.

Browne RM. Per(cyst)ent growth: the odontogenic keratocyst 40 years on. Ann R Coll Surg Engl 1996;78:426.

Chehade A, Daley TD, Wysocki GP et al. Peripheral odontogenic keratocyst. Oral Surg Oral Med Oral Pathol 1994;77:494.

Dabb DJ, Schweitzer RJ, Schweitzer LE, et al. Squamous cell carcinoma arising in recurrent odontogenic keratocyst: case report and literature review. Head Neck 1994;16:375.

Dammer R, Neiderdellmann H, Dammer P, et al. Conservative or radical treatment of keratocysts: a retrospective review. Br J Oral Maxillofac Surg 1997;35:46.

El-Hajj G, Anneroth G. Odontogenic keratocysts: a retrospective clinical and histologic study. Int J Oral Maxillofac Surg 1996;25:124.

Marker P, Brøndum N, Clausen PP, et al. Treatment of large odontogenic keratocysts by decompression and later cystectomy: a long-term follow-up and a histologic study of 23 cases. Oral Surg Oral Med Oral Pathol Oral Radiol Endod 1996;82:122.

Meiselman F. Surgical management of the odontogenic keratocyst: conservative approach. J Oral Maxillofac Surg 1994;52:960.

Mody RN, Bhoosreddy AR. Multiple odontogenic keratocysts: a case report. Ann Dent 1995;54:41.

Neville BW, Damm DD, Brock TR. Odontogenic keratocysts of the midline maxillary region. J Oral Maxillofac Surg 1997;55:340.

Nohl FSA, Gulabivala K. Odontogenic keratocyst as periradicular radiolucency in the anterior mandible: two case reports. Oral Surg Oral Med Oral Pathol Oral Radiol Endod 1996;81:103.

Oikarinen VJ. Keratocyst recurrences at intervals of more than 10 years: case reports. Br J Oral Maxillofac Surg 1990;28:47.

Williams TP, Connor FA Jr. Surgical management of the odontogenic keratocyst: aggressive approach. J Oral Maxillofac Surg 1994;52:964.

## Orthokeratinized Odontogenic Cyst

Crowley TE, Kaugars GE, Gunsolley JC. Odontogenic keratocysts: a clinical and histologic comparison of the parakeratin and orthokeratin variants. J Oral Maxillofac Surg 1992;50:22.

Vuhahula E, Nikai H, Ijuhin N, et al. Jaw cysts with orthokeratinization: analysis of 12 cases. J Oral Pathol Med 1993;22:35.

Wright JM. The odontogenic keratocyst: orthokeratinized variant. Oral Surg Oral Med Oral Pathol 1981; 51:609.

## Nevoid Basal Cell Carcinoma Syndrome

Bale AE. The nevoid basal cell carcinoma syndrome: genetics and mechanism of carcinogenesis. Cancer Invest 1997;15:180.

Chidambaram A, Dean M. Genetics of the nevoid basal cell carcinoma syndrome. Adv Cancer Res 1996; 70:49.

Crean SJ, Cunningham SJ. Gorlin's syndrome: main features and recent advances. Br J Hosp Med 1996; 56:392.

Gorlin RJ. Nevoid basal cell carcinoma syndrome. Dermatol Clin 1995;13:113.

Kimonis VE, Goldstein AM, Pastakia B, et al. Clinical manifestations in 105 persons with nevoid basal cell carcinoma syndrome. Am J Med Genet 1997;69:299.

Ratcliffe JF, Shanley S, Chenevix-Trench G. The prevalence of cervical and thoracic congenital skeletal abnormalities in basal cell naevus syndrome: a review of cervical and chest radiographs in 80 patients with BCNS. Br J Radiol 1995;68:596.

Woolgar JA, Rippin JW, Browne RM. The odontogenic keratocyst and its occurrence in the nevoid basal cell carcinoma syndrome. Oral Surg Oral Med Oral Pathol 1987;64:727.

## Calcifying Odontogenic Cyst

Alcalde RE, Sasaki A, Misaki M, et al. Odontogenic ghost cell carcinoma: report of a case and review of the literature. J Oral Maxillofac Surg 1996;54:108.

Buchner A. The central (intraosseous) calcifying odontodenic cyst: an analysis of 215 cases. J Oral Maxillofac Surg 1991;49:330.

Buchner A, Merrell PW, Hansen LS, et al. Peripheral (extraosseous) calcifying odontogenic cyst. Oral Surg Oral Med Oral Pathol 1991;72:65.

Devin H, Horner K. The radiological features of calcifying odontogenic cyst. Br J Radiol 1993;66:403.

Hirshberg A, Kaplan I, Buchner A. Calcifying odontogenic cyst associated with odontoma: a possible separate entity (odontocalcifying odontogenic cyst). J Oral Maxillofac Surg 1994;52:555.

Hong SP, Ellis GL, Hartman KS. Calcifying odontogenic cyst: a review of ninety-two cases with reevaluation of their nature as cysts or neoplasms, the nature of ghost cells, and subclassification. Oral Surg Oral Med Oral Pathol 1991;72:56.

Johnson A III, Fletcher M, Gold L, et al. Calcifying odontogenic cyst: a clinicopathologic study of 57 cases with immunohistochemical evaluation for cytokeratin. J Oral Maxillofac Surg 1997;55:679.

Raubenheimer EJ, van Heerden WFP, Sitzman F, et al. Peripheral dentinogenic ghost cell tumor. J Oral Pathol Med 1992;21:93.

## Glandular Odontogenic Cyst

Ide F, Shimoyama T, Horie N. Glandular odontogenic cyst with hyaline bodies: an unusual dentigerous presentation. J Oral Pathol Med 1996;25:401.

High AS, Main DM, Khoo SP, et al. The polymorphous odontogenic cyst. J Oral Pathol Med 1996;25:25.

Hussain K, Edmondson HD, Browne RM. Glandular odontogenic cysts: diagnosis and treatment. Oral Surg Oral Med Oral Pathol Oral Radiol Endod 1995;79:593.

Ramer M, Montazem A, Lane SL, et al. Glandular odontogenic cyst: report of a case and review of the literature. Oral Surg Oral Med Oral Pathol Oral Radiol Endod 1997;84:54.

Takeda Y. Glandular odontogenic cyst mimicking a lateral periodontal cyst: a case report. Int J Oral Maxillofac Surg 1994;23:96.

## Carcinoma Arising in Odontogenic Cysts

Eversole LR, Sabes WR, Rovin S. Aggressive growth and neoplastic potential of odontogenic cysts. Cancer 1975;35:270.

Foley WL, Terry BC, Jacoway JR. Malignant transformation of an odontogenic keratocyst: report of a case. J Oral Maxillofac Surg 1991;49:768.

Manganaro AM, Cross SE, Startzell JM. Carcinoma arising in a dentigerous cyst with neck metastasis. Head Neck 1997;19:436.

Schwimmer AM, Aydin F, Morrison SN. Squamous cell carcinoma arising in residual odontogenic cyst: report of a case and review of literature. Oral Surg Oral Med Oral Pathol 1991;72:218.

Yoshida H, Onizawa K, Yusa H. Squamous cell carcinoma arising in association with an orthokeratinized odontogenic keratocyst: report of a case. J Oral Maxillofac Surg 1996;54:647.

## Ameloblastoma

Feinberg SE, Steinberg B. Surgical management of ameloblastoma: current status of the literaature. Oral Surg Oral Med Oral Pathol Oral Radiol Endod 1996;81:383.

Gardner DG. Some current concepts on the pathology of ameloblastomas. Oral Surg Oral Med Oral Pathol Oral Radiol Endod 1996;82:660.

Leider AS, Eversole LR, Barkin ME. Cystic ameloblastoma: a clinicopathologic analysis. Oral Surg Oral Med Oral Pathol 1985;60:624.

Nastri AL, Wiesenfeld D, Radden BG, et al. Maxillary ameloblastoma: a retrospective study of 13 cases. Br J Oral Maxillofac Surg 1995;33:28.

Philipsen HP, Ormiston IW, Reichart PA. The desmo-and osteoplastic ameloblastoma: histologic variant or clinicopathologic entity? Case reports. Int J Oral Maxillofac Surg 1992;21:352.

Reichart PA, Philipsen HP, Sonner S. Ameloblastoma: biologic profile of 3677 cases. Oral Oncol Eur J Cancer 1995;31B:86.

Robinson L, Martinez MG. Unicystic ameloblastoma: a prognostically distinct entity. Cancer 1977;40:2278.

Small IA, Waldron CA. Ameloblastomas of the jaws. Oral Surg Oral Med Oral Pathol 1955;8:281.

Thompson IOC, Ferreira R, van Wyk CW. Recurrent unicystic ameloblastoma of the maxilla. Br J Oral Maxillofac Surg 1993;31:180.

Waldron CA, El-Mofty SA. A histopathologic study of 116 ameloblastomas with special reference to the desmoplastic variant. Oral Surg Oral Med Oral Pathol 1987;63:441.

Williams TP. Management of ameloblastoma: a changing perspective. J Oral Maxillofac Surg 1993;51:1064.

## Peripheral (Extraosseous) Ameloblastoma

Baden E, Doyle JL, Petriella V. Malignant transformation of peripheral ameloblastoma. Oral Surg Oral Med Oral Pathol 1993;75:214.

Batsakis JG, Hicks MJ, Flaitz CM. Peripheral epithelial odontogenic tumors. Ann Otol Rhinol Laryngol 1993;102:322.

El-Mofty S, Gerard NO, Farish SE, et al. Peripheral ameloblastoma: a clinical and histologic study of 11 cases. J Oral Maxillofac Surg 1991;49:970.

Gurol M, Burkes EJ Jr. Peripheral ameloblastoma. J Periodontol 1995;66:1065.

Hernandez G, Sanchez G, Caballero T, et al. A rare case of a multicentric peripheral ameloblastoma of the gingiva: a light and electron microscopic study. J Clin Periodontol 1992;19:281.

Zhu EX, Okada N, Takagi M. Peripheral ameloblastoma: case report and review of literature. J Oral Maxillofac Surg 1995;53:590.

## Malignant Ameloblastoma and Ameloblastic Carcinoma

Califano L, Maremonti P, Boscaino A, et al. Peripheral ameloblastoma: report of a case with malignant aspect. Br J Oral Maxillofac Surg 1996;34:240.

Corio RL, Goldblatt LI, Edwards PA, et al. Ameloblastic carcinoma: a clinicopathologic assessment of eight cases. Oral Surg Oral Med Oral Pathol 1987;64:570.

Elzay RP. Primary intraosseous carcinoma of the jaws: review and update of odontogenic carcinomas. Oral Surg Oral Med Oral Pathol 1982;54:299.

Houston G, Davenport W, Kewaton W, et al. Malignant (metastatic) ameloblastoma: report of a case. J Oral Maxillofac Surg 1993;51:1152.

Lau SK, Tideman H, Wu PC. Ameloblastic carcinoma of the jaws. Oral Surg Oral Med Oral Pathol Oral Radiol Endod 1998;85:78.

## Adenomatoid Odontogenic Tumor

Courtney RM, Kerr DA. The odontogenic adenomatoid tumor: a comprehensive review of 21 cases. Oral Surg Oral Med Oral Pathol 1975;39:424.

Hicks MJ, Flaitz CM, Batsakis JG. Adenomatoid and calcifying epithelial odontogenic tumors. Ann Otol Rhinol Laryngol 1993;102:159.

Kearns GJ, Smith R. Adenomatoid odontogenic tumor: an unusual cause of gingival swelling in a 3-year-old patient. Br Dent J 1996;181:380.

Philipsen HP, Reichart PA, Zhang KH, et al. Adenomatoid odonogenic tumor: biologic profile based on 499 cases. J Oral Pathol Med 1991;20:149.

## Calcifying Epithelial Odontogenic Tumor

Basu MK, Matthews JB, Sear AJ, et al. Calcifying epithelial odontogenic tumor: a case showing features of malignancy. J Oral Pathol 1984;13:310.

Franklin CD, Pindborg JJ. The calcifying epithelial odontogenic tumor: a review and analysis of 113 cases. Oral Surg Oral Med Oral Pathol 1976;42:753.

Hicks MJ, Flaitz CM, Wong MEK, et al. Clear cell variant of calcifying epithelial odoontogenic tumor: case report and review of the literature. Head Neck 1994;16:272.

Krolls SO. Calcifying epithelial odontogenic tumor: a survey of 23 cases and discussion of histomorphologic variations. Arch Pathol 1974;98:206.

Pindborg JJ. A calcifying epithelial odontogenic tumor. Cancer 1958;11:838.

## Sqamous Odontogenic Tumor

Baden E, Doyle J, Mesa M, et al. Squamous odontogenic tumor: report of three cases including the first extraosseous case. Oral Surg Oral Med Oral Pathol 1993;75:733.

Leider AS, Jonker LA, Cook HE. Multicentric familial squamous odontogenic tumor. Oral Surg Oral Med Oral Pathol 1989;68:175.

Philipsen HP, Reichart PA. Squamous odontogenic tumor (SOT): a benign neoplasm of the periodontium: a review of 36 reported cases. J Clin Periodontol 1996;23:922.

Pullon PA Shafer WG Elzay RP, et al. Squamous odontogenic tumor: report of six cases of a previously undescribed lesion. Oral Surg Oral Med Oral Pathol 1975;40:616.

Stoll C, Barelton G, Winter W, et al. An asymptomatic enlargement of the mandible causing marked root resorption. J Oral Maxillofac Surg 1997;55:740.

## Ameloblastic Fibroma

Dallera P, Bertoni F, Marchetti C, et al. Ameloblastic fibroma: a follow-up of six cases. Int J Oral Maxillofac Surg 1996;25:199.

Hansen LS, Ficarra G. Mixed odontogenic tumors: an analysis of 23 new cases. Head Neck Surg 1988; 10:330.

Regezi JA, Kerr DA, Courtney RM. Odontogenic tumors: analysis of 706 cases. J Oral Surg 1978;36:771.

Trodahl JN. Ameloblastic fibroma: a survey of cases from the Armed Forces Institute of Pathology. Oral Surg Oral Med Oral Pathol 1972;33:547.

Zellen RD, Preskar MH, McClary SA. Ameloblastic fibroma. J Oral Maxillofac Surg 1983;40:513.

## Ameloblastic Fibro-Odontoma

Kitano M, Tsuda-Yamada S, Semba I, et al. Pigmented ameloblastic fibro-odontoma with melanophages. Oral Surg Oral Med Oral Pathol Oral Radiol Endod 1994;77:271.

Miller AS, Lopez CF, Pullon PA, et al. Ameloblastic fibro-odontoma. Oral Surg Oral Med Oral Pathol 1976;41:354.

Miyauchi M, Takata T, Ogawa I, et al. Immunohistochemical observations on a possible ameloblastic fibro-odontoma. J Oral Pathol Med 1996;25:93.

Philipsen HP, Reichart PA, Praetorius F. Mixed odontogenic tumors and odontomas: considerations on interrelationship: review of the literature and presentation of 134 new cases of odontomas. Oral Oncol 1997;33:86.

Slootweg PJ. An analysis of the inter-relationships of the mixed odontogenic tumors: ameloblastic fibroma, ameloblastic fibro-odontoma and odontoma. Oral Surg Oral Med Oral Pathol 1981;51:266.

## Ameloblastic Fibrosarcoma

Dallera P, Bertoni F, Marchetti C, et al. Ameloblastic fibrosarcoma of the jaws: report of five cases. J Craniomaxillofac Surg 1994;22:349.

Müller S, Parker DC, Kapadia SB, et al. Ameloblastic fibrosarcoma of the jaws: a clinicopathologic and DNA analysis of five cases and review of the literature with discussion of its relationship to ameloblastic fibroma. Oral Surg Oral Med Oral Pathol Oral Radiol Endod 1995;79:469.

Nogueira T de O, Carvalho YR, Rosa LE, et al. Possible malignant transformation of an ameloblastic fibroma to ameloblastic fibrosarcoma: a case report. J Oral Maxillofac Surg 1997;55:180.

Tajima Y, Utsumi N, Suzuki S, et al. Ameloblastic fibrosarcoma arising de novo in the maxilla. Pathol Int 1997;47:564.

Park HR, Shin KB, Sol MY, et al. A highly malignant ameloblastic fibrosarcoma: report of a case. Oral Surg Oral Med Oral Pathol Oral Radiol Endod 1995;79:478.

## Clear Cell Odontogenic Carcinoma

De Aguiar MC, Gomez RS, Silva EC, et al. Clear-cell ameloblastoma (clear-cell odontogenic carcinoma): report of a case. Oral Surg Oral Med Oral Pathol Oral Radiol Endod 1996;81:79.

Eversole LR, Duffey DC, Powell NB. Clear cell odontogenic carcinoma: a clinicopathologic analysis. Arch Otolaryngol Head Neck Surg 1995;121:685.

Hansen LS, Eversole LR, Green TL, et al. Clear cell odontogenic tumor-a new histologic variant with aggressive potential. Head Neck Surg 1985;8:115.

Muramatsu T, Hashimoto S, Inoue T, et al. Clear cell odontogenic carcinoma in the mandible: histochemical and immunohistochemical observations with a review of the literature. J Oral Pathol Med 1996;25:516.

Piattelli A, Sesenna E, Trisi P. Clear cell odontogenic carcinoma: report of a case with lymph node and pulmonary metastases. Eur J Cancer B Oral Oncol 1994;30B:278.

## Odontoma

Budnick SN. Compound and complex odontomas. Oral Surg Oral Med Oral Pathol 1976;42:501.

Castro GW, Houston G, Weyrauch C. Peripheral odontoma: report of case and review of literature. ASDC J Dent Child 1994;61:209.

Giunta JL Kaplan MA. Peripheral, soft tissue odontomas: two case reports. Oral Surg Oral Med Oral Pathol 1990;69:406.

Kaugars GE, Miller ME, Abbey LM. Odontomas. Oral Surg Oral Med Oral Pathol 1989;67:172.

## Odontogenic Fibroma

Daley TD, Wysocki G.P. Peripheral odontogenic fibroma. Oral Surg Oral Med Oral Pathol 1994;78:329.

Dunlap C, Barker B. Central odontogenic fibroma WHO type. Oral Surg Oral Med Oral Pathol 1984; 57:390.

Gardner DG. The central odontogenic fibroma: an attempt at clarification. Oral Surg Oral Med Oral Pathol 1980;50:425.

Handlers JP, Abrams AM, Melrose RJ, et al. Central odontogenic fibroma: clinicopathologic features of 19 cases and review of the literature. J Oral Maxillofac Surg 1991;49:46.

Kaffe I, Buchner A. Radiologic features of central odontogenic fibroma. Oral Surg Oral Med Oral Pathol 1994;78:811.

## Odontogenic Myxoma

Lamberg MA, Calonius BPE, Mäkinen JEA, et al. A case of malignant myxoma (myxosarcoma) of the maxilla. Scand J Dent Res 1984;92:352.

Lombardi T, Lock C, Samson J, et al. S100, alpha-smooth muscle actin and cytokeratin 19 immunohistochemistry in odontogenic and soft tissue myxomas. J Clin Pathol 1995;48:759.

Moshiri S, Oda D, Worthington P, et al. Odontogenic myxoma: histochemical and ultrastructural study. J Oral Pathol Med 1992;21:401.

Muzio LL, Nocini P, Favia G, et al. Odontogenic myxoma of the jaws: a clinical, radiologic, immunohistochemical, and ultrastructural study. Oral Surg Oral Med Oral Pathol Oral Radiol Endod 1996;82:426.

Peltola J, Magnusson B, Happonen RP, et al. Odontogenic myxoma: a radiographic study of 21 tumors. Br J Oral Maxillofac Surg 1994;32:298.

White DK, Chen S, Mohnac AM, et al. Odontogenic myxoma: a clinical and ultrastructural study. Oral Surg Oral Med Oral Pathol 1975;39:901.

# chapter 13
# DERMATOLOGIC DISEASES

### Figs. 13.1 and 13.2

Hereditary hypohidrotic ectodermal dysplasia is a genetic disorder characterized by defective formation of various ectodermally derived structures. It is most commonly inherited as an X-linked recessive trait, although autosomal-dominant and autosomal-recessive transmission also rarely may occur. Affected individuals have a marked reduction or absence of sweat glands resulting in the inability to tolerate heat. Severe fever may occur during infancy and early childhood and can be fatal. The skin is soft and dry, with wrinkling and hyperpigmentation often occurring around the eyes. The scalp hair is sparse, fine, and blond, with eyebrows, eyelashes, and other body hair being sparse or absent. There is often frontal bossing and a depressed nasal bridge. Many patients have atopic disease.

The lips are often protuberant and may exhibit pseudorhagades, or fissures. Hypoplasia of the mucoserous glands may lead to xerostomia and chronic rhinitis. The most characteristic oral finding is hypodontia or, in some cases, total anodontia. The teeth that do develop are typically malformed and conical in shape. Taurodontism is a common radiographic finding. Female carriers of the trait may show these tooth anomalies to a milder degree because of partial expression of the condition (Lyon hypothesis).

Treatment of the dental defects depends on the severity of the disease; removable prosthetic replacement is the most common treatment modality, including the use of complete dentures, partial dentures, or overdentures. In the child, the prostheses must be remade periodically to accommodate the growth of the dental arches. Osseointegrated dental implants also have been used with success.

## HEREDITARY HEMORRHAGIC TELANGIECTASIA (RENDU-OSLER-WEBER DISEASE)

### Fig. 13.3

Hereditary hemorrhagic telangiectasia is an autosomal-dominant disorder characterized by multiple vascular defects throughout the body in the form of telangiectasias and arteriovenous malformations. Weakness of the vascular wall and surrounding connective tissue predisposes patients to hemorrhagic episodes. Epistaxis is usually the earliest and most common symptom, often beginning in childhood. Cutaneous telangiectasias may become evident in the second and third decades, with oral lesions characteristically involving the lips and tongue. Oral and gastrointestinal tract bleeding may occur, as well as hemoptysis and intracranial hemorrhage. Treatment for hereditary hemorrhagic telangiectasia may require blood transfusions, laser ablation of skin and mucosal lesions, and surgical resection or embolotherapy of pulmonary and intracranial arteriovenous malformations. Epistaxis can be treated with septal dermoplasty and laser ablation.

### Figure 13.1
### HEREDITARY HYPOHIDROTIC ECTODERMAL DYSPLASIA
Patient exhibiting frontal bossing and sparse, fine, blond hair. (Courtesy of Drs. Charles Hook and Bob Gellin.)

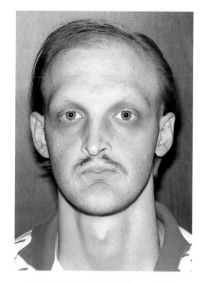

### Figure 13.2
### HEREDITARY HYPOHIDROTIC ECTODERMAL DYSPLASIA
Patient from Figure 13.1 exhibiting hypodontia and conical-shaped teeth. (Courtesy of Drs. Charles Hook and Bob Gellin.)

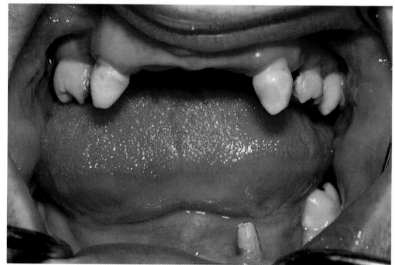

### Figure 13.3
### HEREDITARY HEMORRHAGIC TELANGIECTASIA
Telangiectasias of lips.

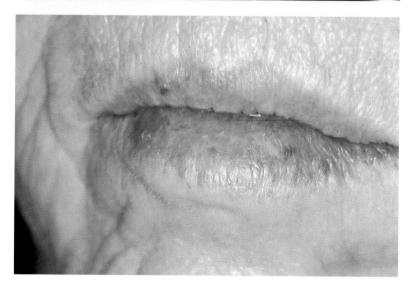

## Figs. 13.4, 13.5, and 13.6

Pachyonychia congenita is a rare genetic syndrome inherited as an autosomal-dominant trait, although occasional cases have appeared to exhibit autosomal-recessive inheritance. At birth, or shortly thereafter, the fingernails and toenails become thickened, elevated, and tubular in shape with accumulation of a yellowish brown, horny material on the undersurface. This material causes the nails to project upward along the free edge. Recently, a late-onset form of the condition has been described (pachyonychia congenita tarda). The nails may have to be surgically removed or later may become hypoplastic. Hyperkeratosis of the palms and soles may occur during the first few years of life, with development of painful bullae that can burst and become infected. Palmar and solar hyperhidrosis also may be seen, as can follicular keratosis of the knees and elbows.

The principal oral manifestation is the development of white, hyperkeratotic lesions, especially in areas of increased trauma. The dorsum of the tongue and the buccal mucosa along the occlusal plane are the most common sites involved. These lesions are not predisposed to malignant degeneration. Neonatal teeth and angular cheilitis also have been reported.

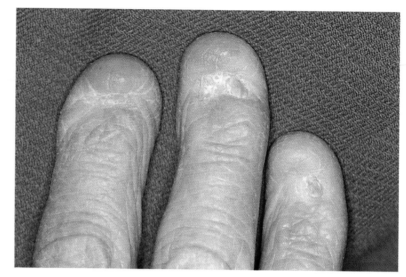

► **Figure 13.5**
**PACHYONYCHIA CONGENITA**
Hyperkeratosis of the soles. (Courtesy of
Dr. Lou Young.)

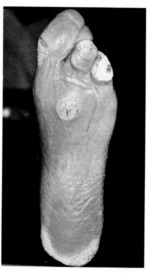

► **Figure 13.6**
**PACHYONYCHIA CONGENITA**
Hyperkeratotic lesions on the lateral
tongue. (Courtesy of Dr. John Lenox.)

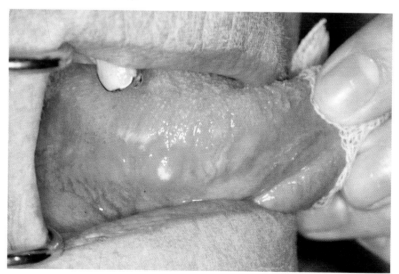

## WHITE SPONGE NEVUS

**Fig. 13.7**

White sponge nevus is a rare, autosomal-dominant abnormality of squamous epithelial differentiation that affects mucosal surfaces but not skin. Typically, spongy white plaques with a folded or corrugated surface occur bilaterally on the buccal mucosa and may also be seen at other oral mucosal sites. Lesions may be present at birth or first be noted in childhood or adolescence. Extraoral lesions may involve the vagina, labia, anorectal mucosa, and nasal cavity. Diagnosis often can be made on the basis of clinical appearance and family history. Cytologic smears, or sometimes biopsy, may help confirm the diagnosis. White sponge nevus is a benign condition, and no treatment is necessary. Interestingly, the lesions may improve with the use of systemic antibiotics, such as penicillin or tetracycline, or after application of topical tetracycline.

## DARIER'S DISEASE (KERATOSIS FOLLICULARIS)

**Figs. 13.8 and 13.9**

Darier's disease is a rare genodermatosis inherited as an autosomal-dominant trait. The disease usually first manifests itself during childhood or adolescence with the development of red to yellowish brown papules behind the ears, around the nose, and on the neck, chest, back, and extremities. These papules become hyperkeratotic and crusty, eventually producing greasy plaques that may become secondarily infected and exude an offensive odor. Hyperkeratotic, papular lesions often involve the palms and soles and may become so severe that the patient has difficulty walking. The nails often are splintered and fissured and may exhibit longitudinal discoloration or subungual hyperkeratosis. The disease typically worsens during the summer months. Management includes frequent cleansing with antibacterial soaps and systemic antibiotics when necessary. Systemic retinoids often are helpful but may not be tolerated because of undesirable side effects.

Oral involvement has been reported in 15 to 50% of patients with Darier's disease. Rough, gray–white papules occur on the hard palate and gingiva and, less commonly, on the tongue and buccal mucosa. The palatal lesions may resemble papillary hyperplasia or nicotine stomatitis. No treatment is indicated for the mucosal lesions. Intermittent obstructive sialadenitis of the major salivary glands has been reported in some patients, probably secondary to squamous metaplasia of the ductal lining. In rare instances, this sialadenitis may become severe enough to necessitate excision of the affected gland.

► **Figure 13.7**
**WHITE SPONGE NEVUS**
Thickened white plaque of the buccal mucosa.

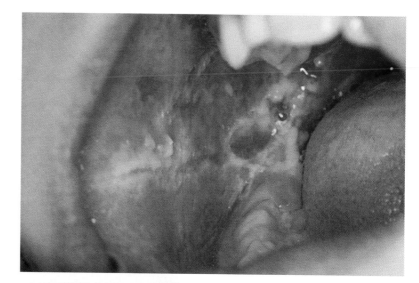

► **Figure 13.8**
**DARIER'S DISEASE**
Crusted, hyperkeratotic lesions of the leg and foot. (Courtesy of Weathers DR, Olansky S, Sharpe LO. Darier's disease with mucous membrane involvement. Arch Dermatol 1969;100:50–53.)

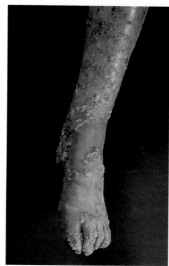

► **Figure 13.9**
**DARIER'S DISEASE**
Papular lesions of the palate. (Courtesy of Weathers DR, Olansky S, Sharpe LO. Darier's disease with mucous membrane involvement. Arch Dermatol 1969:100:50–53.)

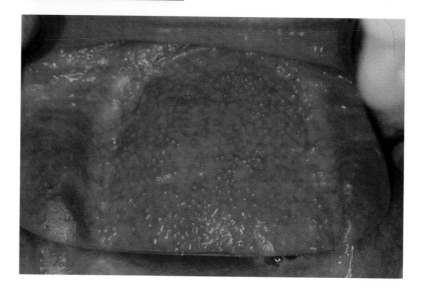

## Figs. 13.10 to 13.12

Tuberous sclerosis is a rare syndrome characterized by epilepsy, mental retardation, and hamartomatous growths in multiple organ systems. Although this syndrome is inherited as an autosomal-dominant trait, about 50 to 75% of cases have no family history and apparently represent new mutations. The earliest skin sign is the presence of congenital white, hypopigmented, ash-leaf–shaped macules on the trunk and limbs. Later, during the first decade, angiofibromas slowly develop, appearing as pink to red nodules most prominent in the nasolabial folds, cheeks, forehead, and scalp. These angiofibromas were once termed "adenoma sebaceum" in the mistaken belief that they represented tumors of the sebaceous glands. Subungual fibromas may elevate the nail bed. Orange-peel–like shagreen patches may occur in the lumbar area.

Numerous smooth, hard masses of glial tissue and ganglion cells occur in the brain and are responsible for the related mental retardation and epilepsy. The name "tuberous sclerosis" is derived from these potato-like tumors of the central nervous system. Intracranial calcifications, renal angiomyolipomas, cardiac rhabdomyomas, and other hamartomatous lesions may be seen.

Fibromatous lesions of the anterior gingiva and other oral mucosal sites have been reported in 11 to 56% of patients. Intrabony fibrous or myxomatous tumors of the jaws also may occur. Generalized gingival hyperplasia secondary to anticonvulsant therapy may be seen. Pitting defects of the enamel have been described in 90% of patients; identification of these pits can be aided with the use of dental plaque disclosing solution.

Management of tuberous sclerosis often is directed primarily at controlling the associated seizures. Facial angiofibromas can be removed for cosmetic reasons. In general, patients have a slightly reduced life span, with death sometimes related to complications of central nervous system and kidney disease.

**Figure 13.10**
**TUBEROUS SCLEROSIS**
Angiofibromas of the face. (Courtesy of
Dr. E. R. Costich.)

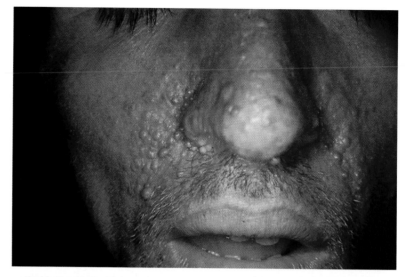

**Figure 13.11**
**TUBEROUS SCLEROSIS**
Intracranial calcifications.

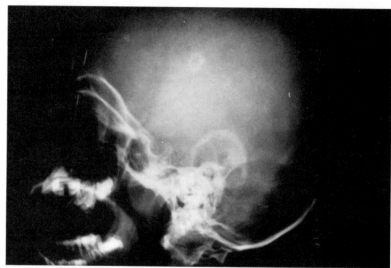

**Figure 13.12**
**TUBEROUS SCLEROSIS**
Fibrous lesion of the gingiva.

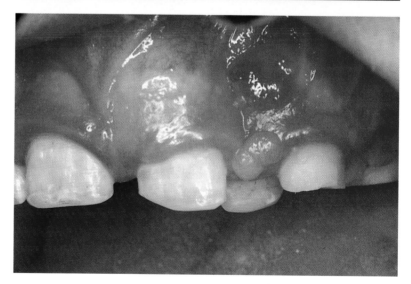

## DYSKERATOSIS CONGENITA

### Figs. 13.13 and 13.14

Dyskeratosis congenita is a rare syndrome that is characterized by multiple defects of ectodermal structures plus bone marrow hypofunction. More than 80% of reported cases have occurred in males, and the condition is believed to be transmitted most frequently as an X-linked recessive trait. However, autosomal-dominant and autosomal-recessive transmission also are believed to occur, which accounts for sporadic cases seen in female patients.

Despite the disease's name, clinical manifestations typically are not congenital but begin to be noticed between 5 and 10 years of age. Reticulated hyperpigmentation is seen on the skin, especially the face, neck, upper arms, and chest. The nails become dystrophic, with longitudinal ridging and splitting. The palms and soles exhibit hyperhidrosis (excessive sweating), frequently in association with hyperkeratosis. Progressive bone marrow failure occurs in half of all cases, causing thrombocytopenia, anemia, and leukopenia. Other frequent findings include alopecia, dysphagia, and obstruction of the nasolacrimal duct.

Oral involvement may begin with the development of vesiculoerosive lesions on the tongue and buccal mucosa. The dorsum of the tongue may exhibit atrophy of the papillae and become smooth and shiny. The most significant oral feature is the frequent development of leukoplakia, which may involve the tongue, buccal mucosa, and labial mucosa. These leukoplakic lesions can undergo malignant transformation at an early age. Patients also have a predisposition to other malignancies, especially carcinomas of the gastrointestinal system. Rapidly progressive periodontal disease has been reported.

Because of the potential complications related to bone marrow failure and development of malignancy, the average life span for more severely affected patients is 32 years. The pancytopenia may be treated with bone marrow transplantation or administration of granulocyte colony-stimulating factor and erythropoietin.

## PEUTZ-JEGHERS SYNDROME

### Fig. 13.15

Peutz-Jeghers syndrome is a rare autosomal-dominant condition characterized by multiple hamartomatous gastrointestinal polyps and mucocutaneous melanin pigmentation. The pigmented lesions are often congenital and are most common on the labial mucosa and perioral skin. They present as round to oval macules 1 to 5 mm in diameter, and are light brown to blue–black. Similar lesions may occur around the eyes, the nose, on the hands and feet, and intraorally. The intestinal polyps are most common in the small intestine, often leading to abdominal pain from small-bowel intussusception. Patients are at increased risk for carcinomas of the gastrointestinal tract, uterus, ovary, pancreas, and possibly breast. These tumors may develop at a young age, and close medical evaluation and monitoring are recommended. If desired, cosmetic removal of the pigmented lip lesions can be accomplished with laser ablation.

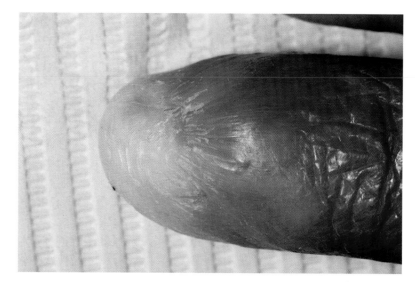

► **Figure 13.14**
**DYSKERATOSIS CONGENITA**
Atrophy of the dorsal tongue mucosa.

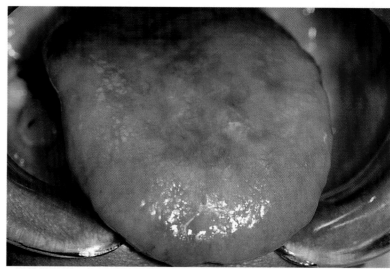

► **Figure 13.15**
**PEUTZ-JEGHERS SYNDROME**
Macular pigmentation of the lips.
(Courtesy of Dr. Ahmed Uthman.)

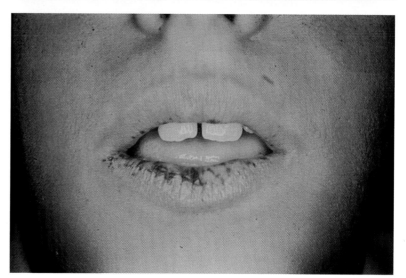

## MELANOTIC MACULE (FOCAL MELANOSIS)

**Figs. 13.16 and 13.17**

The term melanotic macule has been used to describe a benign pigmented lesion of the oral cavity characterized by an increase in melanin pigmentation along the basal cell layer of the epithelium. The melanotic macule is typically a well-circumscribed flat area of pigmentation that most frequently exhibits a brown color but also may appear black, blue, or gray. Most lesions are less than 1 cm in diameter, although occasional cases may be larger. Most occur as single lesions, but multiple lesions can be seen. The most common location is the vermilion border of the lip, with a predilection for the midportion of the lower lip. The gingiva, buccal mucosa, and palate are the most common intraoral locations. The melanotic macule is most common in young and middle-aged adults, and females are affected more frequently than males.

Treatment usually consists of surgical excision to rule out the possibility of early melanoma, although long-standing lesions exhibiting no evidence of change may be followed clinically, especially those on the lips. Biopsy is recommended especially for pigmented lesions of the hard palate–maxillary gingiva complex because this is the most common site for oral melanoma. Labial melanotic macules have been treated successfully with the use of a Q-switched ruby laser, which causes selective damage to pigmented cells in the tissue.

## ORAL MELANOACANTHOSIS (ORAL MELANOACANTHOMA)

**Fig. 13.18**

Oral melanoacanthosis is a rare pigmented lesion that probably represents a reactive hyperplasia of melanocytes in response to local trauma. It is most common in young adults and occurs almost exclusively in blacks. Oral melanoacanthosis often has a sudden onset, sometimes exhibiting rapid growth over a period of several weeks to months. The buccal mucosa is the most common location, and bilateral involvement may occur. Lesions have been described as dark blue, brown, or black and range from less than 5 mm in diameter to extensive lesions several centimeters in size. The pigmentation often resolves spontaneously after removal of irritating factors or incomplete excision.

**Figure 13.16**
**MELANOTIC MACULE**
Pigmented lesion on the lower lip.

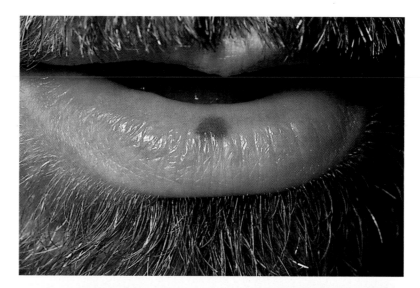

**Figure 13.17**
**MELANOTIC MACULE**
Flat, pigmented lesion of the maxillary gingiva.

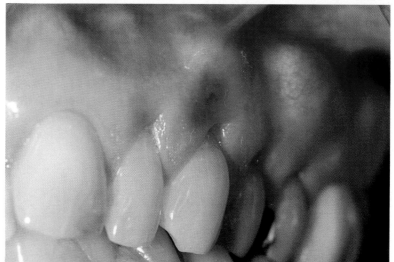

**Figure 13.18**
**ORAL MELANOACANTHOSIS**
Pigmented lesion of the buccal mucosa.

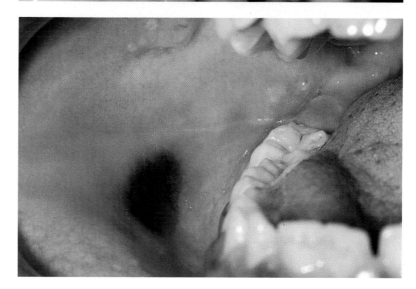

# ERYTHEMA MIGRANS (GEOGRAPHIC TONGUE, BENIGN MIGRATORY GLOSSITIS, ECTOPIC GEOGRAPHIC TONGUE, MIGRATORY STOMATITIS)

## Figs. 13.19, 13.20, and 13.21

Erythema migrans is a common inflammatory condition that usually affects the tongue, where it is known as "geographic tongue" or "benign migratory glossitis." Most studies indicate that the prevalence of geographic tongue is in the range of 1 to 3% of the population. The condition occurs at all ages, and women are affected almost twice as often as men. Concomitant fissured tongue also may be present. The cause of erythema migrans is unknown, although a family history or association with stress or atopy may be seen. An increased prevalence of certain histocompatibility antigens has been reported in affected patients, supporting the theory that genetic influences play a role in the pathogenesis of this condition. Because of their histopathologic similarities and cases showing coexistence of both conditions, it has been suggested that erythema migrans may represent an oral manifestation of psoriasis. Although the relationship between these two conditions is still debated, one study did show a significantly increased prevalence of erythema migrans in patients with psoriasis.

Geographic tongue typically affects the dorsal and lateral surface of the tongue, presenting as red patches caused by loss of the filiform papillae but with preservation of the fungiform papillae. These red patches are usually, but not always, surrounded by an elevated, circinate white or yellow border. The red patches rapidly enlarge and may coalesce, producing large areas devoid of filiform papillae. The filiform papillae rapidly regrow, however, returning the area to its normal appearance. The loss of papillae often begins in another area, resulting in an ever-changing pattern of papillae loss and regrowth, hence the name "benign migratory glossitis." This changing pattern is a rapid process; daily differences can be noted in the maplike pattern. Most patients are without symptoms, although some may experience soreness or sensitivity to spicy foods.

Although involvement of the dorsal and lateral tongue is common, involvement of the ventral tongue and other oral mucosal sites is seen much less frequently. These lesions, however, have the same migrating pattern as the tongue lesions, presenting as atrophic, erythematous patches, usually with a raised, circinate, white border. Extralingual lesions usually occur on the buccal and labial mucosa. Almost all patients with "ectopic geographic tongue" also have typical dorsal tongue involvement.

Erythema migrans is a persistent condition that may exhibit periods of remission and exacerbation. No treatment is indicated, except possibly palliative therapy in some instances when significant tenderness is present. Topical application of corticosteroids, diphenhydramine, or anesthetic agents have been used with variable success.

**Figure 13.19**
**ERYTHEMA MIGRANS**
Loss of filiform papillae with a raised white border. Associated fissured tongue is also present.

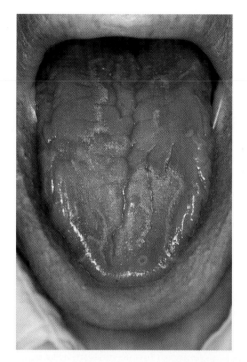

**Figure 13.20**
**ERYTHEMA MIGRANS**
Ventral tongue involvement.

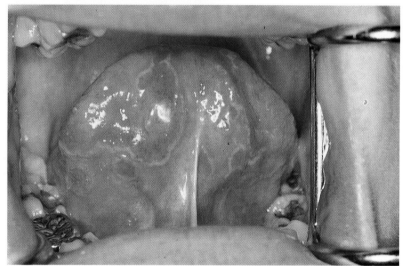

**Figure 13.21**
**ERYTHEMA MIGRANS**
Lesions on the soft palate.

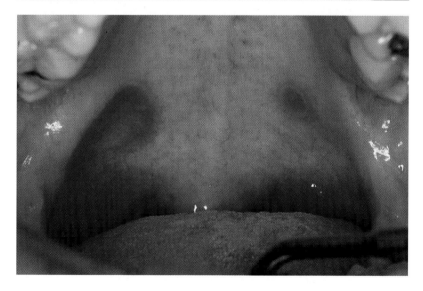

## TRANSIENT LINGUAL PAPILLITIS ("LIE BUMPS")

### Fig. 13.22

Transient lingual papillitis is a common condition that is characterized by the development of enlarged and painful fungiform papillae on the tongue. One or more fungiform papillae become swollen and exhibit a red, white, or yellow color. The lesions typically resolve spontaneously within several hours to days, but periodic recurrences are not unusual. Despite its common occurrence, little was known about this entity until a recent article by Whitaker and colleagues. In their survey, they found that these lesions were reported by 56% of their study population and were most common in young women. A subsequent study, which apparently reported the same entity, showed a familial clustering of cases. The cause is unknown, although it has been speculated that the lesions may result from local trauma or a viral infection. The term "lie bumps" is derived from the popular superstition that these lesions are caused by telling lies. There is no effective treatment in most cases, although some individuals have found relief with over-the-counter mouthrinses or salt water rinses.

## PSORIASIS

### Figs. 13.23 and 13.24

Psoriasis is a common chronic inflammatory skin disorder that is estimated to affect 1 to 3% of the world's population. The cause of psoriasis seems to be multifactorial, but there is a strong genetic influence because one-third of patients with psoriasis have affected relatives. In addition, patients with psoriasis demonstrate an increased frequency of certain histocompatibility antigens. Factors that can exacerbate the disease include psychological stress, infections, alcohol abuse, and certain drugs, such as lithium and beta blockers. A strong association between psoriasis and human immunodeficiency virus infection has been shown.

Psoriasis most frequently has its onset during the second and third decades of life and shows periods of exacerbation and remission. It is characterized clinically by the development of erythematous papules and plaques that are covered by a silvery scale. If the scales are scraped off, one may observe tiny pinpoint areas of bleeding (Auspitz sign). However, eliciting the Auspitz sign is currently discouraged because of the aforementioned possible association with human immunodeficiency virus infection. Lesions are often bilaterally symmetrical and most commonly affect the scalp, elbows, knees, and sites of local trauma (Koebner phenomenon). Itching is not an unusual complaint. More severe forms of the disease may exhibit generalized pustular lesions. A small percentage of patients develop psoriatic arthritis, which may involve the temporomandibular joint. Oral lesions are rare and have been variably described as appearing as white plaques, erythematous patches, or ulcerations. An increased prevalence of erythema migrans has been reported, and some authors believe that this represents an oral manifestation of psoriasis. This association is strongest for pustular forms of the disease. An increased frequency of fissured tongue also is reported.

No treatment may be necessary for mild forms of psoriasis. For moderate cases, topical corticosteroids or coal tar derivatives may be used. Severe cases may require ultraviolet light treatment or systemic drug therapy with methotrexate, retinoids, or cyclosporine. Symptomatic oral lesions may be treated with warm salt water rinses or application of topical anesthetics, antihistamines, or corticosteroids.

▶ **Figure 13.22**
**TRANSIENT LINGUAL PAPILLITIS**
Painful white papules along the anterior margin of the tongue.

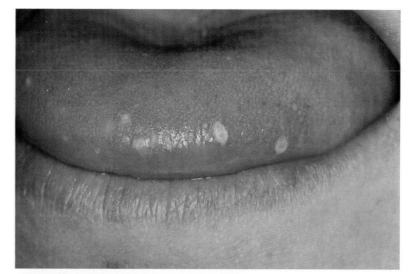

▶ **Figure 13.23**
**PSORIASIS**
Scaly lesions on the elbow.

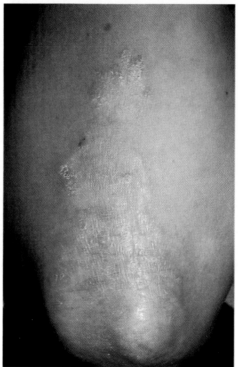

▶ **Figure 13.24**
**PSORIASIS**
Erythematous lesions of the hard palate.

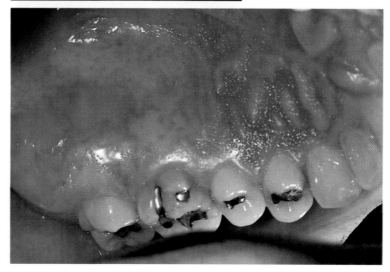

## Figs. 13.25, 13.26, and 13.27

Systemic sclerosis is an unusual disorder of unknown cause that best fits into the category of autoimmune collagen-vascular diseases. Although the term "scleroderma" describes well the principal and most obvious site of involvement in most patients, the term "systemic sclerosis" better denotes the multisystem nature of the disorder.

Systemic sclerosis usually has its onset in middle age and is more common in females than in males. There is thickening and induration of the skin cause by dermal fibrosis, which may lead to clawlike flexion contractures of the hands and a masklike facial appearance. In long-standing scleroderma, ulcerations develop over pressure points due to trauma. Hyperpigmentation and hypopigmentation of the skin may occur. The fibrosis is not confined to the skin but may involve internal organs such as the lungs, heart, gastrointestinal tract, and kidneys, resulting in loss of normal visceral function. Other common features include Raynaud phenomenon, telangiectasias, soft-tissue calcifications, arthritis, an elevated erythrocyte sedimentation rate, and the presence of antinuclear antibodies in the serum.

Oral manifestations include difficulty opening the mouth and loss of tongue mobility because of perioral and lingual fibrosis. The anterior maxillary teeth often are exposed because of retraction of the lips. Crenations of the buccal mucosa and tongue have been reported. A classic radiographic finding is generalized symmetric widening of the periodontal ligament space, which occurs to at least some degree in almost all patients. Bony erosions may occur at the angle of the mandible, or they may destroy the coronoid and condylar processes. Xerostomia and dysphagia are also common findings. The salivary changes are similar to those seen in Sjögren syndrome.

Systemic sclerosis pursues an unpredictable course, but is typically a progressive disorder with no cure. Patients with diffuse involvement may exhibit rapid progression of their disorder, with death occurring within several years after onset. In other patients, the disease is less severe, with slow progression over a period of many years or periods of rapid spread and quiescence. The 5-year survival has been reported to be between 50 and 70%; 40 to 60% of patients survive for 10 years. Internal organ complications include pulmonary fibrosis, heart failure, renal insufficiency, and hypertension. Death usually results from complications of internal organ involvement. Renal disease formerly was the leading cause of morbidity and mortality, but since the advent of angiotension-converting enzyme inhibitor therapy for kidney disease, pulmonary complications are now the primary cause of death in patients with systemic sclerosis.

**Figure 13.25**
**SYSTEMIC SCLEROSIS**
**(A)** Fibrosis of the skin resulting in a masklike facial expression. **(B)** The fibrosis has caused marked atrophy of the mandibular ramus. Note the widened periodontal ligament space around the mandibular molar.

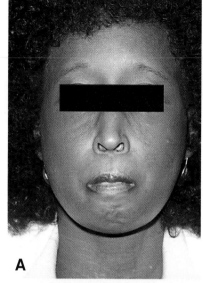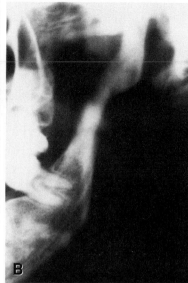

A  B

**Figure 13.26**
**SYSTEMIC SCLEROSIS**
Fibrosis of the hands with flexion contractures and blunting of digits.

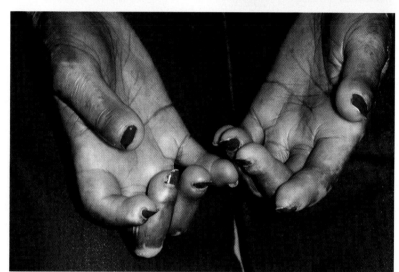

**Figure 13.27**
**SYSTEMIC SCLEROSIS**
Symmetric widening of the periodontal ligament space.

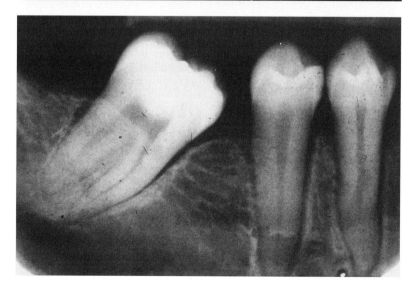

## CREST SYNDROME

**Fig. 13.28**

The CREST syndrome is a clinical variant of systemic sclerosis. The term "CREST" is an acronym for the five major components of the disorder: calcinosis cutis, Raynaud phenomenon, esophageal dysfunction, sclerodactyly, and telangiectasias. The telangiectasias often are most prominent on the face and lips and also can be seen intraorally. Although considered a variant of systemic sclerosis, the CREST syndrome is often less severe than the more common systemic variety.

## LUPUS ERYTHEMATOSUS

**Figs. 13.29 and 13.30**

Lupus erythematosus (LE) is an autoimmune disorder that usually has its onset in young adults and is considerably more common in women than in men. Chronic cutaneous LE (CCLE) primarily affects only the skin and mucous membranes, whereas systemic LE (SLE) affects the skin and multiple other tissues and organs. A third form of the disease, subacute cutaneous LE, has clinical features intermediate between SLE and CCLE.

Skin involvement is most common in areas of sun exposure. In SLE, patients often present with an erythematous rash in a butterfly distribution across the bridge of the nose and malar areas. Other features that may be seen in SLE include Raynaud phenomenon, arthritis, proteinuria, pericarditis, pleuritis, psychosis, convulsions, anemia, leukopenia, thrombocytopenia, and circulating antinuclear antibodies. The characteristic skin manifestation of CCLE is the development of discoid lesions, which present as elevated, erythematous, indurated plaques with an adherent scale and central atrophy and scarring. Although the term "discoid LE" sometimes has been used synonymously with CCLE, it should be emphasized that discoid skin lesions may be seen in all forms of the disease.

Oral lesions occur in 10 to 40% of patients with LE and seem to be more common in those with SLE. The most characteristic lesion consists of a central atrophic, speckled, erythematous area surrounded by a slightly elevated border exhibiting radiating white striae and telangiectasias. These lesions are most common on the buccal mucosa and may mimic lichen planus. Later stages can be indistinguishable from oral leukoplakia. Other oral manifestations include scaling lip lesions, erythema, nonspecific ulcers, and secondary Sjögren syndrome (see Figs. 8.5 and 8.6).

Management of LE depends on the extent and severity of the disease. Treatment usually consists of antimalarial drugs, topical and systemic corticosteroids, or both. The prognosis for CCLE is excellent, with only about 5% of cases progressing to systemic involvement. In SLE, the most common cause of death is renal failure, although most cases can be controlled with appropriate medications. The 5-year survival rate for SLE is approximately 95%, but survival drops to around 75% after 15 years.

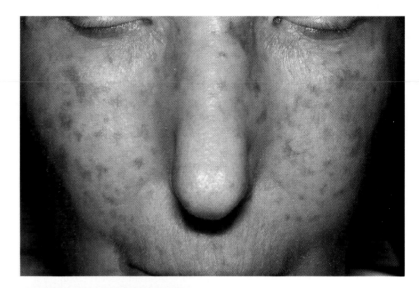

▶ **Figure 13.28**
**CREST SYNDROME**
Facial telangiectasias.

▶ **Figure 13.29**
**SYSTEMIC LUPUS ERYTHEMATOSUS**
Lesions of the malar area.

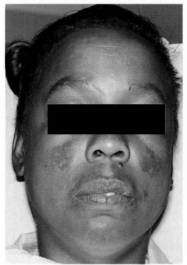

▶ **Figure 13.30**
**CHRONIC CUTANEOUS LUPUS ERYTHEMATOSUS**
Speckled erythematous lesion with peripheral radiating white striae on the buccal mucosa.

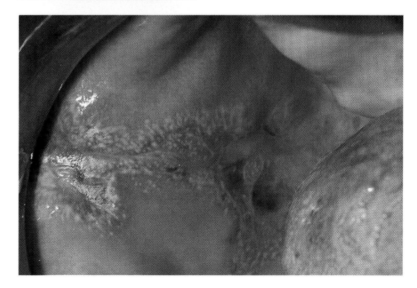

## Figs. 13.31, 13.32, and 13.33

The term "pemphigus" refers to a group of autoimmune disorders characterized by development of vesiculobullous lesions on the skin and mucous membranes. It is most common in middle-aged adults and affects both sexes equally. An increased prevalence has been noted in Ashkenazi Jews. Patients with pemphigus develop autoantibodies directed toward an antigen on the surface of squamous epithelial cells, destroying the intercellular attachments and resulting in intraepithelial blister formation. Although several clinical variants are recognized, pemphigus vulgaris is the most common form and the type most likely to exhibit oral manifestations.

On the skin, the primary lesions of pemphigus vulgaris are vesicles and bullae that can arise on normal skin or on an erythematous base. These blisters are fragile and rupture easily, producing painful, raw, denuded areas. In later stages of the disease, extensive areas of epidermis may be sloughed. Scaling and crusting of the ulcerated areas are common. A characteristic feature is the Nikolsky sign, which is the ability to elicit the formation of a bulla by the application of firm lateral pressure on normal-appearing skin.

Oral involvement in pemphigus vulgaris is extremely common: more than 90% of patients develop oral lesions at some time during the course of their disease. In fact, the mouth is the most common presenting site for lesions of pemphigus vulgaris, with some studies showing more than half of all cases originating there. The oral lesions often have a slow, insidious onset with symptoms present for many months before a diagnosis is made or skin lesions develop. Lesions may be found anywhere but are most common on the palate, buccal mucosa, and gingiva. Although the oral lesions are vesiculobullous in nature, intact blisters rarely are seen; patients usually exhibit collapsed bullae, ulcers, or widespread areas of erosion. Gingival involvement may produce "desquamative gingivitis." Pain and resultant weight loss are common complaints.

Diagnosis is established by biopsy and immunofluorescent studies. Titers on indirect immunofluorescence often correlate to the severity of the disease. Before the advent of systemic corticosteroid therapy, pemphigus vulgaris was fatal in 60 to 90% of the patients because of general debilitation, malnutrition, and protein loss. Even today, pemphigus vulgaris is a serious disease, with a mortality of approximately 10%. Many of these deaths arise from complications of corticosteroid therapy. Other immunosuppressive drugs, such as azathioprine, also are frequently used to reduce the amount of systemic corticosteroids needed.

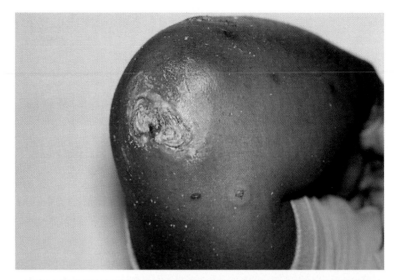

▶ **Figure 13.32**
**PEMPHIGUS VULGARIS**
Ulcer at the commissure.

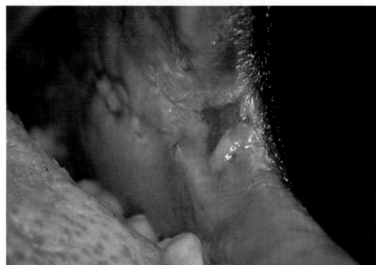

▶ **Figure 13.33**
**PEMPHIGUS VULGARIS**
Extensive ulcerative lesions of the buccal
mucosa and soft palate.

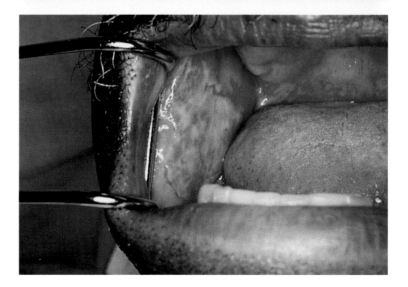

## PARANEOPLASTIC PEMPHIGUS (NEOPLASIA-INDUCED PEMPHIGUS)

### Figs. 13.34 and 13.35

Paraneoplastic pemphigus is a recently recognized vesiculobullous disorder that arises secondary to an underlying malignancy, most frequently non-Hodgkin's lymphoma or chronic lymphocytic leukemia. It is believed that antibodies that are produced against the tumor cross-react against antigens of the adhesion complex of the epithelium.

Paraneoplastic pemphigus presents a variable clinical and histopathologic picture that can be confused with other vesiculobullous disorders. The condition often has a rather sudden onset, with the development of multiple blisters and ulcers affecting the skin and oral mucosa. In some instances, the skin lesions are papular and pruritic, resembling lichen planus. The oral lesions can affect any location but frequently involve the lips to produce hemorrhagic crusting that may mimic erythema multiforme. Ocular involvement can produce scarring lesions similar to mucous membrane pemphigoid.

The diagnosis of paraneoplastic pemphigus is made on the basis of light microscopy, direct immunofluorescence, indirect immunofluorescence, and, sometimes, immunoprecipitation studies. The indirect immunofluorescence should be performed on transitional-type epithelium, which shows a highly specific pattern of antibody deposition in the intercellular areas of the epithelium. Treatment usually consists of systemic immunosuppressive medications such as prednisone and azathioprine. Unfortunately, patients usually have a poor prognosis, with death resulting from complications of the vesiculobullous lesions or the underlying malignancy. However, occasional long-term survivors have been described.

## CHRONIC ULCERATIVE STOMATITIS

### Fig. 13.36

Chronic ulcerative stomatitis is a recently described condition with clinical and light microscopic features that mimic erosive lichen planus. However, both direct and indirect immunofluorescent studies demonstrate specific autoantibodies directed against the nuclei of stratified squamous epithelial cells. The condition is most common in middle-aged and older women who present with chronic symptoms of desquamative gingivitis or ulcerations of the buccal mucosa or tongue. Associated Wickham's striae may be present, as well as lichenoid skin lesions. Unfortunately, unlike lichen planus, chronic ulcerative stomatitis is less responsive to topical and systemic corticosteroid therapy. Hydroxychloroquine has been reported to be successful in controlling the lesions in some patients.

### Figure 13.34
**PARANEOPLASTIC PEMPHIGUS**
Crusting, hemorrhagic lip lesions.
(Courtesy of Dr. Carl Allen.)

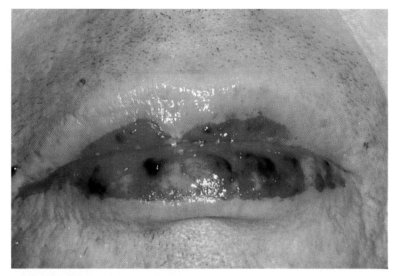

### Figure 13.35
**PARANEOPLASTIC PEMPHIGUS**
Extensive erosive lesions of the buccal
mucosa. (Courtesy of Dr. Carl Allen.)

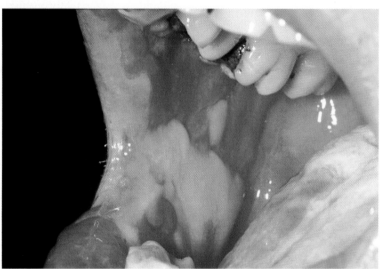

### Figure 13.36
**CHRONIC ULCERATIVE STOMATITIS**
White and red erosive changes on the
dorsal tongue.

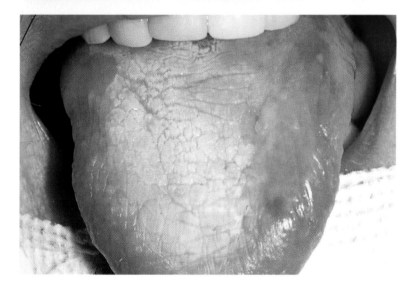

## Figs. 13.37, 13.38, and 13.39

Pemphigoid is an autoimmune disorder characterized by the development of vesiculobullous lesions on the skin or mucous membranes. Patients develop autoantibodies directed toward the epithelial basement membrane zone that result in the formation of subepithelial blisters. Two major forms are recognized: bullous pemphigoid and mucous membrane pemphigoid.

Bullous pemphigoid primarily affects the skin of middle-aged and older adults. It is characterized by the development of tense blisters on the trunk, arms, and legs. Oral lesions have been reported in 8 to 39% of patients.

Mucous membrane pemphigoid primarily affects mucosal surfaces; skin involvement is uncommon. In some sites, the ulcerative lesions may result in scar formation—hence the name "cicatricial" pemphigoid. This condition is most common in middle-aged and older adults and shows a female predilection. The oral cavity is affected in most cases; the eyes are the second most common location. Although lesions may occur anywhere in the mouth, the gingiva is the most commonly affected site, with patients often presenting with a clinical "desquamative gingivitis." As with pemphigus vulgaris, mucous membrane pemphigoid usually has a slow, insidious onset, with lesions present for many months before a diagnosis is made. Patients usually present with painful erythematous or erosive lesions; intact blisters rarely are seen.

Ocular involvement is characterized by conjunctivitis, with patients often complaining of burning and photophobia. As the disease progresses, a mucoid discharge may develop and scarring occurs, resulting in symblepharon formation (adhesions between the lid and eyeball). Inflammation, vascularization, and scarring of the cornea may lead to blindness. Esophageal involvement can produce dysphagia and stricture formation that may require dilatation. Laryngeal lesions may cause pain and hoarseness and can be life-threatening, though this is rare. Nasal, pharyngeal, genital, and anorectal lesions also can occur.

Diagnosis is established by biopsy and immunofluorescent studies. Treatment depends on the severity of the disease but often involves topical or systemic corticosteroids. For desquamative gingival lesions, custom soft acrylic trays can be fabricated to hold the topical corticosteroid in place for longer periods of time. When systemic corticosteroids are needed, azathioprine also may be used to lower the needed corticosteroid dosage. Dapsone may be effective in some patients, as may tetracycline and nicotinamide. In patients who present with only oral disease, an ophthalmologic examination is still recommended to evaluate for the possibility of early ocular disease.

**Figure 13.37**
**MUCOUS MEMBRANE PEMPHIGOID**
Erythematous and erosive gingival lesions ("desquamative gingivitis"). (Courtesy of Dr. Lynn Wallace.)

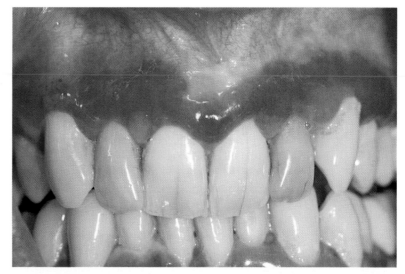

**Figure 13.38**
**MUCOUS MEMBRANE PEMPHIGOID**
Lesions of the palate.

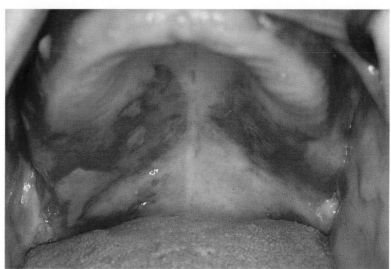

**Figure 13.39**
**MUCOUS MEMBRANE PEMPHIGOID**
Symblepharon formation of the eye.

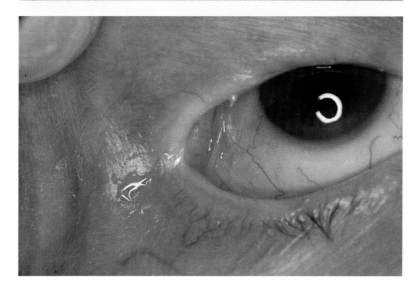

### Figs. 13.40 to 13.54

Lichen planus is an inflammatory disorder of unknown cause that can affect both the skin and the oral cavity. The disease is relatively common and has been estimated to affect approximately 1% of the general population. Although stress has been suggested as a possible etiologic factor, a definite cause-and-effect relationship has not been established. A variety of drugs can cause lichenoid lesions (lichenoid drug reactions) that may be clinically and microscopically indistinguishable from idiopathic lichen planus. The disease most often has its onset in middle-aged adults. Females seem to be affected more often than males, especially with oral lichen planus. Studies show a wide variation in the relative prevalence of oral and skin lesions, which depends on whether the patient was seen primarily in a dermatology clinic or a dental clinic. In patients seen primarily for skin lesions, about 70% also show oral involvement. In patients seen initially for oral lesions, 20 to 40% show skin lesions.

The characteristic skin lesion of lichen planus is a flat-topped, polygonal papule with a red to violet color. The surface of the papule may exhibit a fine scale or lacy white streaks known as "Wickham's striae." Papules may coalesce to form hypertrophic plaques, especially on the lower legs and ankles. In rare instances, bullous lesions can arise. Pruritis, which can be severe, occurs in most cases. The most common sites of involvement are the flexor surfaces of the wrists, the legs, the abdomen, and the back. Lesions may develop in a linear distribution in areas of trauma (Koebner phenomenon). Nail involvement is seen in 6 to 10% of cases, usually producing longitudinal ridging and roughening of the surface. The clinical course of lichen planus of the skin is variable; some patients develop localized lesions, others develop a more generalized eruption.

Oral lesions begin as small white papules that usually coalesce to form an interlacing network of white lines (reticular lichen planus). These interlacing lines also are known as Wickham's striae. Hypertrophic white plaques sometimes occur, especially on the dorsum of the tongue. Erythematous atrophic areas and erosive lesions (erosive lichen planus) are common. In rare instances, intact bullae (bullous lichen planus) are seen. Although lesions may occur anywhere in the oral cavity, the buccal mucosa is involved in 78 to 87% of cases. The gingiva and tongue are also common sites of involvement. Oral lesions tend to be bilateral and symmetric in their distribution. Reticular lichen planus is often asymptomatic, except for a feeling of roughness of the mucosa. Atrophic or erosive lichen planus, however, is usually tender or painful and may interfere with eating. When erosive lesions involve the gingiva, they may present clinically as a "desquamative gingivitis."

Because of its characteristic features, classic reticular lichen planus may not require biopsy, although biopsy is often advisable for atrophic or erosive lichen planus to rule out a dysplastic process or other vesiculoerosive disorder. Oral lichen planus and lupus erythematosus (see Figs. 13.29 and 13.30) can have similar clinical features; therefore, biopsy and immunofluorescent studies may be indicated for oral lichenoid lesions if skin lesions suggestive of lupus erythematosus are present. Biopsy and immunofluorescent studies also may be indicated for lichenoid lesions that are not responsive to therapy.

Oral lichen planus is typically a chronic condition that may exhibit exacerbations and remissions over many years. If the lesions are asymptomatic, no treatment is necessary. For symptomatic atrophic or erosive lesions, treatment usually consists of topical corticosteroids, such as fluocinonide gel. Topical corticosteroid therapy affords only temporary control of the disease, and patients should be advised that the lesions will probably recur and require reapplication of the medication. In rare instances, systemic corticosteroids may be needed to bring the disease under control. A potential complication of corticosteroid therapy is the development of iatrogenic candidiasis, but this usually responds to appropriate antifungal therapy.

Considerable controversy exists concerning the malignant potential of oral lichen planus. A number of series and individual cases have been reported that show carcinoma developing in a small percentage (0.4–2.5%) of patients with oral lichen planus, especially the erosive form. Other authors have questioned this association, however, suggesting that in many cases the original diagnosis actually may have been a hyperkeratotic or dysplastic process with clinical or histopathologic features that mimicked lichen planus. In any case, periodic follow-up of patients with oral lichen planus seems to be prudent.

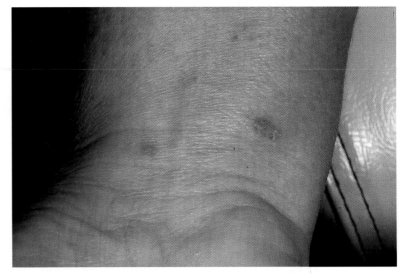

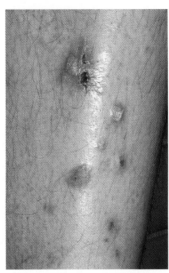

► **Figure 13.42**
**LICHEN PLANUS**
Nail involvement.

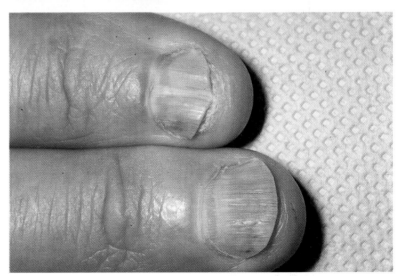

**Figure 13.43**
**LICHEN PLANUS**
White papules and striae on the buccal mucosa.

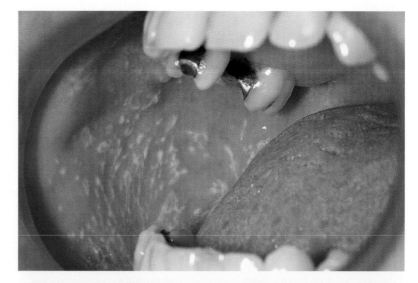

**Figure 13.44**
**LICHEN PLANUS**
White striae on the posterior buccal mucosa.

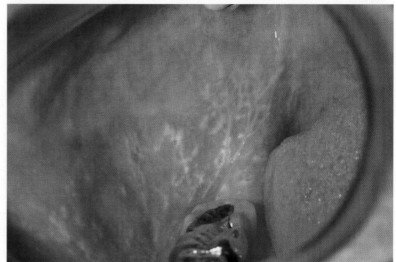

**Figure 13.45**
**LICHEN PLANUS**
Confluent reticular lesions on the buccal mucosa.

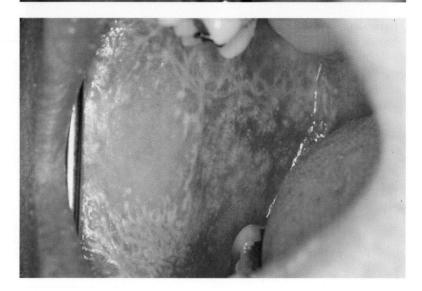

### Figure 13.46
**LICHEN PLANUS**

White papules and plaquelike lesion of the dorsum of the tongue.

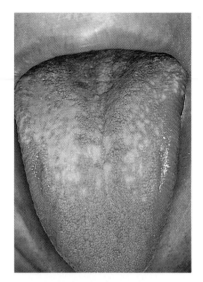

### Figure 13.47
**LICHEN PLANUS**

White papules and striae on the lower lip mucosa.

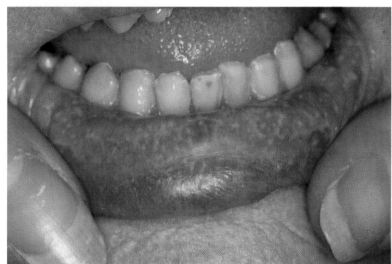

### Figure 13.48
**LICHEN PLANUS**

White plaque with peripheral striae on the hard palate.

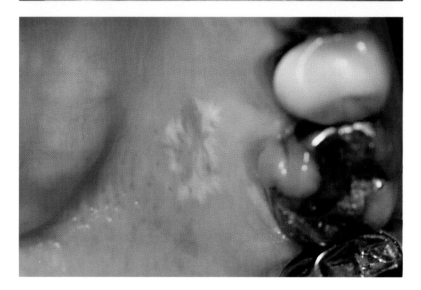

▶ **Figure 13.49**
**LICHEN PLANUS**
Red, erosive gingival lesions
("desquamative gingivitis").

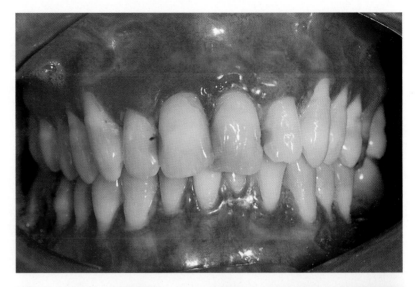

▶ **Figure 13.50**
**LICHEN PLANUS**
Erosive lesions of the mandibular facial
gingiva.

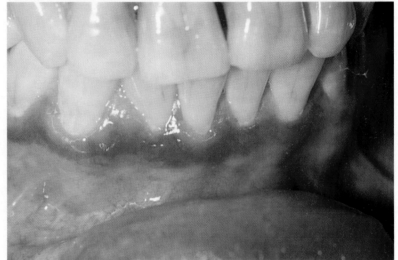

▶ **Figure 13.51**
**LICHEN PLANUS**
Erosive lesion of the palatal gingiva. Note
the peripheral white striae.

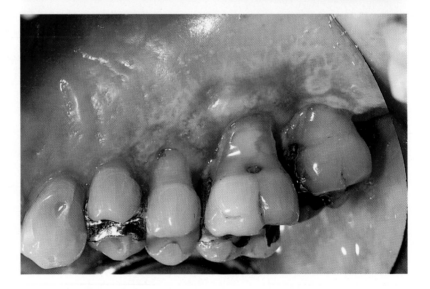

▶ **Figure 13.52**
**LICHEN PLANUS**
Erosive lesion of the buccal mucosa.

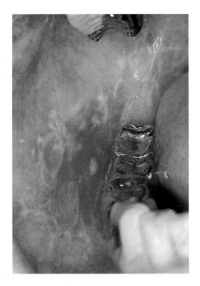

▶ **Figure 13.53**
**LICHEN PLANUS**
Severe erosive lesions of the buccal
mucosa before treatment.

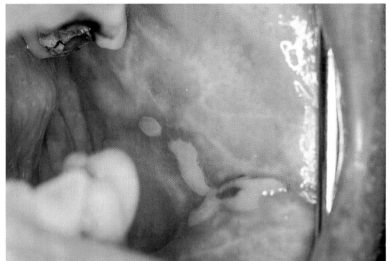

▶ **Figure 13.54**
**LICHEN PLANUS**
Same patient as depicted in Figure 13.53
after 10 days of topical fluocinonide
therapy.

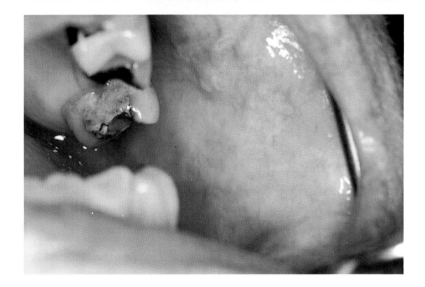

### Figs. 13.55, 13.56, and 13.57

Erythema multiforme is an acute vesiculoerosive disorder of the skin and mucous membranes. It is seen most commonly in young adults but may occur at almost any age. Males are affected more often than females. Although the clinical features of erythema multiforme suggest an immune or allergic reaction, in many instances a specific precipitating agent is never identified. The best-documented precipitating factors include various infections, especially herpes simplex and *Mycoplasma pneumoniae*. Several drugs also have been implicated as causing erythema multiforme, including sulfonamides, penicillins, and cephalosporins. Erythema multiforme has a wide range of severity; the terms "Stevens-Johnson syndrome" and "toxic epidermal necrolysis" (Lyell disease) have been used traditionally for more severe forms of the disease. However, some recent studies have suggested that Stevens-Johnson syndrome and toxic epidermal necrolysis may represent a separate disease process. Such cases are more likely to be triggered by a drug than by an infection.

Skin lesions of erythema multiforme usually begin as round, erythematous papules that enlarge to produce the characteristic iris or target lesions. The target lesion is created by a central area of epithelial necrosis or blister formation surrounded by an erythematous inflammatory zone and a lighter ring of edema at the periphery. These skin lesions may develop anywhere but are most common on the extremities, with a predilection for the extensor surfaces. A nonspecific rash also may be seen. In rare instances, blistering or necrotic lesions may coalesce to produce extensive areas of sloughing (toxic epidermal necrolysis).

Mucosal involvement is commonly seen and may affect the oral cavity, eyes, and genitalia. More severe cases affecting multiple mucosal sites and the skin are referred to as Stevens-Johnson syndrome. Oral lesions are typically sudden in onset and are characterized by multiple painful ulcers and erosions that often cause difficulty in eating and may lead to dehydration. Lesions may occur anywhere in the mouth but are most typical on the lips, where they often result in hemorrhagic crusting. Ocular involvement can be manifested by conjunctivitis, periorbital edema, and photophobia, rarely leading to scarring and permanent visual impairment.

Erythema multiforme is usually a self-limiting process that runs its course in 2 to 4 weeks, although severe cases of Stevens-Johnson syndrome and especially toxic epidermal necrolysis can be life-threatening. Recurrent episodes are not uncommon. Treatment consists of supportive care, including oral topical anesthetic agents and possibly intravenous rehydration if the patient cannot eat. Topical corticosteroids also may be helpful in the management of oral lesions. Systemic corticosteroid therapy has been used traditionally for erythema multiforme, but some authors have questioned the advisability of such treatment, especially for severe forms of Stevens-Johnson syndrome and toxic epidermal necrolysis. Such cases may be managed best in a hospital burn unit. In recurring cases of erythema multiforme that are precipitated by herpes simplex infections, prophylactic acyclovir therapy often is helpful in preventing further outbreaks. Some authors also have reported success using azathioprine or levamisole.

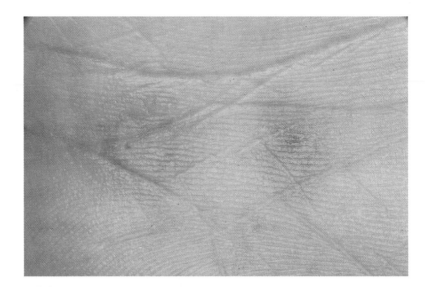

▶ **Figure 13.56**
**ERYTHEMA MULTIFORME**
Hemorrhagic, crusting lesions of the lips
and nostrils.

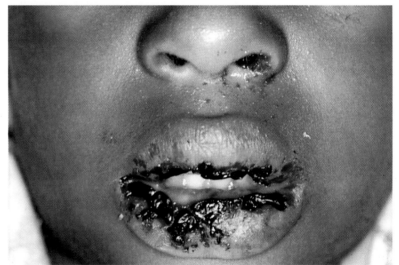

▶ **Figure 13.57**
**ERYTHEMA MULTIFORME**
Ulcers of the buccal mucosa.

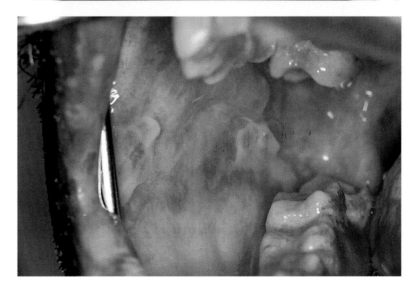

## Figs. 13.58 and 13.59

The term "epidermolysis bullosa" (EB) is used for a group of mechanobullous diseases characterized by the development of blisters in areas of minor trauma. At least 23 distinct forms of the disease have been recognized. Most of these have a hereditary basis, with onset of blistering lesions at birth or within the first few years of life. Epidermolysis bullosa acquisita is not hereditary, however, and appears to be an autoimmune disorder, with lesions typically arising during adolescence or adulthood. The various types are characterized by spontaneous or trauma-induced blister formation caused by degeneration of basal or parabasal epithelial cells (EB simplex), lack of hemidesmosomes (junctional EB), or defects in anchoring fibrils in the connective tissue (dystrophic EB).

A wide range of severity is seen, from EB of Weber-Cockayne, with minor blisters of the hands and feet, to EB letalis, with extensive bullous lesions and shedding of sheets of skin. Scarring occurs in some forms of EB and is especially prominent in recessive dystrophic EB, in which scarring may result in encasement and fusion of fingers and toes, plus flexion contractures. Oral lesions are common in several types of EB and may result in painful erosions and severe scarring. Enamel hypoplasia is a common finding in junctional forms of EB. Rampant dental caries frequently is seen in patients with junctional EB and severe recessive dystrophic EB. Development of squamous cell carcinoma of the tongue has been reported in several cases of recessive dystrophic EB.

The prognosis for EB depends on the specific subtype: EB letalis is usually fatal during the first few months of life because of fluid loss and sepsis; dystrophic recessive EB is often fatal before patients reach adulthood; milder forms of EB are usually compatible with a normal life span.

### Figure 13.58
**EPIDERMOLYSIS BULLOSA**
Scarring vesiculobullous oral lesions.

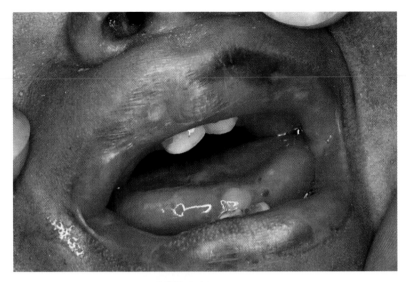

### Figure 13.59
**EPIDERMOLYSIS BULLOSA**
Scarring and fusion of toes.

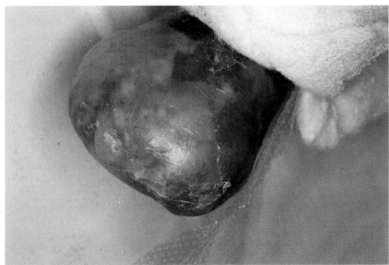

### Hereditary Hypohidrotic Ectodermal Dysplasia

Clarke A, Phillips DIM, Brown R, et al. Clinical aspects of X-linked hypohidrotic ectodermal dysplasia. Arch Dis Child 1987;62:989.

Crawford PJM, Aldred MJ, Clarke A. Clinical and radiographic dental findings in X linked hypohidrotic ectodermal dysplasia. J Med Genet 1991;28:181.

Davarpanah M, Moon JW, Yang LR, et al. Dental implants in the oral rehabilitation of a teenager with hypohidrotic ectodermal dysplasia: report of a case. Int J Oral Maxillofac Implants 1997;12:252.

Kupietzky A, Houpt M. Hypohidrotic ectodermal dysplasia: characteristics and treatment. Quintessence Int 1995;26:285.

Pigno MA, Blackman RB, Cronin RJ Jr. Prosthodontic management of ectodermal dysplasia: a review of the literature. J Prosthet Dent 1996;76:541.

### Hereditary Hemorrhagic Telangiectasia

Flint SR, Keith O, Scully C. Hereditary hemorrhagic telangiectasia: family study and review. Oral Surg Oral Med Oral Pathol 1988;66:440.

Guttmacher AE, Marchuk DA, White RI Jr. Hereditary hemorrhagic telangiectasia. N Engl J Med 1995;333:918.

Haitjema T, Westermann CJJ, Overtoom TTC, et al. Hereditary hemorrhagic telangiectasia (Osler-Weber-Rendu disease): new insights in pathogenesis, complications, and treatment. Arch Intern Med 1996;156:714.

Siegel MB, Keane WM, Atkins JP Jr, et al. Control of epistaxis in patients with hereditary hemorrhagic telangiectasia. Head Neck Surg 1991;105:675.

### Pachyonychia Congenita

Feinstein A, Friedman J, Schewach-Millet M. Pachyonychia congenita. J Am Acad Dermatol 1988;19:705.

Haber RM, Rose TH. Autosomal recessive pachyonychia congenita. Arch Dermatol 1986;122:919.

Maser ED. Oral manifestations of pachyonychia congenita. Oral Surg Oral Med Oral Pathol 1977;43:373.

Paller AS, Moore JA, Scher R. Pachyonychia congenita tarda: a late onset form of pachyonychia congenita. Arch Dermatol 1991;127:701.

Su WPD, Chun SI, Hammond DE, et al. Pachyonychia congenita: a clinical study of 12 cases and review of the literature. Pediatr Dermatol 1990;7:33.

### White Sponge Nevus

Jorgenson RJ, Levin LS. White sponge nevus. Arch Dermatol 1981;117:73.

McDonagh AJG, Gawkrodger DJ, Walker AE. White sponge nevus successfully treated with topical tetracycline. Clin Exp Dermatol 1990;15:152.

Morris R, Gansler TS, Rudisill MT, et al. White sponge nevus: diagnosis by light microscopic and ultrastructural cytology. Acta Cytol 1988;32:357.

Nichols GE, Cooper PH, Underwood PB Jr, et al. White sponge nevus. Obstet Gynecol 1990;76:545.

### Darier's Disease

Adams AM, Macleod RI, Munro CS. Symptomatic and asymptomatic salivary duct abnormalities in Darier's disease: a sialographic study. Dentomaxillofac Radiol 1994;23:25.

Burge SM, Wilkinson JD. Darier-White disease: a review of the clinical features in 163 patients. J Am Acad Dermatol 1992;27:40.

Macleod RI, Munro CS. The incidence and distribution of oral lesions in patients with Darier's disease. Br Dent J 1991;171:133.

Weathers DR, Driscoll RM. Darier's disease of the oral mucosa. Oral Surg Oral Med Oral Pathol 1974;37:711.

### Tuberous Sclerosis

Harrison MG, O'Neill ID, Chadwick BL. Odontogenic myxoma in an adolescent with tuberous sclerosis. J Oral Pathol Med 1997;26:339.

Kwiatkowski DJ, Short MP. Tuberous sclerosis. Arch Dermatol 1994;130:348.

Miyamoto Y, Satomura K, Rikimaru K, et al. Desmoplastic fibroma of the mandible associated with tuberous sclerosis. J Oral Pathol Med 1995;24:93.

Mlynarczyk G. Enamel pitting: a common symptom of tuberous sclerosis. Oral Surg Oral Med Oral Pathol 1991;71:63.

Scully C. Orofacial manifestations in tuberous sclerosis. Oral Surg Oral Med Oral Pathol 1977;44:706.

## Dyskeratosis Congenita

Alter BP, Gardner FH, Hall RE. Treatment of dyskeratosis congenita with granulocyte colony-stimulating factor and erythropoietin. Br J Haematol 1997;97:309.

Anil S, Beena VT, Raji MA, et al. Oral squamous cell carcinoma in a case of dyskeratosis congenita. Ann Dent 1994;53:15.

Drachtman RA, Alter BP. Dyskeratosis congenita: clinical and genetic heterogeneity: report of a new case and review of the literature. Am J Pediatr Hematol Oncol 1992;14:297.

Yavuzyilmaz E, Yamalik N, Yetgin S, et al. Oral-dental findings in dyskeratosis congenita. J Oral Pathol Med 1992;21:280.

## Peutz-Jeghers Syndrome

DePadova-Elder SM, Milgraum SS. Q-switched ruby laser treatment of labial lentigines in Peutz-Jeghers syndrome. J Dermatol Surg Oncol 1994;20:830.

Giardiello FM, Welsh SB, Hamilton SR, et al. Increased risk of cancer in the Peutz-Jeghers syndrome. N Engl J Med 1987;316:1511.

Hizawa K, Iida M, Matsumoto T, et al. Cancer in Peutz-Jeghers syndrome. Cancer 1993;72:2777.

Rodu B, Martinez MG Jr. Peutz-Jeghers syndrome and cancer. Oral Surg Oral Med Oral Pathol 1984;58:584.

## Melanotic Macule

Ashinoff R, Geronemus RG. Q-switched ruby laser treatment of labial lentigos. J Am Acad Dermatol 1992;27:809.

Buchner A, Hansen LS. Melanotic macule of the oral mucosa. Oral Surg Oral Med Oral Pathol 1979;48:244.

Ho KK-L, Dervan P, O'Loughlin S, et al. Labial melanotic macule: a clinical, histopathologic, and ultrastructural study. J Am Acad Dermatol 1993;28:33.

Kaugars GE, Heise AP, Riley WT, et al. Oral melanotic macules: a review of 353 cases. Oral Surg Oral Med Oral Pathol 1993;76:59.

Weathers DR, Corio RL, Crawford BE, et al. The labial melanotic macule. Oral Surg Oral Med Oral Pathol 1976;42:196.

## Oral Melanoacanthosis

Goode RK, Crawford BE, Callihan MD, et al. Oral melanoacanthoma. Oral Surg Oral Med Oral Pathol 1983;56:622.

Heine BT, Drummond JF, Damm DD, et al. Bilateral oral melanoacanthoma. Gen Dent 1996;44:451.

Tomich CE, Zunt SL. Melanoacanthosis (melanoacanthoma) of the oral mucosa. J Dermatol Surg Oncol 1990;16:231.

## Erythema Migrans

Bánóczy J, Szabó L, Csiba Á. Migratory glossitis: a clinical-histologic review of seventy cases. Oral Surg Oral Med Oral Pathol 1975;39:113.

Brooks JK, Balciunas BA. Geographic stomatitis: review of the literature and report of five cases. J Am Dent Assoc 1987;115:421.

Espelid M, Bang G, Johannessen AC, et al. Geographic stomatitis: report of 6 cases. J Oral Pathol Med 1991;20:425.

Fenerli A, Papanicolaou S, Papanicolaou M, et al. Histocompatibility antigens and geographic tongue. Oral Surg Oral Med Oral Pathol 1993;76:476.

Morris LF, Phillips CM, Binnie WH, et al. Oral lesions in patients with psoriasis: a controlled study. Cutis 1992;49:339.

Sigal MJ, Mock D. Symptomatic benign migratory glossitis: report of two cases and literature review. Pediatr Dent 1992;14:392.

### Transient Lingual Papillitis

Lacour J-P, Perrin C. Eruptive familial lingual papillitis: a new entity? Pediatr Dermatol 1997;14:13.

Whitaker SB, Krupa JJ III, Singh BB. Transient lingual papillitis. Oral Surg Oral Med Oral Pathol Oral Radiol Endod 1996;82:441.

### Psoriasis

Hietanen J, Salo OP, Kanerva L, et al. Study of the oral mucosa in 200 consecutive patients with psoriasis. Scand J Dent Res 1984;92:50.

Morris LF, Phillips CM, Binnie WH, et al. Oral lesions in patients with psoriasis: a controlled study. Cutis 1992;49:339.

Ulmansky M, Michelle R, Azaz B. Oral psoriasis: report of six new cases. J Oral Pathol Med 1995;24:42.

Zhu J-F, Kaminski MJ, Pulitzer DR, et al. Psoriasis: pathophysiology and oral manifestations. Oral Dis 1996;2:135.

### Systemic Sclerosis and CREST Syndrome

Marmary Y, Glaiss R, Pisanty S. Scleroderma: oral manifestations. Oral Surg Oral Med Oral Pathol 1981;52:32.

Mitchell H, Bolster MB, LeRoy EC. Scleroderma and related conditions. Med Clin North Am 1997;81(1):129.

Nagy G, Kovács J, Zeher M, et al. Analysis of the oral manifestations of systemic sclerosis. Oral Surg Oral Med Oral Pathol. 1994;77:141.

Rout PGJ, Hamburger J, Potts AJC. Orofacial radiological manifestations of systemic sclerosis. Dentomaxillofac Radiol 1996;25:193.

Velayos EE, Masi AT, Stevens MB, et al. The "CREST" syndrome: comparison with systemic sclerosis (scleroderma). Arch Intern Med 1979;139:1240.

Wood RE, Lee P. Analysis of the oral manifestations of systemic sclerosis (scleroderma). Oral Surg Oral Med Oral Pathol 1988;65:172.

### Lupus Erythematosus

Callen JP. Lupus erythematosus. In: Demis DJ, ed. Clinical dermatology. Philadelphia: Lippincott-Raven, 1992.

Laman SD, Provost TT. Cutaneous manifestations of lupus erythematosus. Rheum Dis Clin North Am 1994;20:195.

Pisetsky DS, Gilkeson G, St Clair EW. Systemic lupus erythematosus: diagnosis and treatment. Med Clin North Am 1997;81(1):113.

Rhodus NL, Johnson DK. The prevalence of oral manifestations of systemic lupus erythematosus. Quintessence Int 1990;21:461.

Schiødt M. Oral manifestations of lupus erythematosus. Int J Oral Surg 1984;13:101.

### Pemphigus Vulgaris

Chrysomallis F, Loannides D, Teknetzis A, et al. Treatment of oral pemphigus vulgaris. Int J Dermatol 1994;33:803.

Korman N. Pemphigus. J Am Acad Dermatol 1988;18:1219.

Lamey PJ, Rees TD, Binnie WH, et al. Oral presentation of pemphigus vulgaris and its response to systemic steroid therapy. Oral Surg Oral Med Oral Pathol 1992;74:54.

Robinson JC, Lozada-Nur F, Frieden I. Oral pemphigus vulgaris: a review of the literature and a report on the management of 12 cases. Oral Surg Oral Med Oral Pathol Oral Radiol Endod 1997;84:349.

Williams DM. Vesiculobullous mucocutaneous disease: pemphigus vulgaris. J Oral Pathol Med 1989;18:544.

### Paraneoplastic Pemphigus

Anhalt GJ, Kim S, Stanley JR, et al. Paraneoplastic pemphigus: an autoimmune mucocutaneous disease associated with neoplasia. N Engl J Med 1990;323:1729.

Camisa C, Helm TN, Liu Y-C, et al. Paraneoplastic pemphigus: a report of three cases including one long-term survivor. J Am Acad Dermatol 1992;27:547.

Helm TN, Camisa C, Valenzuela R, et al. Paraneoplastic pemphigus: a distinct autoimmune vesiculobullous disorder associated with neoplasia. Oral Surg Oral Med Oral Pathol 1993;75:209.

Perniciaro C, Kuechle MK, Colón-Otero G. Paraneoplastic pemphigus: a case of prolonged survival. Mayo Clin Proc 1994;69:851.

## Chronic Ulcerative Stomatitis

Beutner EH, Chorzelski TP, Parodi A, et al. Ten cases of chronic ulcerative stomatitis with stratified epithelium-specific antinuclear antibody. J Am Acad Dermatol 1991;24:781.

Church LF Jr, Schosser RH. Chronic ulcerative stomatitis associated with stratified epithelial specific antinuclear antibodies: a case report of a newly described disease entity. Oral Surg Oral Med Oral Pathol 1992;73:579.

Jaremko WM, Beutner EH, Kumar V, et al. Chronic ulcerative stomatitis associated with a specific immunologic marker. J Am Acad Dermatol 1990;22:215.

Lewis JE, Beutner EH, Rostami R, et al. Chronic ulcerative stomatitis with stratified epithelium-specific antinuclear antibodies. Int J Dermatol 1996;35:272.

## Mucous Membrane Pemphigoid

Lamey P-J, Rees TD, Binnie WH, et al. Mucous membrane pemphigoid: treatment experience at two institutions. Oral Surg Oral Med Oral Pathol 1992;74:50.

Lilly JP, Spivey JD, Fotos PG. Benign mucous membrane pemphigoid with advanced periodontal involvement: diagnosis and therapy. J Periodontol 1995;66:737.

Poskitt L, Wojnarowska F. Minimizing cicatricial pemphigoid orodynia with minocycline. Br J Dermatol 1995;132:784.

Poskitt L, Wojnarowska F. Treatment of cicatricial pemphigoid with tetracycline and nicotinamide. Clin Exp Dermatol 1995;20:258.

Silverman S Jr, Gorsky M, Lozada-Nur F, et al. Oral mucous membrane pemphigoid: a study of sixty-five patients. Oral Surg Oral Med Oral Pathol 1986;61:233.

Vincent SD, Lilly GE, Baker KA. Clinical, historic, and therapeutic features of cicatricial pemphigoid: a literature review and open therapeutic trial with corticosteroids. Oral Surg Oral Med Oral Pathol 1993;76:453.

Williams DM. Vesiculo-bullous mucocutaneous disease: benign mucous membrane and bullous pemphigoid. J Oral Pathol Med 1990;19:16.

## Lichen Planus

Duffey DC, Eversole LR, Abemayor E. Oral lichen planus and its association with squamous cell carcinoma: an update on pathogenesis and treatment implications. Laryngoscope 1996;106:357.

Eisenberg E, Krutchkoff DJ. Lichenoid lesions of oral mucosa: diagnostic criteria and their importance in the alleged relationship to oral cancer. Oral Surg Oral Med Oral Pathol 1992;73:699.

Gorsky M, Raviv M, Moskona D, et al. Clinical characteristics and treatment of patients with oral lichen planus in Israel. Oral Surg Oral Med Oral Pathol Oral Radiol Endod 1996;82:644.

Porter SR, Kirby A, Olsen I, et al. Immunologic aspects of dermal and oral lichen planus: a review. Oral Surg Oral Med Oral Pathol Oral Radiol Endod 1997;83:358.

Silverman S Jr, Gorsky M, Lozada-Nur F. A prospective follow-up study of 570 patients with oral lichen planus: persistence, remission, and malignant association. Oral Surg Oral Med Oral Pathol 1985;60:30.

Thompson DF, Skaehill PA. Drug-induced lichen planus. Pharmacotherapy 1994;14:561.

Vincent SD, Fotos PG, Baker KA, et al. Oral lichen planus: the clinical, historical, and therapeutic features of 100 cases. Oral Surg Oral Med Oral Pathol 1990;70:165.

## Erythema Multiforme

Barone CM, Bianchi MA, Lee B, et al. Treatment of toxic epidermal necrolysis and Stevens-Johnson syndrome in children. J Oral Maxillofac Surg 1993;51:264.

Côte B, Wechsler J, Bastuji-Garin S, et al. Clinicopathologic correlation in erythema multiforme and Stevens-Johnson syndrome. Arch Dermatol 1995;131:1268.

Farthing PM, Maragou P, Coates M, et al. Characteristics of the oral lesions in patients with cutaneous recurrent erythema multiforme. J Oral Pathol Med 1995;24:9.

Lozada-Nur F, Cram D, Gorsky M. Clinical response to levamisole in thirty-nine patients with erythema multiforme: an open prospective study. Oral Surg Oral Med Oral Pathol 1992;74:294.

Nazif MM, Ranalli DN. Stevens-Johnson syndrome: a report of fourteen pediatric cases. Oral Surg Oral Med Oral Pathol 1982;53:263.

Schofield JK, Tatnall FM, Leigh IM. Recurrent erythema multiforme: clinical features and treatment in a large series of patients. Br J Dermatol 1993;128:542.

Stewart MG, Duncan NO III, Franklin DJ, et al. Head and neck manifestations of erythema multiforme in children. Otolaryngol Head Neck Surg 1994;111:236.

## Epidermolysis Bullosa

Harel-Raviv M, Bernier S, Raviv E, et al. Oral epidermolysis bullosa in adults. Spec Care Dent 1995;15:144.

Pearson RW. Clinicopathologic types of epidermolysis bullosa and their nondermatological complications. Arch Dermatol 1988;124:718.

Wright JT, Fine J-D, Johnson LB. Oral soft tissues in hereditary epidermolysis bullosa. Oral Surg Oral Med Oral Pathol 1991;71:440.

Wright JT, Fine J-D, Johnson L. Hereditary epidermolysis bullosa: oral manifestations and dental management. Pediatr Dent 1993;15:242.

Wright JT, Fine J-D, Johnson L. Dental caries risk in hereditary epidermolysis bullosa. Pediatr Dent 1994;16:427.

# chapter 14
# ORAL MANIFESTATIONS OF SYSTEMIC DISEASES

## HYPOPHOSPHATASIA

### Fig. 14.1

Hypophosphatasia is a rare hereditary disease in which there are decreased levels of alkaline phosphatase, an enzyme necessary for proper bone formation. Four types of hypophosphatasia are recognized: perinatal, infantile, childhood, and adult. The severe perinatal and infantile forms are autosomal-recessive traits; evidence suggests that the milder childhood and adult forms could be autosomal dominant. The childhood form is the variety that most often presents with dental manifestations. The affected child initially exhibits low alkaline phosphatase levels, but these levels often rise with age. Secondary to the low levels, there is absence or reduced formation of cementum on the teeth, which results in premature tooth loss because of inadequate periodontal ligament attachment. The deciduous incisors are usually affected first; the posterior deciduous teeth and permanent teeth may form sufficient cementum and not be prematurely lost. Enamel hypoplasia and increased pulp size may also occur. Phosphoethanolamine is usually excreted in the urine. Otherwise, individuals with childhood hypophosphatasia may appear healthy.

## HYPOPHOSPHATEMIC VITAMIN D–RESISTANT RICKETS (X-LINKED HYPOPHOSPHATEMIC RICKETS, FAMILIAL HYPOPHOSPHATEMIC RICKETS)

### Figs. 14.2 and 14.3

Hypophosphatemic vitamin D–resistant rickets is an X-linked–dominant inherited kidney disorder that leads to renal loss of phosphate and subsequent decreased serum phosphate levels (hypophosphatemia). Although it is a rare disease that occurs in 1 of every 20,000 births, it is the most common form of rickets in developed countries. The hypophosphatemia leads to rachitic bone changes that are not responsive to therapeutic doses of vitamin D, hence the name "vitamin D–resistant rickets." Affected patients have a short stature with bowing of the legs. Bone pain also frequently occurs.

Hypophosphatemic vitamin D–resistant rickets cause defects in the mineralization of the dentin, characterized by the presence of large numbers of calcospherites that are separated by irregular zones of interglobular dentin. The pulp chambers are larger in size and often demonstrate pulp horns that extend to the dentinoenamel junction. Multiple dental abscesses can develop in the absence of dental caries, presumably because of bacterial invasion of these abnormally high pulp horns. These dental defects are more severe in males, and affected males also have been shown to be at increased risk for taurodontism and impacted canines.

Systemic treatment for hypophosphatemic vitamin D–resistant rickets usually consists of the administration of calcitriol and phosphate. Appropriate endodontic therapy is indicated for any nonvital teeth that may develop.

### Figure 14.1
### HYPOPHOSPHATASIA
Premature loss of anterior deciduous teeth from lack of cellular cementum development in a 2-year-old male. (Courtesy of Dr. Jackie B. Forbess.)

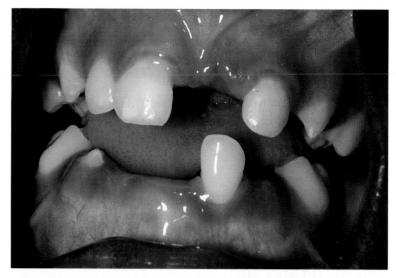

### Figure 14.2
### HYPOPHOSPHATEMIC VITAMIN D–RESISTANT RICKETS
Bilateral fistulas are present on the gingiva overlying the maxillary lateral incisors.

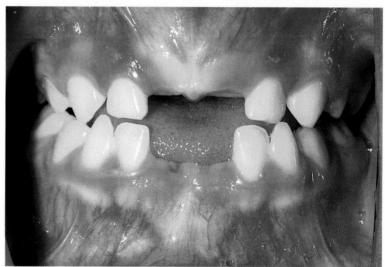

### Figure 14.3
### HYPOPHOSPHATEMIC VITAMIN D–RESISTANT RICKETS
Radiograph showing teeth with large pulp chambers and high pulp horns.

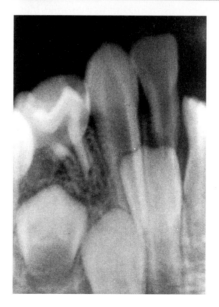

ORAL MANIFESTATIONS OF SYSTEMIC DISEASES

### Fig. 14.4

Diabetes mellitus is a complex endocrine disorder that results in impaired glucose metabolism. It can be caused by a deficiency of insulin, impaired use of insulin, or an error in insulin metabolism. Two forms of the disease are recognized: type I, or insulin-dependent diabetes mellitus, and type II, or non–insulin-dependent diabetes mellitus. Type I diabetes mellitus is more severe and is more likely to be associated with oral manifestations, which may include xerostomia, burning mouth, altered taste, parotid enlargement (sialadenosis), and candidiasis. Diabetic patients also have an increased susceptibility to the development of gingivitis and periodontitis secondary to altered host defenses, lowered resistance to infection, and decreased effectiveness of the healing process. The gingiva may become unusually hyperplastic and erythematous. Patients with uncontrolled diabetes demonstrate more rapidly progressing periodontitis and more periodontal abscesses. Because diabetes without overt systemic symptoms may go undetected for a long time, the oral changes may represent an important early clinical manifestation that can lead to the diagnosis.

## HYPERPARATHYROIDISM

### Figs. 14.5 and 14.6

Increased production of parathyroid hormone results in a generalized disorder of calcium, phosphate, and bone metabolism. Hyperparathyroidism can result from hyperplasia of the parathyroid glands or an adenoma or carcinoma of a parathyroid gland. Primary hyperparathyroidism is usually caused by an adenoma (80–85% of cases), less commonly by hyperplasia of all parathyroid glands (15–20% of cases), and rarely by a carcinoma (less than 1% of cases). Secondary hyperparathyroidism is caused by parathyroid hyperplasia in response to low serum calcium levels, usually as a result of renal failure or severe intestinal malabsorption.

Primary hyperparathyroidism is most commonly seen in middle-aged patients and is more common in females. Renal calculi, nephrocalcinosis, and peptic ulceration are the most common manifestations. Bone disease is present in 10 to 25% of cases. This may consist of generalized skeletal demineralization, development of destructive lytic lesions (brown tumors), or pathologic fractures. Jaw involvement is usually noted only in the more advanced cases but may be the first sign of the disease. A generalized alteration of the trabecular pattern may be seen on dental radiographs, resulting in a ground-glass appearance, but this feature is more common in secondary hyperparathyroidism. This change may be accompanied by a loss of the lamina dura. Loss of lamina dura, however, is not as common or specific as is often stated. Brown tumors also occur in the jaws and radiographically appear as unilocular or multilocular lytic defects. These lesions are histopathologically identical to central giant cell granulomas; it is prudent to rule out hyperparathyroidism in all cases of giant cell granuloma.

Secondary hyperparathyroidism related to chronic renal failure is commonly associated with bony changes known as "renal osteodystrophy" (see Figs. 14.8 and 14.9). Most patients undergoing renal dialysis show evidence of bone disease. The bone lesions can be similar to those seen in primary hyperparathyroidism, but brown tumors are less common and there is an increased frequency of ground-glass changes. Macrognathia (jaw enlargement) also can occur. Primary hyperparathyroidism may be cured by surgical removal of the involved gland or glands, and bone lesions usually resolve. Secondary hyperparathyroidism is treated medically by trying to control the underlying cause.

### Figure 14.4
### DIABETIC GINGIVITIS

Erythematous and hyperplastic gingivitis in a patient with uncontrolled diabetes. (Courtesy of Van Dis ML, Allen CM, Neville BW. Erythematous gingival enlargement in diabetic patients: a report of four cases. J Oral Maxillofac Surg 1988;46:794.)

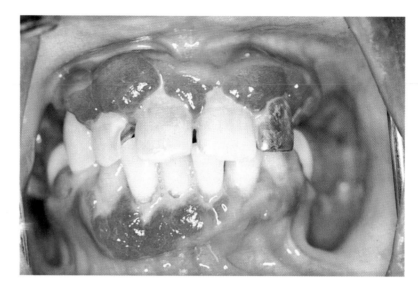

### Figure 14.5
### HYPERPARATHYROIDISM

Panographic radiograph of a 45-year-old female showing a large multilocular radiolucent lesion of the left ascending ramus and a smaller radiolucent lesion in the right premolar area. A biopsy specimen of both lesions showed giant cell granuloma. Further investigations demonstrated that the patient had primary hyperparathyroidism. A parathyroid adenoma was removed, and her blood calcium level returned to normal.

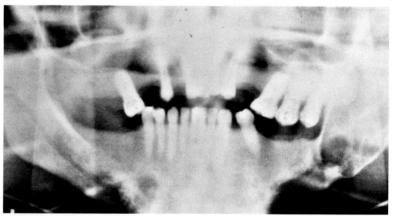

### Figure 14.6
### HYPERPARATHYROIDISM

Brown tumor of hyperparathyroidism presenting as an ulcerated palatal mass in a patient with secondary hyperparathyroidism caused by malabsorption syndrome resulting in chronically low serum calcium levels.

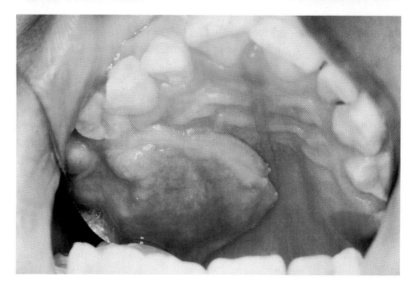

## ADDISON'S DISEASE (PRIMARY HYPOADRENOCORTICISM)

**Fig. 14.7**

Addison's disease, or primary adrenocortical insufficiency, is a rare disorder characterized by inadequate production of cortisol and other adrenal steroids. In the past, tuberculosis was the most common cause of Addison's disease, but today the most frequent cause is idiopathic adrenocortical atrophy, which is probably of autoimmune origin. Many patients also have one or more other autoimmune or endocrine disorders. The most common and characteristic clinical finding is hyperpigmentation of the skin, often along with brown to black macular pigmented lesions affecting the oral mucosa. Other manifestations include weakness, fatigue, weight loss, gastrointestinal tract complaints, hypotension, and electrolyte disturbances in the form of low serum sodium and high serum potassium levels. Addison's disease is managed with corticosteroid replacement therapy. Because the body's need for corticosteroid hormones may increase during times of stress, the corticosteroid dosage may need to be adjusted for certain dental and oral surgical procedures.

## RENAL OSTEODYSTROPHY

**Figs. 14.8 and 14.9**

Chronic renal failure can lead to a variety of clinical problems, especially skeletal changes that are known as "renal osteodystrophy." Because the failing kidneys cannot activate vitamin D, intestinal absorption of calcium is impaired, with a corresponding increase in serum phosphate levels. The phosphatemia causes a secondary reduction in serum calcium levels to maintain a stable calcium/phosphate solubility product. The decreased serum calcium level results in a compensatory increase in parathyroid hormone production (secondary hyperparathyroidism), which results in elevated phosphate excretion, decreased calcium excretion, and increased removal of calcium from the bones. Treatment with long-term renal dialysis and phosphate binders can complicate the clinical picture, resulting in uremic mixed bone disease that shows features of both high-turnover bone (osteitis fibrosa) and low-turnover bone (osteomalacia).

Radiographic alterations of the jaw bones are common in patients undergoing dialysis for chronic renal disease. Bone resorption can result in loss of the lamina dura, thinning of the cortical plates, and blurring of anatomic landmarks such as the mental foramen, inferior alveolar canal, and floor of the maxillary sinus. Frequently, the bony trabecular pattern assumes a ground-glass appearance similar to that of fibrous dysplasia. On occasion, radiolucent osteoclastic brown tumors may develop, but such lesions are more common in patients with primary hyperparathyroidism. Recently, several patients with renal osteodystrophy undergoing dialysis have been described who developed striking enlargement of one or both jaws (macrognathia). Treatment of these patients consists of supplementation of vitamin D and calcium, combined with attempts to decrease phosphate levels. The jaw enlargements may require surgical recontouring.

### Figure 14.7
### ADDISON DISEASE

Diffuse hyperpigmentation of the facial gingiva.

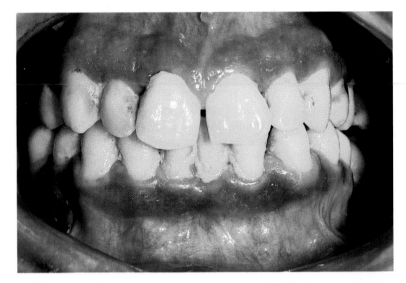

### Figure 14.8
### RENAL OSTEODYSTROPHY

Marked enlargement of the maxilla with obliteration of the palatal vault in a patient on long-term dialysis for renal failure. (Courtesy of Damm DD, Neville BW, McKenna S, et al. Macrognathia of renal osteodystrophy in dialysis patients. Oral Surg Oral Med Oral Pathol Oral Radiol Endod 1997;83:489.)

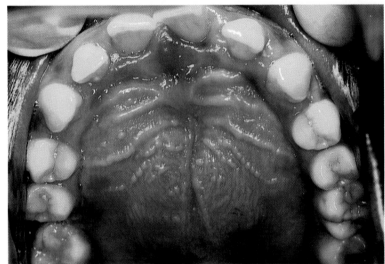

### Figure 14.9
### RENAL OSTEODYSTROPHY

Occlusal radiograph of the patient shown in Figure 14.8. Note the generalized ground-glass appearance of the bone and loss of the lamina dura.

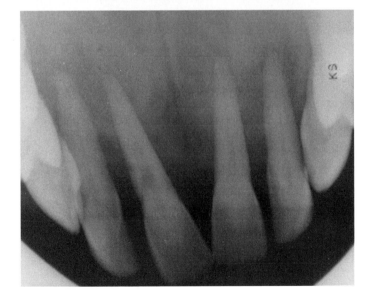

## ENAMEL HYPOPLASIA OF RENAL OSTEODYSTROPHY

### Figs. 14.10 and 14.11

As discussed in the previous section, patients with chronic renal failure may be unable to activate vitamin D, resulting in abnormalities in calcium/phosphate metabolism and secondary hyperparathyroidism. These abnormalities can be associated with bony changes known as "renal osteodystrophy" (see Figs. 14.8 and 14.9). In addition, if the renal failure begins at a young age, enamel hypoplasia may occur on the developing teeth. These hypoplastic areas may correspond to the age of onset of advanced renal failure. Other dental findings associated with renal osteodystrophy include tooth mobility, malocclusion, and development of pulp stones.

## CROHN'S DISEASE (REGIONAL ENTERITIS)

### Fig. 14.12

Crohn's disease is a chronic granulomatous inflammatory disorder that primarily affects the small and large intestine, although any site along the alimentary tract may be affected, including the oral cavity. The bowel inflammation produces clinical symptoms of intermittent diarrhea and abdominal pain and may result in severe malabsorption, fibrosis, and development of fistulous tracts. Oral involvement has been reported in 6 to 20% of cases. The buccal mucosa may exhibit a lobulated, edematous, fissured appearance described as resembling cobblestones. Hyperplastic folds may develop in the mucobuccal fold that resemble an epulis fissuratum. Linear ulcers with hyperplastic borders also can be seen. Some cases of orofacial granulomatosis (see Figs. 6.10 to 6.12) may represent oral manifestations of Crohn's disease. These oral lesions are significant because they may predate the onset of gastrointestinal tract lesions. Aphthous-like ulcerations also have been reported in patients with Crohn's disease, although the significance of this finding is uncertain because these ulcers occur frequently in the general population. Treatment for Crohn's disease consists primarily of systemic steroids, sulfasalazine, or both. Surgical resection of affected segments of intestine may become necessary.

### Figure 14.10
### ENAMEL HYPOPLASIA OF RENAL OSTEODYSTROPHY

Anterior view of patient who demonstrated enamel hypoplasia of bicuspids and second molars secondary to severe renal failure as a child.

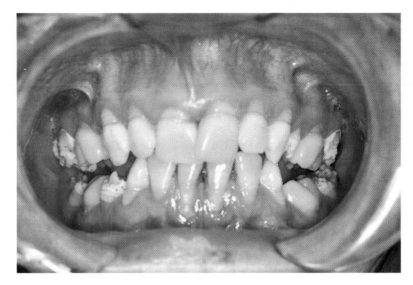

### Figure 14.11
### ENAMEL HYPOPLASIA OF RENAL OSTEODYSTROPHY

Occlusal view of the dentition of the patient described in Figure 14.10. Note the hypoplastic and irregular crowns of the bicuspids and second molars.

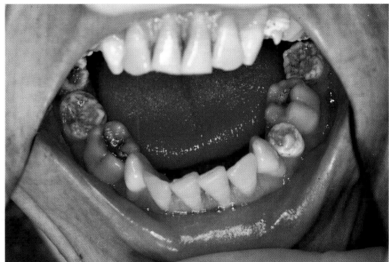

### Figure 14.12
### CROHN'S DISEASE

Hyperplastic fold in the lower labial vestibule. (Courtesy of Dr. Greg W. Dimmich.)

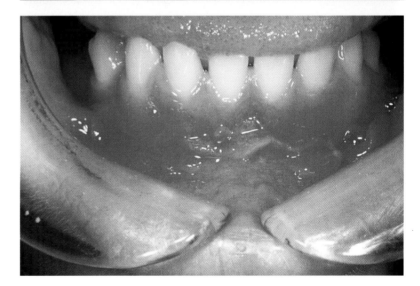

## PYOSTOMATITIS VEGETANS

**Fig. 14.13**

Pyostomatitis vegetans is a rare inflammatory condition of the oral mucosa that exhibits a highly distinctive pattern. The mucosa appears erythematous and edematous, often exhibiting papillary folds and grooves that impart a somewhat pebbly appearance to the surface. The most characteristic feature is the presence of multiple yellow pustules, 2 to 3 mm in diameter, over the mucosal surface; these pustules often coalesce in a linear pattern described as having a "snail-track" appearance. Lesions are most common on the facial gingiva, vestibule, and buccolabial mucosa. Surprisingly, discomfort is often not a prominent feature. The significance of pyostomatitis vegetans is that it represents an oral sign of inflammatory bowel disease. Most patients have ulcerative colitis, but a few cases have been associated with Crohn's disease. Liver dysfunction also has been reported in some affected patients. The oral lesions often rapidly disappear with systemic corticosteroid therapy, but they may recur when the medication is withdrawn. Topical corticosteroids also have been used with some success.

## VITAMIN B COMPLEX DEFICIENCY

**Figs. 14.14 and 14.15**

It has long been recognized that a deficiency of various vitamins, especially B complex, can result in the development of characteristic oral lesions. Oral manifestations may result from deficiency of a single B vitamin or a group of B vitamins and have been associated with deficiencies of niacin, riboflavin, folic acid, pyridoxine, and vitamin B12. Vitamin B12 deficiency results in a megaloblastic anemia and may arise from inadequate dietary intake, gastric atrophy with loss of intrinsic factor production (pernicious anemia), or gastrointestinal tract surgery limiting its absorption (see Figs. 11.4 to 11.6).

The most characteristic oral manifestations of B complex deficiency involve the lips and tongue. Angular cheilitis, or cracking and fissuring at the commissures, is a common finding. Another classic feature is atrophy of the tongue papillae, which may result in a smooth, glossy, bald appearance. The tongue can be pale or bright red and can swell or shrink. The tongue surface may become ulcerated, and a burning sensation is often reported.

A deficiency of niacin results in the disease known as "pellagra" (from the Italian words for "rough skin"). In addition to the above-mentioned oral manifestations, classic pellagra is characterized by the three Ds: dermatitis, diarrhea, and dementia. The skin changes consist of rough, scaly, hyperpigmented lesions that are most prevalent in areas of exposure to sunlight or trauma. Neurologic symptoms can include weakness, anxiety, depression, or delirium. Near the end of the 19th century and the beginning of the 20th century, there was an outbreak of pellagra in the southern United States that resulted from economic depression after the Civil War and diets that relied heavily on cheap, nonnutritious cornmeal. Pellagra is rare in the United States today, but it still may be encountered in some less-developed parts of the world.

### Figure 14.13
**PYOSTOMATITIS VEGETANS**
Yellow pustular lesions of the buccal mucosa.

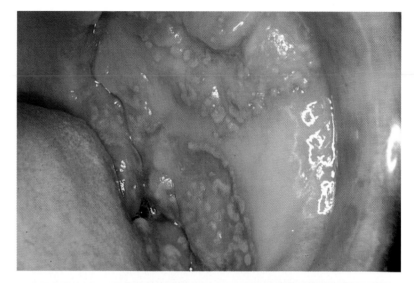

### Figure 14.14
**PELLAGRA**
Atrophic "bald" tongue.

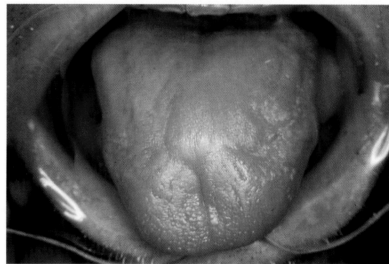

### Figure 14.15
**PELLAGRA**
Rough skin on the neck and chest in areas exposed to sun.

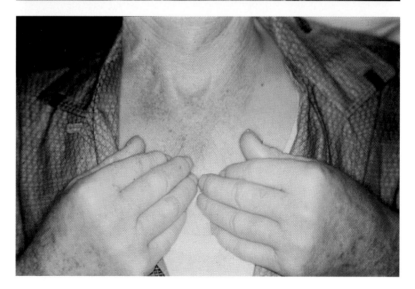

## AMYLOIDOSIS

### Fig. 14.16

Amyloidosis refers to a group of disorders characterized by deposition of a protein material (amyloid) in body tissues. Widespread deposits may occur in the absence of underlying disease (primary amyloidosis), in association with multiple myeloma, or secondary to a variety of chronic inflammatory conditions such as tuberculosis, osteomyelitis, or rheumatoid arthritis. Hereditary and localized forms of amyloidosis are also recognized. Oral involvement occurs in about 25% of cases of myeloma-related and primary amyloidosis, usually affecting the tongue and gingiva. Nodular deposits in the tongue typically produce macroglossia, with indentations often observed along the lateral border from pressure against the teeth. These amyloid nodules may be associated with secondary ulceration or submucosal hemorrhage. The prognosis for patients with systemic primary and myeloma-associated amyloidosis is poor, with a mean survival time of 4 to 15 months; most patients die of heart failure, renal failure, or multiple myeloma. Patients with secondary amyloidosis may do better if the underlying inflammatory disease can be controlled. Because of its limited nature, the prognosis for localized amyloidosis is good.

## ACANTHOSIS NIGRICANS

### Figs. 14.17 and 14.18

Acanthosis nigricans is an uncommon dermatosis that can be divided into malignant and benign forms. In the malignant type, the skin changes are a sign of underlying malignant disease, usually gastric or other abdominal adenocarcinoma. These carcinomas are highly malignant, and the prognosis is poor. In the benign form, acanthosis nigricans may be hereditary, drug induced, or associated with a variety of other diseases, a number of which are characterized by tissue resistance to the action of insulin. The term "pseudo-acanthosis nigricans" is sometimes used for cases associated with obesity.

Skin involvement is most common in the intertriginous areas, especially the axillae and neck. These lesions are characterized by hyperpigmentation and epidermal hyperplasia resulting in velvety thickening or verrucous changes. Oral involvement has been reported in 25 to 50% of patients with malignant acanthosis nigricans, and it is probably encountered less frequently in the benign forms. Hyperplastic, pebbly, or verrucalike lesions may be seen on the lips, especially the upper lip and commissures. Intraoral lesions also may occur, usually involving the tongue. Unlike skin lesions, oral lesions usually do not exhibit hyperpigmentation.

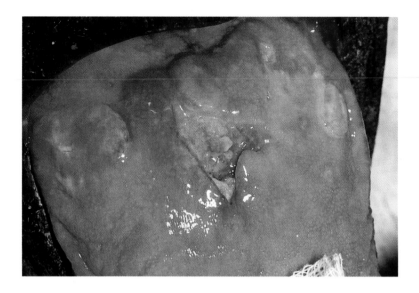

**Figure 14.16**
**AMYLOIDOSIS**

Nodularity and ulceration of the dorsum of the tongue.

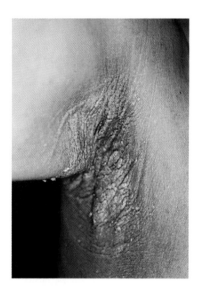

**Figure 14.17**
**ACANTHOSIS NIGRICANS**

Rough, hyperpigmented lesion of the axilla. (Courtesy of Hall JM, Moreland A, Cox GJ, et al. Oral acanthosis nigricans: report of a case and comparison of oral and cutaneous pathology. Am J Dermatopathol 1988;10:68.)

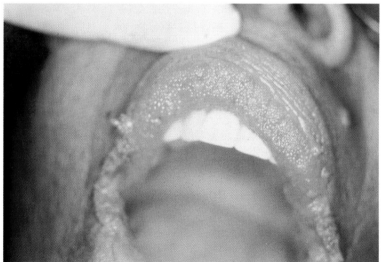

**Figure 14.18**
**ACANTHOSIS NIGRICANS**

Papillary changes of the upper lip. (Courtesy of Hall JM, Moreland A, Cox GJ, et al. Oral acanthosis nigricans: report of a case and comparison of oral and cutaneous pathology. Am J Dermatopathol 1988;10:68.)

### Hypophosphatasia

Chapple ILC. Hypophosphatasia: dental aspects and mode of inheritance. J Clin Periodontol 1993;20:615.

Chapple ILC, Thorpe GHG, Smith GM, et al. Hypophosphatasia: a family study involving a case diagnosed from gingival crevicular fluid. J Oral Pathol Med 1992;21:426.

Macfarlane JD, Swart JGN. Dental aspects of hypophosphatasia: a case report, family study, and literature review. Oral Surg Oral Med Oral Pathol 1989;67:521.

Plagmann H-C, Kocher T, Kuhrau N, et al. Periodontal manifestation of hypophosphatasia: a family case report. J Clin Periodontol 1994;21:710.

### Hypophosphatemic Vitamin D–Resistant Rickets

Berndt M, Ehrich JHH, Lazovic D, et al. Clinical course of hypophosphatemic rickets in 23 adults. Clin Nephrol 1996;45:33.

Carpenter TO. New perspectives on the biology and treatment of X-linked hypophosphatemic rickets. Pediatr Clin North Am 1997;44:443.

Hillmann G, Geurtsen W. Pathohistology of undecalcified primary teeth in vitamin D–resistant rickets: review and report of two cases. Oral Surg Oral Med Oral Pathol Oral Radiol Endod 1996;82:218.

McWhorter AG, Seale NS. Prevalence of dental abscess in a population of children with vitamin D–resistant rickets. Pediatr Dent 1991;13:91.

Seow WK, Needleman HL, Holm IA. Effect of familial hypophosphatemic rickets on dental development: a controlled, longitudinal study. Pediatr Dent 1995;17:346.

### Diabetic Gingivitis

Lamey P-J, Darwazeh AMG, Frier BM. Oral disorders associated with diabetes mellitus. Diabet Med 1992;9:410.

Oliver RC, Tervonen T. Periodontitis and tooth loss: comparing diabetics with the general population. J Am Dent Assoc 1993;124:71.

Rees TD. The diabetic dental patient. Dent Clin North Am 1994;38:447.

Van Dis ML, Allen CM, Neville BW. Erythematous gingival enlargement in diabetic patients: a report of four cases. J Oral Maxillofac Surg 1988;46:794.

### Hyperparathyroidism

Al Zahrani A, Levine MA. Primary hyperparathyroidism. Lancet 1997;349:1233.

Silverman S Jr, Ware WH, Gilooly C Jr. Dental aspects of hyperparathyroidism. Oral Surg Oral Med Oral Pathol 1968;26:184.

Smith BR, Fowler CB, Swane TJ. Primary hyperparathyroidism presenting as a "peripheral" giant cell granuloma. J Oral Maxillofac Surg 1988;46:65.

Solt DB. The pathogenesis, oral manifestations, and implications for dentistry of metabolic bone disease. Curr Opin Dent 1991;1:783.

### Addison's Disease

DeRosa G, Corsello SM, Cecchini L, et al. A clinical study of Addison's disease. Exp Clin Endocrinol 1987;90:232.

Kong M-F, Jeffcoate W. Eighty-six cases of Addison's disease. Clin Endocrinol 1994;41:757.

Ziccardi VB, Abubaker AO, Sotereanos GC, et al. Precipitation of an addisonian crisis during dental surgery: recognition and management. Compend Contin Educ Dent 1992;13:518.

### Renal Osteodystrophy

Chow MH, Peterson DS. Dental management for children with chronic renal failure undergoing hemodialysis therapy. Oral Surg Oral Med Oral Pathol 1979;48:34.

Damm DD, Neville BW, McKenna S, et al. Macrognathia of renal osteodystrophy in dialysis patients. Oral Surg Oral Med Oral Pathol Oral Radiol Endod 1997;83:489.

De Rossi SS, Glick M. Dental considerations for the patient with renal disease receiving dialysis. J Am Dent Assoc 1996;127:211.

Nadimi H, Bergamini J, Lilien B. Uremic mixed bone disease: a case report. Int J Oral Maxillofac Surg 1993;22:368.

## Crohn's Disease

Basu MK, Asquith P. Oral manifestations of inflammatory bowel disease. Clin Gastroenterol 1980;9:307.

Bernstein ML, McDonald JS. Oral lesions in Crohn's disease: report of two cases and update of the literature. Oral Surg Oral Med Oral Pathol 1978;46:234.

Halme L, Meurman JH, Laine P, et al. Oral findings in patients with active or inactive Crohn's disease. Oral Surg Oral Med Oral Pathol 1993;76:175.

Lisciandrano D, Ranzi T, Carrassi A, et al. Prevalence of oral lesions in inflammatory bowel disease. Am J Gastroenterol 1996;91:7.

Plauth M, Jenss H, Meyle J. Oral manifestations of Crohn's disease: an analysis of 79 cases. J Clin Gastroenterol 1991;13:29.

Williams AJK, Wray D, Ferguson A. The clinical entity of orofacial Crohn's disease. Q J Med 1991;79:451.

## Pyostomatitis Vegetans

Calobrisi SD, Mutasim DF, McDonald JS. Pyostomatitis vegetans associated with ulcerative colitis: temporary clearance with fluocinonide gel and complete remission after colectomy. Oral Surg Oral Med Oral Pathol Oral Radiol Endod 1995;79:452.

Healy CM, Farthing PM, Williams DM, et al. Pyostomatitis vegetans and associated systemic disease: a review and two case reports. Oral Surg Oral Med Oral Pathol 1994;78:323.

Neville BW, Smith SE, Maize JC, et al. Pyostomatitis vegetans. Am J Dermatopathol 1985;7:69.

Storwick GS, Prihoda MB, Fulton RJ, et al. Pyodermatitis-pyostomatitis vegetans: a specific marker for inflammatory bowel disease. J Am Acad Dermatol 1994;31:336.

## Vitamin B Complex Deficiency

Dreizen S. Oral indications of the deficiency states. Postgrad Med 1971;49:97.

Judd LE, Poskitt BL. Pellagra in a patient with an eating disorder. Br J Dermatol 1991;125:71.

Lanska DJ. Stages in the recognition of epidemic pellagra in the United States: 1865-1960. Neurology 1996;47:829.

Zaki I, Millard L. Pellagra complicating Crohn's disease. Postgrad Med J 1995;71:496.

## Amyloidosis

Al-Hashimi I, Drinnan AJ, Uthman AA, et al. Oral amyloidosis: two unusual case presentations. Oral Surg Oral Med Oral Pathol 1987;63:586.

Geist JR, Geist S-MR, Wesley RK. Diagnostic procedures in oral amyloidosis. Compend Contin Educ Dent 1993;14:924.

Kyle RA, Bayrd ED. Amyloidosis: review of 236 cases. Medicine 1975;54:271.

Stimson PG, Tortoledo ME, Luna MA, et al. Localized primary amyloid tumor of the parotid gland. Oral Surg Oral Med Oral Pathol 1988;66:466.

## Acanthosis Nigricans

Hall JM, Moreland A, Cox GJ, et al. Oral acanthosis nigricans: report of a case and comparison of oral and cutaneous pathology. Am J Dermatopathol 1988;10:68.

Schwartz RA. Acanthosis nigricans. J Am Acad Dermatol 1994;31:1.

Sedano HO, Gorlin RJ. Acanthosis nigricans. Oral Surg Oral Med Oral Pathol 1987;63:462.

Tyler MT, Ficarra G, Silverman S Jr, et al. Malignant acanthosis nigricans with florid papillary oral lesions. Oral Surg Oral Med Oral Pathol Oral Radiol Endod. 1996;81:445.

# INDEX